PRACTICAL CLINICAL NEUROLOGY

John K. Wolf, M.D.
Associate Professor of Neurology
State University of New York
Upstate Medical Center;
Chief
Division of Neurology
Crouse-Irving Memorial Hospital
Syracuse, New York

 Medical Examination Publishing Co., Inc.
an *Excerpta Medica* company

Garden City, New York

Cover Illustration (Fig. 14-1) courtesy of S.U.N.Y. Upstate Medical Center.

Copyright © 1980 by
MEDICAL EXAMINATION
PUBLISHING CO., INC.
an **Excerpta Medica** company

Library of Congress Card Number
79-91846

ISBN 0-87488-728-3

January, 1980

Printed in the United States of America

SIMULTANEOUSLY PUBLISHED IN:

Europe   : HANS HUBER PUBLISHERS
                             Bern, Switzerland

Japan   : IGAKU-SHOIN Ltd.
                             Tokyo, Japan

South and East Asia : TOPPAN COMPANY (S) Pte. Ltd.
                             Singapore

United Kingdom   : HENRY KIMPTON PUBLISHERS
                             London, England

Preface

*"A strong wind is of little use unless you
know where you are going."*
(Greek Fisherman's Proverb)

The prime requirement for the professional is a firm basis in the scientific aspects of medical practice. I have attempted to provide such information in the text and I have also discussed subjective issues in the practice of medicine, as these require the attention of each practitioner. "Ethical" and interpersonal issues are matters largely of attitude and belief rather than of fact. Because we rarely discuss them either orally or in print, all of us are left to resolve them largely in isolation from other members of the profession.

The doctor's first job is to make an accurate diagnosis. Second, he must educate the patient and family about the diagnosis and about options for treatment. Next, he must give the best possible advice based upon a knowledge both of medicine and of the patient himself. Finally, the doctor's behavior reflects the fact that this relationship may last for the rest of the patient's life, through some good times and through some very bad times; and that the doctor may well preside at the patient's death. This means that communication must be as honest and direct as possible within the bounds of kindness and tact. The goals of this professional relationship are to avoid trouble where possible, and to prepare the patient and family for trouble that is inevitable.

This is not a controversial philosophy of medical practice, and yet we apply it in diverse manners as we practice our individual art. My discussions of management and philosophy are included as concrete examples of ethical and interpersonal issues to show one way to apply these thoughts and feelings to the practice of medicine, and to stimulate the reader to examine his own beliefs and to seek his own solutions to similar problems.

I have written this book for the clinician who is not a neurologist, so that he may be able to understand his neurological patient's complaints, and to plan his clinical evaluation. Medical students, house officers, and graduate physicians may also find useful information within. Neurological nurses and nursing students may find that various sections will help them to better understand their patients' disease processes.

I have stressed the clinical use of neuroanatomy in diagnosis, emphasized new developments in the scientific aspects of neurology, described in detail various neurological procedures that the clinician does himself, and explained many plans for patient management. Laboratory examinations are discussed without details of interpretation if the clinician has no primary responsibility for them.

The book reflects great changes in the specialty of neurology. The chapter on slow viral infections could not have been written 20 years ago, and during the next 20 years it may expand to include many diseases that are now to be found in other sections. The chapter on cerebrovascular disease reflects our continuing frustration with the treatment of atherosclerosis, but it also provides modern information about potentially useful techniques for the prevention of stroke. Sections on seizure disorders, movement disorders, headache, and myasthenia gravis reflect great changes in management techniques and in medicinal and surgical treatments for neurological diseases that have greatly improved the lot of many neurological patients.

On the other hand, chapters on clinical neuroanatomy could have been written 50 years ago, because that information was hammered out by the careful observations of doctors and anatomists who have gone before us. The treatment of acute infections of the nervous system has been intentionally omitted in this book, since these diseases are now the province of a new kind of specialist in the treatment of infectious diseases. The diagnosis of brain tumors is merely another problem in cerebral localization, greatly simplified with brain scanning and CT scanning; their treatment is a neurosurgical problem, and their identification a matter for neuropathology, so there is no chapter that deals specifically with these entities.

In regard to references, I have in most instances relied heavily upon published symposia. The reader can borrow a single informative volume without long library searches, as it is my opinion that busy practitioners do not have the time to delve into the neurological literature.

Some references, like the article in Chapter 4 by Suttie, are included because they are old favorites of mine. I hope some readers will be challenged by them as I have been in the past. When there are recent advances, I have provided specific references because the reader may want to examine the original literature, but I have not provided a comprehensive literature review. Once in the library, the reader may trace the references back to the original articles without difficulty.

John K. Wolf, M.D.

Acknowledgements

I did not write this book alone. After each chapter had been completed, my wife, Mitzi, civilized it before it ever saw the light of day. She was my severest critic and has always given me my greatest encouragement.

My chairman, Dr. Gilbert S. Ross, read the entire manuscript. His suggestions for the improved presentation of neurological information were concise and extremely helpful. He and Dr. Richard P. Schmidt, my University President and colleague, encouraged me to take the sabbatical leave in order to write the book in the first place.

My parents, Doctors John and Theta Wolf, also read the entire manuscript. Because they themselves are authors and medical lay-people, their suggestions have greatly improved the readability of the text.

Doctors Edward G. Bell and Eugene F. Binet read the portions of the manuscript that pertain to their areas of specialization, nuclear medicine and neuroradiology. I have incorporated their corrections and leaned heavily on their advice. Without their help, those portions would have been woefully inadequate.

Two of our neurological nurses, Ms. Mary Kaye Caufield and Ms. Beverly Ianuzi, reviewed the material on nursing management in stroke; and our occupational therapist, Ms. Kathleen Rake, reviewed the material on O.T. and P.T. Their corrections lend their professional authority to this book.

The expressive line drawings are the product of Mrs. Delilah Cohn who demanded anatomical accuracy and combined it with the simplicity that allows easy understanding. Mrs. Julie Hammack completed Figure 8-1 after Mrs. Cohn left on maternity leave.

Mildred Knowles and Gary McConnell learned with us how to portray a flowing examination in still photographs. Their professional approach to medical photography has allowed us to show some of the action.

My secretary, Mrs. Karen Reese, untiringly typed, re-typed, and determined the format of the manuscript in addition to her daily work. She even served as the model for our screening neurological examination patient. I cannot be accused of overworking her though, because during the preparation of the manuscript, she and her husband conceived an entirely different project and they plan to rush into print long before this book is published!

Above all, the reader's thanks should go to Dr. Bruce Dearing, University Professor for the Humanities at the Upstate Medical Center. Bruce *volunteered* to read this manuscript, spent untold hours studying it, and many more hours discussing it with me. He showed me something of the elegance of the English language, and he helped me to provide clarity and accuracy that would have been lacking without his advice. If the text is readable, much of the credit belongs to Bruce Dearing.

Lastly, I want to thank two people who guided this work from me to you. Publishers are supposed to edit an author's work, but my publisher provided me with help from two superior people— Laura Lavé, the production manager, and Helen Powers, the editress. These two women made highly significant contributions to English usage within the text and also determined how we should set special type throughout the book.

Almost to a woman, my readers have complained that the text has a sexist flavor—it does not. I have used the masculine pronoun throughout for simplicity, not for gender. Female readers who feel strongly about the matter are encouraged to insert an "s" in front of every "he." I have not discovered a simple way to change the "hims" to "hers," and for this, I offer my apologies.

Contents

To my wife, Mitzie, with love
and with thanks for your contributions
to all our projects!

CHAPTER 1

The Diagnostic Interview

INTRODUCTION

Each symptom of neurological dysfunction provides information that can help the clinician to draw logical conclusions about the location of a disease process and even about the pathological diagnosis. Even though the complexity of the nervous system is unmatched, it is orderly, and its symptoms are predictable. Later, when we consider special areas of neurological diagnosis, we shall examine the diagnostic symptoms that originate from each anatomical system. At this point, however, we shall consider the entire diagnostic interview rather than the specifics of neurological diagnosis.

Like other clinicians, my ideas about the diagnostic interview have a personal flavor. They are derived from nearly 20 years of listening to histories and performing examinations. Let the reader consider these ideas, try some of them for himself, and decide how he may use them in his own practice.

NEUROLOGICAL HISTORY

For convenience, we shall consider the events of the presenting complaint, the history of the neurological illness, and the neurological examination. In addition, we shall emphasize cues that can alert the clinician to abnormalities of his patient's mental status, and finally we shall present a brief formal mental status examination to help him to identify those abnormalities.

We shall not emphasize the general past medical history, because if the clinician is alert, that portion of the interview is of little help in the analysis of current problems. In fact, the physician who makes it a practice to use the past medical history to help him to determine the cause of current complaints will stub his diagnostic toe when his patient develops a new disease. Instead, he should listen to current complaints, predict for himself which portions of past history are pertinent to the current problem, and then ask specifically for that historical information.

Presenting Complaint

Throughout this volume, we shall emphasize that neurological symptoms relate to anatomical damage, and that accurate pathological diagnosis depends upon an understanding of both the pathologic anatomy and the cadence of the illness. The diagnostic journey begins with a consideration of the anatomical implications of the presenting complaint.

For instance, if the patient complains of a loss of vision, anatomical considerations are strictly limited to those parts of the body that can produce visual loss: the structures of the globe and orbit, the optic nerve, chiasm and tracts, the visual radiations, and the occipital cortex. The damage must be there somewhere even if the ultimate cause is a systemic disease like temporal arteritis.

When the patient delivers his presenting complaint, the physician can begin to think about anatomical implications and then apply the same kind of analysis to all subsequent symptoms in order to develop a mental picture of his patient's diseased anatomy. Should this patient's history contain a complaint of double vision in addition to visual loss, the anatomical considerations for that complaint are quite distinct from the anatomy of vision; but if there is only a single lesion, its location must be within or immediately behind the orbit, because these are the only locations where both the visual system and the system for the control of eye movements travel together. If the examiner reaches this conclusion after he has taken the history, he can predict that there will be visual loss in one eye only, or visual loss characteristic of a chiasmatic lesion, and that the double vision will relate to peripheral nerve, not brainstem dysfunction. Then he may compare his *predictions* with the results of the *examination*. This kind of reasoning is central to the analytic process of the diagnostic interview.

Five Pathological Processes

Five pathological processes form the basis for most diseases: vascular, neoplastic, infectious, toxic-metabolic, and "degenerative" diseases. Occasionally, the history actually suggests that there is no progressive disease, and then the clinician should be reminded of two additional causes of disability which really are not diseases at all: congenital malformation or birth damage, and previous trauma of some other kind.

Sometimes, it is necessary to bend a diagnosis to fit these catagories. Is a subdural hematoma a neoplasm? It certainly is a tumor. In what category does normal pressure hydrocephalus belong? What is a seizure? Additionally, diseases are not always faithful to their original pathological processes. Recently, as a result of new research, a number of "degenerative" diseases have become infectious ones. Nonetheless, the classification is useful to help organize the clinician's thoughts.

After the clinician has analyzed the anatomical implications of the history, he can begin to limit the diagnostic possibilities by deciding whether the disease is likely to be focal, multifocal, or diffuse in nature. Table 1-1 outlines the usual pathological processes which accompany focal, multifocal, or diffuse symptoms. It also indicates the second critically important aspect of accurate diagnosis; namely, the *cadence* of each process. Neoplasm and stroke usually appear in a completely different cadence even though both produce focal symptoms. Neoplastic and "degenerative" processes are both slowly progressive, but the anatomical distributions are completely different. The history of a neurological illness provides the clinician with the anatomical basis for a diagnosis related to his patient's complaints, as well as with a notion of the cadence of the disease, thus narrowing his diagnostic considerations when he has finished taking the history.

History of the Neurological Illness

The Patient's Initial Presentation

Try this: After the patient has given his presenting complaint and you have asked him to start at the beginning and to tell how his trouble developed, remain silent but attentive. Do not interrupt to

TABLE 1-1

The Five Pathological Processes

Pathologic Process	Pathologic Anatomy	Cadence	
	Distribution	Onset	Course
1. Vascular	Focal or multifocal	Sudden	Stable or improving
2. Neoplasm: Primary neoplasms Metastatic neoplasms	Focal Focal or multifocal	Gradual More rapid	Relentlessly progressive Relentlessly progressive
3. Infection	Focal, multifocal, or diffuse usually accompanied by specific signs	Variable, usually not sudden	Variable, usually self-limited, sometimes progressive
4. Degenerative	Diffuse	Gradual	Progressive
5. Toxic-metabolic	Diffuse (may be focal)	Variable	Depends on the specific metabolic defect

ask questions. Allow him to give his history unhindered. Think continuously about the anatomical implications of each significant complaint and listen to the cadence of the disease. Note which questions of anatomy and cadence still remain unanswered as he speaks. Notice *how* he presents his history. Time the performance by the clock.

When the neurological patient is allowed to give his history without interruption, he usually presents a cogent account of his illness in less than five minutes. At the end of his presentation, he falters, then stops. This is a definite transition because, like other lecturers, he has given all the information he thinks is pertinent.

As we shall see in a later section, the five-minute rule provides early evidence of disordered mentation. If the patient talks longer, or if he fails to make sense, the clinician must be prepared to intervene, because information from a demented or aphasic patient may not be pertinent. The situation is similar if the patient has functional mental abnormalities.

Not all of the information presented in the initial presentation will be pertinent to the patient's disease, and the patient may have left out facts that are of great importance to the physician. Nonetheless, the patient with a presenting complaint of visual loss has probably answered a number of questions. Did it occur in one eye only or in the left field of vision? Were there other neurological symptoms? How fast and how often did the symptom occur? Did permanent disability appear suddenly or gradually? If the clinician has been alert, he probably has a limited number of other specific questions that need to be clarified in order for him to establish with certainty the history of the onset and course of the disease. These questions must be answered during the detailed inquiry.

The Detailed Inquiry

Inexperienced interviewers inevitably fail to conduct a detailed inquiry because they have not yet distinguished between a diagnostic interview and a social conversation. During social intercourse, people ask questions and receive imprecise or irrelevant answers, but the conversation continues uncritically. During the diagnostic interview, specific pieces of information are still missing, and must be found if the diagnosis is to be accurate. If a patient's "blackout lasted only a few moments," was he blind or unconscious? How long is a few moments? The difference between 20 seconds and five minutes of unconsciousness helps to distinguish between syncope and seizure. A visual blackout of five seconds suggests severely increased intracranial pressure, but 20 minutes suggests vascular disease.

The interviewer may have to ask his questions several times and in several different ways. He must persist until he *knows* the answers, or *knows* that they are not available. Often, he must interrogate family members or witnesses, and such questioning is especially important if the patient cannot talk for himself or if there was a spell of unconsciousness. Describe what happened. How did he behave during the spell and as he awoke? Was he confused, sleepy, paralyzed, incontinent? Did he bite his tongue? What was his color? How do you *know* these things?

This is an inappropriate line of questioning during a social conversation, but it is essential during the detailed inquiry if the interviewer is to distinguish between various diagnostic possibilities. Once the physician has finished his careful interrogation, he may review what he thinks he knows about the history in concise terms, so his patient and family may have a chance to clarify any areas of residual misunderstanding.

Like the initial presentation, the detailed inquiry usually requires fewer than five minutes, although it may continue much longer if the problem is exceedingly complex. When the clinician has finished these first few minutes of the interview, he has taken into account the patient's age, the cadence of the illness, and if he uses them, he has thought about which one of the pathologic processes is the most likely cause of the trouble. He probably has already named the disease; certainly, he has satisfied himself about important items of past history that are pertinent to his proposed diagnosis.

Lastly, he has made predictions to himself about the results of neurological and general physical examinations. These predictions allow him to use the examination as a challenge to his diagnosis, rather than as a routine to be performed and recorded. The examinations may prove him wrong, but there is no better time to learn that. If he was wrong in his analysis of history, he is probably wrong about the entire problem, and he has a fresh chance to think it through again and to correct his mistakes before he does any damage.

Behavioral Considerations

The Five-Point Rule About Abnormal Mental Status

Unlike normal individuals, abnormal patients do not give a sequential, understandable story within five minutes. They may remain silent or ramble; their language may be unintelligible; and the history may be irrelevant and interminable. These are pathologic methods of presentaion, which *leave the clinician uninformed,* and by this characteristic they may be used to help him to make the diagnosis of a pathological mental status.

Five kinds of abnormal mental status are associated with an unintelligible initial presentation: two – dementia and aphasia – are caused by organic disease, the other three – hysteria, malingering, and psychosis (usually schizophrenia or depression) – are functional disorders. Let us examine how each of these affects the patient's ability to give a concise history and how they may be diagnosed.

Dementia and Aphasia. Many organic diseases produce dementia or aphasia, but the pathological process may not be evident at the beginning of the interview. Because dementia is usually caused by diffuse cerebral disease, and aphasia is more often caused by focal pathology, the clinical distinction between the two can greatly help the clinician to arrive at an accurate diagnosis.

The term *dementia* relates to a general deterioration of all spheres of intellectual competence. These include recent and remote memory, higher mental functions, calculation, and abstract reasoning. As dementia progresses, the patient eventually loses orientation to time, place, and even to his own identity.

The demented patient's conversation consists primarily of brief answers to direct questions. He does not engage in the normal give and take of ideas. He cannot take an idea from the examiner's question and amplify it as normal people do. His fund of knowledge is deficient. His family may try to talk for him as they would for a small child. The history he gives is brief and wrong. He is awake but not alert. His answers may be strikingly slowed, yet his language structure is likely to be intact.

The *amnestic syndrome* is defined as an isolated inability *to make new permanent memories*. While this syndrome is quite distinct from dementia, patients with the amnestic syndrome also leave the doctor uninformed after they have given a history, so this condition belongs with the five-point rule. Usually, the amnestic patient also has a degree of dementia, but this is not universally true. The patient with a pure amnestic syndrome talks well, calculates flawlessly, can interpret proverbs adequately, and can tell how a cow and a cat are similar. But 10 minutes after the examiner has left his room, the patient does not remember that he was ever there. His world is limited to his more-or-less intact remote memories and to the time span of his immediate memory mechanisms, which have a duration of 10 minutes or less. This sharp dichotomy between his relatively intact current mentation and his dismal failure to make new permanent memories allows the diagnosis to be made. Patients with this syndrome usually confabulate, but confabulation is a common human activity and is not truly a diagnostic criterion for the amnestic syndrome. Korsakoff's psychosis is the prototype amnestic syndrome, but there are several other conditions, unrelated to alcholism, which produce the same symptoms (pp 206).

The term *aphasia* relates to a group of syndromes caused by destruction of cerebral language functions, which are usually located in the left hemisphere. There is a large and fascinating neurological literature concerning the various kinds and manifestations of aphasia and their relationship to higher mental functions. Aphasiologists are able to make accurate localizing predictions simply on the basis of an aphasia examination, but the non-neurological clinician is unequipped to do this, and there are simpler ways to determine cerebral localization. In general, the reader may remember a distinction between *fluent aphasia* and *non-fluent aphasia*.

A patient with non-fluent aphasia has few verbal productions, and all are difficult, both for him and for the examiner. He has more trouble speaking than he does understanding, and some patients with non-fluent aphasia understand perfectly. They mispronounce words and are usually aware that their language is faulty. Non-fluent aphasia is accompanied by (right) facial paresis, at least, and usually there is hemiparesis. Non-fluent aphasia is usually caused by a lesion of frontal portions of the language mechanism.

There are several kinds of fluent aphasia, depending on the location of the causative lesion in the temporal or parietal lobes, but patients with fluent aphasias share the ability to produce verbalizations effortlessly. They usually appear to be unaware of their language defect. They are unintelligible to the examiner even though they carry on a conversation in normal tones and frequently normal cadences of speech. They are likely to produce language that sounds initially like word salad, filled with several kinds of neologisms. Even careful neurological examination may fail to disclose other abnormalities in some cases, but most patients with fluent aphasia have associated sensory loss, visual field defects, and at least reflex changes on the (right) side.

Aphasia may be difficult to distinguish from dementia and even from psychosis unless the examiner is alert to the problem. If the diagnosis of aphasia is unclear, it is often helpful to inquire about the patient's nonverbal behavior, as distinct from his verbal productions. One family had been told that the father was becoming senile because he did not talk right. Further questioning about nonverbal behavior revealed that he was running his own dry goods store and making money at it! Although he could not converse with his family and customers, he singlehandedly made correct change, checked inventory, and ordered new stock. This was not dementia. Investigation disclosed a focal, left temporal lobe lesion.

If the patient talks fluently, but unintelligibly, it may be difficult initially to determine whether his disturbance is aphasic or psychotic. However, the nonverbal behavior of the aphasic patient is not pathological in psychiatric terms, even though he may not respond normally to people who talk to him. Aphasic neologisms relate to language structure and pronunciation difficulties, not to tortured thought processes and misperceptions of motivation or emotion. Aphasic patients usually have focal, right-sided abnormalities and cooperate with the examination, while psychotic patients usually have normal neurological examinations and may not be able to cooperate with the examiner. If a clinician remembers that a diagnostic problem may arise and makes the effort, he will usually have no trouble with the distinction.

Hysteria and Malingering. For this volume, the term *hysteria* means that the patient has complained to a doctor about physical symptoms that have no basis in organic disease. The diagnosis of *malingering* indicates evidence that the patient is deliberately lying. This distinction is largely of medicolegal importance and usually has little significance to the office diagnosis. Unless there is clear evidence of prevarication, the clinician should avoid accusing the patient of malingering. He may use the more inclusive term "hysterical" in the context of this volume without the hazards associated with a false accusation.

Some hysterical patients do present their history briefly, and in sequential fashion, so their diagnosis must be based upon the complete absence of physical abnormalities that could be directly related to the specific history of disability. However, most hysterical and malingering patients offer confusing stories for organic disease because the disease does not exist. Additionally, if they are not interrupted, they offer an interminable story complicated by embellishments and comments. I have identified four characteristic methods of hysterical presentation that leave the clinician uninformed. These characteristics allow the physician to apply the five-minute–five-point rules to his differential diagnosis as he takes the history.

The first is the *shopping list approach.* Instead of giving a sequential history of developing disability, the patient presents a list of symptoms and detailed comments about each one. There may be no direct comments about related disability, or the description of disability does not directly relate to the symptoms. Unless he is interrupted, his presentation may last *much* longer than five minutes!

A second hysterical presentation is closely related to the first. Instead of a list of symptoms, the patient presents a list of the previous physicians he has consulted and their sequential incorrect diagnoses. If a patient still has no accurate diagnosis, his chance of actually possessing a progressive, crippling organic disease diminishes in direct proportion to the number of competent physicians he has consulted and to the elapsed time since the onset of his illness.

Inappropriate emotional tone is also an indication of hysteria and is the third diagnostic clue. The reader has undoubtedly already learned that *la belle indifférence* to ostensibly overwhelming disability suggests hysteria. The converse is also true. If a patient demands instant attention to some terrible symptom that has plagued him without change for the past five years, the diagnosis is just as certainly hysteria as though he were indifferent.

Inappropriate emotional tone occurs among professionals too, when they encounter an hysterical patient. When emergency room personnel request immediate consultation, the consultant usually finds a seriously ill patient awaiting him. If, instead, the patient is perfectly stable and calm, but the emergency room professionals and family are at their wits end, the disorder is usually not organic. How often are the personnel of an active emergency room upset by a seriously ill patient? They are busy, not upset.

Physicians may use their own, as well as others' inappropriate emotional responses in formulating a diagnosis. Doctors are usually not annoyed when their patients talk about symptoms. They are frequently angry with hysterical patients, and this fact may be used as an accurate aid to diagnosis if it is recognized.

The fourth hysterical presentation carries more pitfalls for the clinician, but it emphasizes an important characteristic of hysterical symptoms: their *unusual* nature. A presenting complaint *ostensibly within the doctor's area of specialization* that is completely new to him is likely to be hysterical. Naturally, the orthopedist is unfamiliar with the usual complaints in the practice of hematology, but it must be an unusual patient whose orthopedic complaint is totally unfamiliar to the orthopedist.

The human body is complex, but it is orderly, and it becomes sick and damaged in predictable and recurrent patterns. On the other hand, the human personality is infinitely complex and unpredictable. Hysterical symptoms are often as complex and unpredictable as the personalities that generate them, and their unusual character can alert the diagnostician. To illustrate: An engineer presented with the complaint of decreased visual acuity in his *far peripheral visual field!* The normal visual acuity in that location is less than 20/400, and his neurological examination and visual fields were perfectly normal.

This criterion, the *unusual* nature of hysterical complaints, is dangerous. It must be used with extreme caution, because an unrecognized complaint may actually be a routine part of office practice in some other speciality. Patients may be damaged by a missed diagnosis if the physician diagnoses hysteria using this criterion alone without further supplemental evidence.

Psychosis. It is sometimes hard to determine that a patient is *psychotic.* As we have mentioned, schizophrenic neologisms may resemble fluent aphasia. The depressed patient with psychomotor retardation may appear demented, especially if he is elderly. When the clinician asks about behavioral changes, he may find a history of weeping spells, sleeplessness, agitation, and hallucinations. The physical examination should be normal. Depressed and schizophrenic people frequently develop hysterical symptoms, and the underlying mental illness may remain undiagnosed. This is a tragic failure of medical practice because psychosis and its consequent hysterical symptoms are eminently treatable. It is imperative that every clinician learn to identify significantly depressed or psychotic patients when they come to him under any guise.

If he cannot determine that the patient is actually psychotic, the clinician will not go far astray if he has applied the five-minute–five-point rule correctly. He will have ruled out dementia and aphasia and now need only distinguish between an hysterical symptom of serious mental illness and more restricted hysterical complaint. At this point, he should know how to refer the patient to psychiatric consultation for more accurate assessment and effective treatment.

FORMAL NEUROLOGICAL EXAMINATION

If used intelligently, the careful physical examination becomes an independent diagnostic tool. As the clinician completes his detailed inquiry, he has a picture of his patient's disease, which may be confirmed or denied during the physical examination. If the predictions are borne out, his diagnosis is strengthened. If they are not, he has an opportunity to recognize that he is in error, and he can immediately begin again and correct his mistakes. Once he has formed opinions based on the combined evidence from the history and physical examinations, he can consider how he must use the laboratories to confirm his diagnosis. Like the history and physical examination, clinical laboratories offer independent assessments of the same nervous system from different points of view. Each produces highly reproducible results, and the eventual diagnosis rests upon the clinician's ability to correlate information from all sources.

Chapter 15 describes the techniques and thought processes needed for a very rapid but complete neurological screening examination. However, since this book is first about the nervous system, and second, about some of the ways it is affected by disease, and *not* about "how to do examinations," I counsel the student to refer to that chapter only after reading the rest of the book.

It is important that the student understand the material in at least the first six chapters, so he can use this knowledge in the development of techniques that would allow him to converse intelligently with this marvelous organ and find out what is wrong with it. Without that prior knowledge, he must learn to examine sick people by rote; and he will miss the joy that comes with understanding, and more importantly, the diagnosis!

MENTAL STATUS EXAMINATION

A reproducible examination of higher mental functions is a valuable tool. It should help the clinician to distinguish between dementia and the amnestic syndrome, and should help him to diagnosis hysteria and malingering. It may also provide more information about psychosis and aphasia.

This mental status examination does not provide detailed information about the type of psychosis, because that special information is more important to psychologists and psychiatrists. It does help to determine the presence of psychosis through *identification* of disordered thought processes and abnormal emotional tone. These may be observed during any portion of the diagnostic interview, but they often become more evident during the formal mental status examination if the clinician has experience with the normal answers to his questions. The psychotic patient may know where he is and know the date. He may be able to subtract serial sevens well. His interpretations of proverbs may be concrete, colorful, or highly unusual. He may not remember items from the specific tests of memory, but he may display unusually acute memories of chance events that assumed heightened importance to him during the examination.

People often first recognize that they forget names when they reach 40 or 50, and they become concerned that they are becoming senile. This concern becomes an hysterical symptom if they are not suffering from dementia, and if they are so worried that they come to the doctor about it. It is one form of the "Oh my God, I'm falling apart!" syndrome, which can occur at almost any age and may be identified during the formal mental status examination. Such a patient may give the examiner a detailed description of how he first learned that he was dementing and a list of all the things he forgets. Then, as the formal mental status examination begins, he may not be able to tell where he is or subtract 7 from 100, and he may not remember anything from the immediate or the delayed recall items in the examination. Such failure is the intellectual equivalent of hysterical hemiplegia, which is first displayed during the physical examination of a patient who has walked into the consultation room unassisted.

In such cases, it is imperative that the clinician establish during the initial part of the interview, when he is "not examining mental status," that the patient's memory and higher mental functions are really normal. He can do this by steering the conversation into other channels and discussing current events or some other topic of interest to the patient, or he can simply become aware of the mental processes he is observing during the patient's spontaneous conversation. Once the patient has flunked the formal mental status examination, the clinician can discuss the discrepancy between his function during the two distinct portions of the interview, reassure him that this does not represent dementia, and challenge him to do the formal mental status examination again. Usually, doctor and patient can demonstrate that the performance during the second formal mental status examination is greatly improved or normal, even when new items are introduced. Then the patient can leave his consultation greatly relieved and "cured" of his hysterical concern.

Suggested Sequence for Examination

It is unnecessary to perform a mental status examination for patients whose mentation is clearly normal or whose diagnosis is unquestioned. This examination should be used to differentiate mental status abnormalities when the diagnosis is unclear. It should be performed in the same way each time so that the examiner can learn the range of normal responses. As he begins, the clinician should give the patient an explanation that this is going to be a more formal test of his mental function. The tasks may appear foolish, but his cooperation is essential. The simplest problems are presented first; more complex ones appear as the examination proceeds. The examination also contains several items for immediate recall and short-term memory that are introduced in memorable fashion. It begins innocuously:

"What is today's date?"   (Day, date, year)
"Where are we now?"   (Town, building, floor, room)
"How would you get home from here?"

"Who is the President?"

This last question provides an opportunity to test further details of remote and more recent memory. Answers depend upon the breadth of the patient's interest and his comprehension of complex events. The entire population is exposed to certain issues surrounding the President and the federal government. Questions about public events may involve a current presidency and details of its history, issues of energy conservation, or any other burning issue that affects both the physician and the patient. The advantage of testing memory for public events is that *the physician also knows the answers*. He cannot evaluate the accuracy of a response to questions about the patient's third grade teacher. Push your patient to the limits of his knowledge here, and then move on.

"Now I want to test your ability to calculate. What is 7 from 100?"
"Good. Keep going."

Without repetition of the assignment (subtraction by seven) normal people continue the task as far as they are allowed to go. Even normal people may make an occasional mistake of subtraction. Demented people make more mistakes. More importantly, they forget the task, and may end up subtracting by five or stopping in confusion. When the examiner is satisfied that he knows how the task is being performed, he terminates the subtraction sharply after some specific number, for example, 44.

"Stop!"
"Now count backward by one from 20."
"20, 19, 18, 17, 16-"
"Stop!"

Two memorable numbers have been sharply introduced. The patient is not warned that these numbers will reappear later in the examination to test whether a recent memory has been made. Use of these numbers also has the advantage that they are known to the examiner. Short-term memory items about the patient's breakfast menu cannot be evaluated for accuracy.

Another test of immediate recall and recent memory should be added at this point because the examination must continue for at least ten minutes before recent memory can be tested. Some examiners assign five things to get at the store. This task is disjointed, and some normal people fail. Also, there is clear warning that the five things will be reintroduced, and the patient may concentrate on them as the examination proceeds. This author is partial to a "Cowboy Story" whose plot is not evident till the end. The reader may prefer his own story.

"Listen carefully now, because I am going to tell you a story. I want you to tell it back to me when I am finished.

"Cowboy Joe and his dog, Rex, drove a herd of cattle from Dallas to Abilene. They sold their cattle and came home rich! The cowboy decided to take a vacation so he and his dog got on a train and rode to San Francisco, where the cowboy left his dog in a motel and went downtown shopping. He bought a whole new outfit: new hat, new vest, new chaps, new boots, new gun and holster. When he got home, the dog did not recognize him and barked – until the cowboy spoke."

"Now repeat the story to me as well as you can."

The examiner may assess immediate recall as the patient retells the story this time. Telling the story fixes in the patient's mind those facts he did acquire. He is not warned that the story will recur, and the rest of the examination proceeds while immediate recall is converted into a recent memory.

Proverbs are useful because most Americans have heard common American proverbs.

"People in glass houses. . . ."
"Still waters. . . ."
"Don't count your chickens. . . ."
– and many others. Normal people give responses related to the abstract meanings of each proverb. They talk about people with foibles, or complex silent people, or plans for the future. Demented people are more concrete. They talk about greenhouses, rivers, and broken eggs. The patient should have at least one chance to improve a poor answer.

"Is there any other meaning that you can think of?"

Psychotic people may give a concrete interpretation initially, but their second response may be unique – related to special associations they have to the words or to the examiner himself.

Similarities are given in the order of ascending difficulty.

"How are these things similar?"

	Demented	Normal
1. Dog & Cat	Four legs, hair	Domestic animals Pets, mammals
2. Cat & Cow	Not similar Four legs, hair	Domestic animals Mammals
3. Cow & Fly	Not similar Four legs Cow has flies	Both members of the animal kingdom
4. Fly & Daisy	Not similar	Both living things

These similarities are not immutable. Each examiner will develop his own sequences of increasing difficulty. Some *normal* people need a clue for the last pair of similar things:

"How are a fly and a daisy similar in a way that a daisy and a stone are not?"

The next transition may be abrupt:

"What was the last number you said to me?" (16)

"What number did you reach when you subtracted by sevens?" (44)

"Tell me the cowboy story again."

Normal people remember these things. Demented people may or may not, depending on the extent of their dementia. The person with amnestic syndrome has no notion where the questions originated.

The cowboy story is especially useful in this respect. Normal people may not repeat the story verbatim when they first tell it, but they do not lose information for the second telling. Demented people lose many facts on the first telling and may not even make a coherent story of it. Ten minutes later, more facts have disappeared. The amnestic patient has performed well to this point. He knew where he was, gave a fair account of past events, subtracted sevens well, and told the cowboy story well the first time through. However, when he is asked to tell the cowboy story again, he does not remember that there ever was a cowboy! Worried people become very anxious as the cowboy story unfolds. Their response on first telling may be terribly inadequate. After they have calmed down, the second telling is no worse and may actually improve some.

Having completed his history, his neurological and general physical examinations, and his mental status examination, the physician is in possession of a clear diagnosis or perhaps several related possibilities. The laboratory examinations can help him to distinguish which one is accurate.

CHAPTER 2

Special Laboratory Examinations

Clinical laboratories are best used when they are asked to provide independent assessment of the clinical situation once the clinician has thought through the problems presented by the history and by the physical examination. If he fails to formulate precise questions for the laboratories, he will frequently find that the diagnosis is still in doubt once their results become available.

However, if the history, the physical examination, and the laboratory investigations are viewed as three independent diagnostic modalities, they establish a firm diagnosis when their results all point in the same direction, and they allow the clinician to recognize errors in his analysis of the case when they do not. The clinician may enhance the values of individual laboratory examinations through close consultation with laboratory specialists.

RADIOLOGY

The radiology department offers a wide range of special examinations: plain skull and spine radiography, myelography, cerebral angiography, pneumoencephalography, and computed tomography.

Plain Skull Radiography

Plain skull radiographs disclose the bony structure of the head and demonstrate some calcifications within the brain. Tomography of the skull improves the resolution of subtle abnormalities, especially at the base of the skull; however, most diseases of the brain are not associated with intracranial calcification, so a negative report does not exclude intracranial disease.

Plain skull radiographs are frequently useful in demonstrating metastases to the calvarium, and secondary signs of convexity meningioma are occasionally visible. If the pineal is heavily calcified, it, too, is visible and may be shifted away from the midline. Calcified tumors are occasionally visible on plain skull radiographs, but now there are much more sensitive procedures which supercede the plain skull radiograph for the evaluation of intracranial calcifications.

Plain Spine Radiography

Because the bony spine closely surrounds the spinal cord and nerve roots, bony lesions, or lesions which also damage bone, frequently cause spinal cord or nerve root compression. This is especially true in the cervical region, where the spinal cord is large in relation to the size of the spinal canal. Cervical spondylosis is a common disease which often impinges on neural structures.

However, the normal process of aging produces radiographic changes of cervical spondylosis in most people, so the clinician and radiologist must examine the cervical spine radiographs together in order to correlate the clinical history with the radiographic changes. If the clinician has predicted the presence of abnormalities, and there is radiographic evidence of disease *in the predicted location,* he has strong confirmation for the accuracy of his diagnosis.

Primary tumors of the bone, of the spinal cord, or its nerve roots are frequently evident on plain spine radiographs because of the damage they do to the adjacent pedicle or to the neural foramen. Occasionally, even the vertebral body is eroded. In patients with metastatic cancer to the vertebral column, the bone scan is usually a more sensitive examination than plain spine radiography, because abnormalities can be detected earlier and the scan demonstrates dissemination of disease throughout the bony skeleton more adequately. Multiple myeloma is the exception to this rule, because frequently the bone scan is normal while plain spine and rib radiographs disclose disseminated disease.

Spine radiographs are seldom helpful in patients suspected of having herniated lumbar disc, because the disc itself is not calcified, and disc disease is not well correlated with bone changes. The plain spine films are performed in such cases to help rule out other causes for the patient's symptoms. If the patient has an appropriate history and localizing abnormalities on the physical examination, the myelogram is the diagnostic procedure of choice to evaluate disc disease.

Myelography

An iodinated contrast agent is usually used to examine the spinal subarachnoid space. Mass lesions, which distort the subarachnoid space, may be visualized and their location identified for surgery. Myelography does not identify lesions that are positioned far laterally in the neural foramen or outside the spinal canal. Lesions which do not alter the shape of visualized structures, such as those of multiple sclerosis or amyotrophic lateral sclerosis, are also not visualized during myelography.

Myelography is frequently performed incorrectly because the clinician has failed to tell the radiologist where to look. The techniques for lumbar, thoracic, cervical, and complete myelography differ, so it is important that the radiologist and clinician consult with each other before the procedure.

Myelography is not indicated simply for the complaint of back pain, if there is no localizing abnormality on the neurological examination. Many patients have functional back pain. Some of these have irrelevant myelographic abnormalities, and the myelogram or the subsequent surgery is likely to make them worse. On the other hand, patients with multiple sclerosis and amyotrophic lateral sclerosis frequently need myelography, despite the clinician's prediction that it will be normal, because they and the physician need to be certain that there is no treatable structural disease causing the symptoms.

The physician must be decisive when he orders a myelogram. First, he must decide within narrow limits where to look for the lesion, and convey this information to the radiologist. The clinician should specify that the contrast material be taken to a considerably higher level than originally requested if no lesion is found. In that circumstance, it is helpful for the clinician to be present during the myelogram, so that he and the radiologist may decide together how the study should proceed.

Second, if a structural lesion is found where the clinician expected it, he must be prepared to recommend surgery. Myelography is not a procedure that should be done for diagnosis only, without thought of surgical intervention. For this reason, it is frequently appropriate to involve the surgeon *before* the study.

Third, if the study fails to demonstrate the area of concern, the clinician must be ready to recommend that it be repeated immediately. Such a myelogram is not negative; it is inadequate. Not infrequently, easy diagnoses are missed because an inadequate study was accepted as normal. This is a pitfall that must be avoided at all cost!

Conversely, the clinician may not assume that every abnormality is significant. He must correlate the myelographic results with his history and physical examination, and if the myelogram does not "fit," the myelogram itself or the physician's prior conclusions, should be regarded as suspect. For instance, the patient with back pain, weakness of peronei, anterior tibial and extensor hallucis longus muscles, a nearly normal ankle jerk, and sensory loss on the lateral surface of the leg has an L5 root syndrome. A disc protusion at the L5-S1 disc space is a common myelographic abnormality, but in this case, it is irrelevant because it cannot explain the patient's symptoms. A lesion at the L3-4 interspace is unexpected, but it might be the cause. On the basis of his findings, the clinician had predicted a herniated disc at the L4-5 interspace, and if it is there on the myelogram, surgery will be beneficial. The physician who is not used to making this kind of prediction on the basis of his history and physical examination, should request consultation before he orders myelography.

Myelography is usually not a particularly painful, dangerous, nor difficult examination. Cervical myelography is uncomfortable, especially if the table must be tilted in the head-down position for long periods of time to allow the contrast medium to fill the cervical subarachnoid space. During this time, the head must be held in extreme extension to prevent the contrast medium from spilling into the middle cranial fossa. Despite his discomfort, the patient must be warned to hold still during this part of the examination. The consequences of a sudden movement at that time may be myelographic contrast medium in the middle cranial fossa, headache, and permanent evidence of contrast medium in subsequent skull radiographs. Patients with a history of allergy to iodine or radiographic contrast media may have an allergic reaction during the study. Preparations to handle such a reaction must be made in advance.

The water-soluble myelographic contrast agent, metrizamide (Amipaque®), has recently been released for general use. Because it is water-soluble, this agent leaves the subarachnoid space by bulk flow with spinal fluid and does not need to be removed after the procedure.

In high concentration, metrizamide provides excellent contrast for lumbar and even cervical myelograms. However, its most dramatic value occurs in low concentration where the agent may be used with the CT scanner to outline spinal cord and brainstem structures, providing anatomical detail that cannot be matched by any other procedure.

Occasionally patients have suffered seizures from this contrast agent, so we have recommended that the patient who is scheduled for metrizamide myelography receive 200 mg of phenobarbital by mouth on the evening before his examination and another 100 mg I.M. early the next morning before the study.

Metrizamide is an extremely expensive agent, and this factor may limit its general use where iodinated oil myelography could provide comparable results.

Cerebral Angiography

This is a special procedure that examines the blood vessels of the neck and head. It may identify inflammatory or mass lesions that distort these vessels, and it discloses evidence of atherosclerotic disease in the great vessels of the neck and in small arteries of the brain. It is an invasive study with infrequent but potentially serious consequences, so it should be ordered only by neurologists, neurosurgeons, and vascular surgeons. Like myelography, cerebral angiography may be thought of as a prelude to surgery, even though it discloses many lesions that are not amenable to surgical treatment.

The study is usually performed by passing a radiopaque catheter from the femoral artery into the abdominal and thoracic aorta, and then placing the catheter selectively in the arteries that lead to the head.

After the catheter is properly placed, iodinated contrast medium is injected and radiographs are obtained, using a serial film changer. The patient will feel warmth within his head and hear the noise of the film changer as the films are exposed, but he must remain still during this portion of the examination so that the radiographs will be sharp.

There is a small but real risk of serious complications from angiography. These include stroke, heart attack, and even death. Bleeding into the groin occurs but it is usually of no consequence. Occasionally, a thrombus forms in the femoral artery which must be removed surgically. Allergic reactions to the contrast material can occur, and if the patient gives a history of such a reaction, or is allergic to iodine or seafoods, special precautions must be taken before the study is performed.

Despite these dire warnings, angiography is generally a safe and exceedingly useful diagnostic tool, whose actual risk in skilled hands is small, and whose diagnostic benefits are large. The clinician should recommend angiography to his patient if the specialist and radiologist agree that it is the best test available to arrive at the correct diagnosis.

Pneumoencephalography

The pneumoencephalogram outlines the cerebral ventricular system and sulci with air. It provides exquisite delineation of these structures, especially if it is used in conjunction with tomography. Since the advent of computed tomography, the pneumoencephalogram is not used as much as formerly, but it occasionally plays an important role in the diagnosis of posterior fossa lesions where the computed tomographic studies and nuclear brain scans are less revealing.

Pneumoencephalography should only be ordered by neurologists and neurosurgeons. If the study is performed in the presence of a mass lesion in the brain, there is danger of transtentorial herniation and death. The study is invasive and potentially a preoperative procedure, and therefore not for general use.

Patients undergoing pneumoencephalography are strapped securely into a special sommersaulting chair. The study begins with a lumbar puncture. Then aliquots of air are injected into the subarachnoid space, and radiographs are exposed in many different projections. The patient should be warned that he will certainly develop a severe headache during the procedure, and that he may vomit. Afterward, he may have headaches for several days and may not fully recover for several weeks.

When performed properly, pneumoencephalography is a safe procedure. There are no allergic reactions except to preoperative medications. Complications from the stress of the examination, such as heart attack and stroke, are possible but very uncommon.

Computed Tomography (CT)

CT scanners are becoming universally available. Computed tomography has allowed more accurate and earlier diagnosis of brain and body disease without potentially hazardous invasive procedures and costly hospitalization. The machine uses a highly columnated x-ray beam to produce a computer-generated image of a brain slice. The diagnostic value of a small dose of radiation has been vastly magnified by this technological advancement. Because CT scans do not depend upon the photographic characteristics of x-ray films, they are more sensitive to small differences in radio density than other x-ray methods. At its present best resolution, the CT scan can distinguish between normal gray and white matter. It easily detects fresh blood and clearly distinguishes brain from cerebral spinal fluid. Edema shows darkly lucent by comparison to normal brain, and the pineal is almost always visualized.

During the CT scan, iodinated contrast medium is usually injected intravenously to demonstrate vascular structures. This procedure, called enhancement, routinely discloses normal arterial and venous structures. Vascular lesions emerge dramatically during enhancement, and even the acute lesions of multiple sclerosis are occasionally visible. These have never before been visualized during life! Since the CT scan does not depend upon changes in brain physiology, both active and static structural lesions are clearly visualized.

There are limitations to computed tomography. Small posterior fossa abnormalities may be missed because of the density of the adjacent petrous bones. Lesions which have the same attenuation coefficient as normal brain are invisible (i.e., some subacute subdural hematomas). Lastly, lesions smaller than 0.5 cm in diameter are poorly visualized unless they are calcified or enhance strongly.

CT scanning is safe. Apart from an occasional allergic reaction to iodinated contrast agent, there is no morbidity. Outpatients may be rescanned frequently, and the results are available for immediate examination.

NUCLEAR MEDICINE

By utilizing small doses of a radioactive isotope attached to specific carrier molecules, the modern department of nuclear medicine provides unique information about the biological characteristics of many tissues. Because of the small dose of radioactivity, the photon yield is several orders of magnitude lower than that used to generate a radiographic image. Each portion of the detection apparatus designed to increase the quality of the image lowers the total available signal; so, by comparison to the radiology department, the detection devices are working close to the level of background radiation noise.

Nuclear Brain Scan

Technetium-99m is presently the radionuclide of choice for brain scanning. Its emission energy of 140 KeV provides 8-13 cm. of tissue penetration and allows the resultant images to reflect activity which is located to one or the other side of the brain. Its half-life is only six hours. This rapid decay allows the use of a larger dose of the isotope without danger to the patient. The gamma camera has largely replaced the rectilinear scanner in modern laboratories, because of its greater speed and sharper images.

As a result, the modern brain scan provides information about cerebral blood flow to the brain during the first passage of the radiopharmaceutical agent through the brain. It also detects tissues which have increased permeability to the radiopharmaceutical at one hour, or several hours after injection. Repeated studies over several weeks disclose information about the changing biological characteristics of some lesions and allow for evaluation of treatment. ^{99m}Tc is chemically active and may be attached to many carrier molecules, thus providing the investigator with a wider range of biological specificity.

The "flow study" is performed by injection of the radiopharmaceutical as a bolus into the antecubital vein. As radioactivity first reaches the neck and head, the gamma camera records its changing location during the first circulation through arteries, capillaries, and veins. The accumulated scintillations from each period of 1 1/2 to 2 seconds may be photographed, giving an incomplete but useful notion of the distribution of cerebral blood flow. Decreased blood flow caused by obstruction in a major artery of the brain, or a subdural hematoma on the surface; or increased cerebral blood flow in a vascular tumor or arteriovenous malformation may both be seen on the flow study.

Brain images in at least four projections are taken immediately after the flow study and again one or several hours later. Changes in the distribution of the radiopharmaceutical over the period of the study provide information about the biological activity of target tissues. Biologically avid tissues, like normal parotid gland and metastatic cancer, concentrate the radiopharmaceutical progressively despite its continued excretion from the blood. Such tissues may be visible on initial images but become relatively more prominent several hours later. Less avid tissues, like normal Sylvian vessels and arteriovenous malformations, are prominently detected on the flow study and initial images, but they fade as the vascular pool activity decreases.

The brain scan demonstrates changing characteristics of ischemic stroke over the period of many weeks. If a scan is performed immediately after the stroke, there may be an asymmetry of blood flow, but static images are normal. During the next few days to several weeks, a static imaging abnormality appears in the region of stroke which remains for several months but eventually fades, leaving only the asymmetry of blood flow.

The nuclear brain scan shares with the CT scan a complete absence of morbidity. It is easy for the patient, easily repeated, and it provides unique diagnostic information. For these reasons, the brain scan and CT scan have become the primary neurological screening tools, and have largely replaced the skull x-ray and all but the specialized uses of EEG.

Gamma Cisternogram

The gamma cisternogram discloses pathways of bulk spinal fluid flow around the spinal cord and brain. Technetium-99m–labeled inulin, DTPA or albumin, Iodine-131–labeled human serum albumin, or Ytterbium-169–labeled DTPA is injected into the lumbar subarachnoid space via lumbar puncture, and its migration is followed over the next 48 hours. During the first four to six hours, the radio-pharmaceutical migrates upward into the cisterns at the base of the brain. Under normal circumstances, it continues to ascend sym-metrically through the Sylvian fissues and over the convexities of the brain before it exits over the Pacchionian granulations near the vertex of the skull. Normally, none of the radioactivity is detectable within the ventricular system.

In patients with dilated ventricles due to cerebral atrophy and in those with normal pressure hydrocephalus, radioactivity appears prominently within the ventricles and may not migrate freely over the convexities. Sometimes the radioactivity leaves the ventricles promptly, but other times it remains for 48 hours or more. This phenomenon has been termed "stasis". The abnormalities are easy to detect. However, it is difficult to determine their significance. The problem relates to the treatment of normal pressure hydrocephalus.

Normal Pressure Hydrocephalus

Hakim and Adams[3] first reported the syndrome of occult hydro-cephalus with normal spinal fluid pressure in 1965. The symptoms were progressive dementia, ataxia, and incontinence. The pneumo-encephalogram disclosed dilated ventricles without passage of air over the convexities of the brain. The authors postulated that the syndrome was caused by extraventricular obstruction to the flow of spinal fluid. They reported that their patients responded dramatical-ly to shunting procedures which channeled the spinal fluid directly into the venous system.

Since Hakim and Adams' first paper, investigators have been at-tempting to learn how to predict which patients will improve after a shunt and which will not. There has been no unanimity of opinion. Recently, Belloni et al.[1] found that a combination of typical pneu-moencephalographic findings and typical abnormalities in the gam-ma cisternogram provided the best prediction for improvement. In doubtful cases, 24-hour recordings of CSF pressure added weight to the prognosis for improvement. The physical and mental status of the patient was irrelevant except when there was depression of con-sciousness. On the other hand, in an apparently equal study, Jacobs et al.[4] concluded that the clinical presentation is most important while laboartory examinations were unreliable predictors of improvement. Shinkin et al.[5] have seriously questioned the notion that obstruction to spinal fluid flow is actually a major etiological

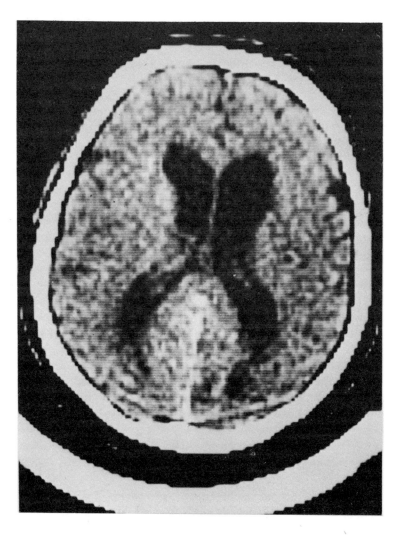

Figure 2-1. *CT scan of patient with normal pressure hydrocephalus. Note marked enlargement of lateral ventricles without significant cerebral atrophy. Courtesy of Dr. Alfred S. Berne, Crouse-Irving Memorial Hospital, Syracuse, New York.*

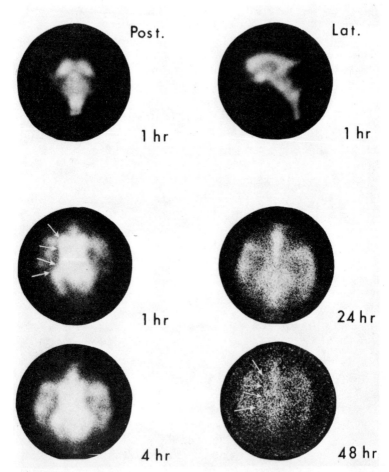

Figure 2.2. ⁹⁹ᵐ*Tc gamma cisternogram of same patient. Courtesy of Dr. Edward G. Bell, Crouse-Irving Memorial Hospital, Syracuse, New York. Above, the lateral ventricles are strongly visualized at one-hour without evidence of flow over the cerebral convexities. Below, four vertex views disclose "stasis" of the radiopharmaceutical agent within the ventricles, even at 48 hours. Even though this patient had an absolutely typical history, and strong CT and gamma cisternographic evidence for normal pressure hydrocephalus, he showed no improvement after his shunt.*

factor in the production of the syndrome. They have suggested that there may be an alteration of brain chemistry, which is corrected in some cases by shunting procedures, and may account for improvement when it occurs.

What recommendations can one make in light of this conflicting evidence? First, it seems certain that patients with gradually progressing dementia whose cortical atrophy is commensurate with the increase in ventricular size, are not candidates for a shunt.[2] This is the picture of Alzheimer's disease, and there is no effective treatment. If a pneumoencephalogram is done and shows air over the convexities, or if a CT scan shows a typical picture of cerebral atrophy, and if the gamma cisternogram shows normal patterns of flow, the diagnosis of Alzheimer's disease would be confirmed.

It also seems certain that there are patients who do improve after a shunt, but it is difficult to identify them in advance. If a patient is developing dementia, incontinence, and ataxia, and the examinations reveal hydrocephalus out of proportion to the amount of cortical atrophy, or a typically abnormal gamma cisternogram, CT scan, and pneumoencephalogram, a shunt should be recommended as a last resort which might halt the progression of a relentless disease.

Lastly, some patients develop hydrocephalus and mental and motor abnormalities after subarachnoid hemorrhage, head trauma, or meningitis. This probably occurs because of scarring in the basal cisterns with obstruction of the foramina of Magendie and Luschka, or because of direct obstruction of the Pacchionian granulations. We cannot make definite predictions about the results of shunting in such patients either, but having been normal previously, they should be given the benefit of treatment until we develop better predictive examinations.

ELECTROENCEPHALOGRAM (EEG)

Despite the development of powerful diagnostic tools like the CT and nuclear brain scans, the EEG is still useful in certain instances: 1) diagnosis of seizure type, 2) determination of death, 3) follow-up after trauma, and 4) diagnosis and prognosis of certain slow viral infections. It has been superseded by the CT and nuclear brain scans for the diagnosis and localization of structural cerebral disease and because of this, has ceased to be a routine screening procedure in neurology.

Seizure Type

An abnormal EEG is not diagnostic of a seizure disorder. That is the function of the clinical history. A carefully performed EEG can strengthen the clinical diagnosis, and more importantly, the EEG is the best laboratory examination to establish the type of seizure disorder present. This subject will be discussed more fully in the chapter on seizure disorder (see 180 ff).

Determination of Death

Standards are being established for the determination of death in patients with irreversible coma. In several states in this country, laws have been enacted which permit a determination of death after criteria of current medical practice are met, even though the heart still beats. The medical definition of death is still evolving, but clinical signs include absence of respiratory or cardiovascular function, absence of brainstem and deep tendon reflexes, absence of all reaction to outside stimuli. Highly specific EEG criteria have also evolved. None of these criteria may be applied if the patient has hypothermia or is in the acute stages of drug overdose.

The role of the EEG in the determination of death is a medicolegal one. The electroencephalographer must arrange for proper instrumentation and protocol to perform a death recording. Without these precautions, it would be hazardous for a physician to use the results of EEG in his determination of death.

Follow-Up After Trauma

There are sequential changes in the EEG after head trauma which can help document that a given accident produced brain damage and indicate whether the electrical activity is returning toward normal. Sequential tracings, performed by a competent laboratory, may be used as evidence in court.

Slow Viral Infections

Most recently, EEG has become helpful in the diagnosis of several slow viral infections (see subacute sclerosing panencephalitis p. 261 and Creuzfeldt-Jakob disease pp. 254 ff.). Abnormal discharges with regular periodicity develop in these diseases and become more frequent as death approaches.

The EEG is useful in proportion to the care given to its recording and interpretation. The electrodes must be positioned correctly and applied with a minimum of electrical resistance, then tested to be sure they are correctly applied. The recording should consist of at least 30 minutes of unactivated EEG, recorded from various combinations of electrodes. Photic stimulation and forced hyperventilation are routinely performed. A well-run laboratory has facilities for sleep recordings and other special examinations. Finally, the technician and the electroencephalographer need special training in the modern aspects of electroencephalography. The usefulness of the EEG is seriously diminished by inattention to detail at any stage. The individual clinician must evaluate the EEG laboratory available to his patients and determine for himself whether its quality warrants the spending of their money.

ELECTROMYOGRAPHY (EMG) AND NERVE CONDUCTION VELOCITY (NCV)

EMG and NCV help to distinguish the anatomical origin of symptoms from the motor unit: the anterior horn cells of the spinal cord, peripheral nerve, myoneural junction, and the muscle itself. The EMG uses intramuscular needle electrodes to detect the electrical activity of resting and contracting muscle. The NCV is performed with a surface stimulation electrode and a surface recording electrode to determine nerve conduction velocity and characteristics of neuromuscular transmission.

A number of clinical questions are definitely resolved after competent electrical examination. Amyotrophic lateral sclerosis frequently begins with weakness and wasting in hands and arms. It may be confused with spinal cord involvement due to cervical spondylosis. The EMG can disclose abnormal motor units in the lower extremities of such a patient and establish the diagnosis of diffuse motor neuron disease.

Myasthenia, polymyositis, and psychoneurosis all produce symptoms of weakness. The electrical characteristics of each are quite different.

Nerve entrapments, such as carpal tunnel syndrome and tardy ulnar palsy, are common. The electrical changes in these conditions are clearly evident before definitive physical findings appear, and surgery may be performed with confidence if the history and nerve conduction velocity findings correspond well. On the other hand, if the symptoms of median nerve dysfunction result from a generalized neuropathy, producing more disturbing symptoms from the median nerve than elsewhere, the nerve conduction velocity in other nerves discloses a widespread abnormality and can lead toward a more productive medical evaluation.

The examination is electrically complex, but the patient's part is simple. Apart from the modest pain of the intramuscular electrodes, or the momentary pain of maximal nerve stimulation during examination of the myoneural junction, there is little discomfort, and the procedure is completely safe. In the hands of a careful operator, the EMG and NCV provide exquisite accuracy of diagnosis.

LUMBAR PUNCTURE

There are still clearly identifiable uses for the lumbar puncture in spite of the development of sophisticated radiographic and nuclear medicine procedures. Although these have largely superseded lumbar puncture in neurologic diagnosis, the clinician should know when and how to do it.

Indications for Lumbar Puncture

1) To inject material into the subarachnoid space as in spinal anesthesia, myelography, pneumoencephalography, gamma cisternography, and occasionally for intrathecal therapy.

2) To examine the CSF for bacteria, cells, blood, and other components in order to:

Establish the specific diagnosis of meningitis

Establish the specific diagnosis of subarachnoid hemorrhage

Aid in the diagnosis of several diseases:

Neurosyphillis, for positive FTA or VDRL

Multiple sclerosis, where an elevation in CSF gamma globulin strengthens the clinical diagnosis

Guillain-Barré syndrome where elevated CSF protein
strengthens the clinical diagnosis

Subacute sclerosing panencephalitis where rising titers of
measles antibodies over several weeks confirm the clinical
diagnosis

3) To determine the CSF pressure if it is in dispute. Drusen of
the optic disc are normal, but they may be invisible and resemble the
funduscopic appearance of papilledema. Normal CSF pressure
rules out papilledema.

Technique for the Performance of Lumbar Puncture

The lumbar puncture needle is constructed with a short bevel
which deviates less drastically in its course through the tough connective tissues of the back than a long beveled needle. Use of the
smaller bore, #21 needle, produces a smaller dural hole and may
reduce postspinal headache, but the inexperienced operator may
prefer the #18 needle because it is less flexible and easier to insert
into the midline structures.

The patient lies on his side with his knees drawn up toward the
chest to widen the interspaces. He is positioned with hips and back
vertical so the needle may be introduced horizontally toward the
midline. *Failure to be certain that the back is vertical commonly allows the operator to insert his needle laterally, where it hits bone instead of dura.*

The exposed surface of the back is washed with disinfectant, and
unsterilized areas, including the bedsheets in front of the operator,
are draped. The puncture is easier if sterile areas of the back are left
exposed, rather than covered with a sterile sheet. Then, the operator
can more easily maintain his orientation to anatomical landmarks.

Any interspace below L2-3 is acceptable. Higher interspaces are
avoided because the spinal cord lies under those areas and may be
damaged. The L4-5 interspace lies directly between the two superior iliac crests and is most easily identified.

Local anesthetic should be used unless the patient is allergic to
it. If he is, injectable diphenhydramine (Benedryl®) is an effective

substitute. Patients are anxious about lumbar puncture, and prevention of pain is important. An intradermal wheal is raised in the center of the selected interspace, and anesthetic is then injected with a 1–1 1/2 inch needle into deeper tissues, but not into the subarachnoid space, since injection of local anesthetic there would produce spinal anesthesia!

The spinal needle is then introduced *into the same puncture site.* The bevel of the spinal needle should be perpendicular to the spine, facing the left or the right side of the patient, since dural fibers course along the length of the spine and will not be damaged as the needle penetrates the dura in this orientation. The spinal needle is aimed slightly cephalad and advanced in the midline about halfway to the lumbar sac. This distance will vary from patient to patient. If the needle is released and observed at this point, the operator will see that it has deviated slightly away from the bevel. This may be corrected by rotating the bevel 180° and advancing the needle directly into the lumbar sac. *Rotation of the needle at the halfway point is an important step that will make difficult lumbar punctures easier and help the operator to hit the dural sac in the midline instead of the spinal lamina laterally.*

The stylet should be firmly in place as the needle is advanced. This helps to prevent pieces of skin and surface bacteria from accompanying the tip into the subarachnoid space. The tip may "pop" as it penetrates the dura; if it does not, the stylet may be removed at various depths to ascertain whether spinal fluid appears. Occasionally, after a successful puncture, the bevel lies against a nerve root, preventing free flow spinal fluid. Rotation of the needle corrects this immediately.

Pitfalls to Avoid

1) Needle hits bone without penetrating the lumbar sac: Is the hub pointing toward the midline? If it is not, the patient may be repositioned and the puncture performed again. It is important to retract the needle tip *all the way* to the subcutaneous tissues before readvancing it. Otherwise, only the hub is redirected and the tip hits bone again. The bevel should *always be rotated 180°* at the midpoint of insertion to cancel deviation of the tip away from the midline as it is advanced.

Does the patient have scoliosis? Some patients with severe scoliosis have developed enough spinal rotation that the operator may miss the interspace completely unless he is careful to feel the posterior spinous processes before he begins.

Is the interspace opened as fully as possible? Some patients arch their backs even with knees to chest. They must be helped to relax and allow the back to curve toward the operator. Occasionally, it is helpful to have the patient sit up, bending over the edge of the bed, legs dangling, arms clasping the knees. If the puncture is performed in this position, the patient lies on his side again after the needle reaches the subarachnoid space, before opening pressure is taken.

It is very important to use only *one* puncture hole. If the needle is not positioned just right the first time, it may be withdrawn to the subcutaneous tissues. Then both needle and skin are moved *together* to the correct location. If this is not done, the result may be a circle of many individual needle holes, all within a centimeter of each other around several different interspaces. This has been called the "hamburger syndrome." When the family of such a patient examines his back after the procedure and sees all the puncture sites, they may exclaim, "They made hamburger out of Jake!" Lumbar puncture is a trying procedure for patients and families. They do not need this extra stress.

2) Errors of opening pressure measurement: Elevated spinal fluid pressure is a serious finding. Incorrectly recorded spinal fluid pressure is confusing. The opening pressure must be taken with the patient stretched out and relaxed. A crying child, a straining adult, or a patient whose knees are still against his chest will all normally have high pressure readings. The patient should be told that the needle is in, that he may stretch out carefully and relax. He is asked to take five deep breaths. This blows off some CO_2 and causes intracranial vasoconstriction. The resultant transient drop in CSF pressure documents that the needle is in the correct space. The pressure returns to baseline in 30-60 seconds, and at this point, an accurate reading may be taken and recorded. Closing pressure has no value in modern neurological practice.

3) Bloody tap: Like elevated spinal fluid pressure, the presence of blood in the CSF is serious. A bloody tap is of no consequence. The operator must document *unequivocally* which of the two occurred. If the CSF does not become clear of blood after the first few drops, the laboratory cell count will record the presence of RBCs. In that case, it is important to document that the blood is fresh by

showing that there is no xanthochromia. The fluid must be delivered to the laboratory *immediately* and *immediately* spun down. Blood from a bloody tap can produce slight xanthochromia during the first hour after the LP while the fluid is lying on the ward awaiting attention. Normal spinal fluid cannot be distinguished from water. Xanthochormic spinal fluid can be.

4) CSF collection: Lumbar puncture is not particularly hazardous or painful, but patients are anxious about the procedure, so it should not be repeated needlessly. The physician should plan beforehand what studies he needs and be certain that he has taken enough fluid before he removes the needle. He should collect a total of at least 10 cc, using four collection tubes. The amount of fluid removed makes no difference to the patient's comfort unless that amount is too little, and he needs a second lumbar puncture!

5) Laboratory determinations:

Sugar. A blood sugar drawn simultaneously with the lumbar puncture is vitally important if there is the slightest doubt about the presence of meningitis or the cause of coma. Normally, the CSF sugar is at least half as high as the blood sugar. Bacterial meningitis causes a relative decrease in this figure. The diagnosis of hypoglycemia can be missed until the results of spinal fluid sugar are available. If a simultaneous blood sugar is drawn, the resultant low value prevents further confusion.

Protein and cells. Normal values of CSF protein are established on the first cubic centimeter removed. Spinal fluid protein should be performed on the first tube which is free of gross blood. Cells should be counted on the last tube collected.

Cultures. Bacterial cultures are easy to perform and should be ordered routinely. If they are not performed and then needed later, the information is not available. If the diagnosis of fungal meningoencephalitis is in question, large quantities of CSF may be needed because there are few organisms free in the spinal fluid. Thirty to 60 cc of fluid should be taken on several occasions, spun down, and cultured in special media.

Special Studies. The operator must decide in advance whether he needs special studies. If he does, he needs to be certain he has enough fluid for them to be performed. The gamma globulin or electrophoresis for oligoclonal bands, measles antibodies, FTA, and fungus cultures all take specified fluid volumes. Those volumes must be available to the laboratory or the answers will not appear on the chart.

If there are clear indications for lumbar puncture, it should be performed immediately and with care for the acquisition of accurate results. Under these circumstances, the lumbar puncture may be a valuable neurological tool.

The clinician's special skill involves his ability to coordinate the results of all special studies in order to arrive at an accurate diagnosis by the most direct route and with least discomfort to his patient. As he gains insight into the special uses of individual studies, he can become more effective as a diagnostician and derive increasing pleasure from his job.

REFERENCES

1. Belloni, G., di Rocco, C., Focacci, C., Galli, G., Maira, G., Rossi, G.F.: Surgical Indications in Normotensive Hydrocephalus. A Retrospective Analysis of the Relations of Some Diagnostic Findings to the Results of Surgical Treatment. Acta Neurosurg. 33:1-21, 1976.
2. Gunasekera, L., Richardson, A.E.: Computerized Axial Tomography in Idiopathic Hydrocephalus. Brain 100:749-754, 1977.
3. Hakim, S., Adams, R.D.: The Special Clinical Problem of Symptomatic Hydrocephalus with Normal Cerebrospinal Fluid Pressure: Observations of Cerebrospinal Fluid Dynamics. J. Neurol. Sci. 2:307-327, 1965.
4. Jacobs, L., Conti, D., Kinkel, W.R., Manning, E.J.: "Normal Pressure" Hydrocephalus. Relationsship of Clinical and Radiographic Findings to Improvement Following Shunt Surgery. J.A.M.A. 235:510-512, 1976.
5. Shinkin, H.A., Greenberg, J.O., Grossman, C.B.: Ventricular Size After Shunting for Idiopathic Normal Pressure Hydrocephalus. J. Neurol., Neurosurg. Psychiat. 38:833-837, 1975.

CHAPTER 3

Disorders of Voluntary Movement

INTRODUCTION

The clinician who sees patients with neurological disorders needs some knowledge of the complexities of brain function and of the anatomy of neurological symptoms, because he must always keep in mind the functional neuroanatomy of his patients' complaints if he is to define the pathology behind their diseases. Brain function is not to be understood as a simple sum of all neuronal activity. Instead, there is an unfathomed interaction by which all regions of the nervous system cooperate to provide more precise motor control, and more intricate higher mental functions than could be expected from the simple summation of nerve impulses. Fortunately, clinical neurology is much simpler because deficit symptoms are subject to analysis in terms of damaged fiber bundles and neuronal colonies, so our analysis of the normal control of movement and of neurological symptoms, can also represent a simplification of the actual nature of brain function. If the anatomical discussion is still unclear, the serious student should consult an additional textbook of neuroanatomy to clarify unfamiliar neuroanatomical terms and to solidify his knowledge.

In the four succeeding chapters, we shall continue our examination of functional neuroanatomy as it applies to deficit symptoms in vision and control of eye movements; then we shall consider diseases of the motor unit and the movement disorders.

If the material in this chapter appears difficult, do not give up in despair. If you master this material, subsequent topics will be easier. No small part of the joy of being a neurologist is that the specialty is so large that one person cannot master it, and there is always something new to learn. If you, gentle reader, can sample some of this "joy" as you struggle through this material and come away from the experience with new and useful knowledge, it may stimulate you to return for more!

THE ANATOMY OF COORDINATED MOTOR ACTIVITY

When we consider body movements, we frequently think of discharges from the motor strip to spinal cord levels in simplistic terms. In reality, the brain is much more complex. Before it ever initiates a movement, the brain has been primed by activity indicating the position of the entire body, velocities of movement, probable dangers in the outside environment; and it is in possession of information about the progress of movements already initiated. As a movement starts, it is constantly monitored and redirected. All major systems of the brain except the corticospinal system direct a large portion of their influence upward toward *cortical* levels in order to perform continuously monitored smooth movements.

Selective inhibition is the prime determinant of precise movement. All parts of the central nervous system selectively inhibit activity in other parts in order to focus a precise motor response to outside stimuli. Seven great systems form the basis for normal movements, and all seven work together to produce a smoothly coordinated discharge to spinal levels: 1) the cerebral cortex; 2) the basal ganglia, gray matter in the depths of the brain; 3) the reticular formation, the diffuse sensory-motor system centered in the brainstem; 4) the vestibular system, functioning to maintain spacial orientation; 5) the cerebellum, providing coordination of motor and sensory information; 6) conscious and unconscious proprioception, providing information about position and movement of joints and tendons; and 7) the visual system. We shall discuss the visual system in later chapters.

Once a corticospinal discharge reaches spinal levels, normal motor activity depends further on the structure and function of anterior horn cells in the spinal cord, the peripheral nerves, and the muscles themselves. Malfunction of any link in the chain results in disintegration of finely coordinated movements. Let us examine the anatomical interrelations between these systems before we consider specific complaints and physical abnormalities which result from disease in each one.

Descending fibers in the internal capsule originate primarily in the cortex. As they pass the caudate nucleus, putamen, globus pallidus, and substantia nigra, they send collaterals to these nuclei. Information is passed from the globus pallidus via the thalamus back to prefrontal regions of the cortex. In each nucleus, it is modified in an unknown manner. When they reach the brainstem, fibers of the internal capsule pass through the belly of the pons, then into the medulla, where they cross to the opposite side and eventually synapse at segmental levels of the spinal cord. We shall come back to segmental events in a few moments.

As the nerve fibers of the corticospinal system pass through the pons, some collaterals synapse with neurons in the belly of the pons; these project into the cerebellum via the middle cerebellar peduncle. These connections are called the cortico-pontine-cerebellar system, whose function is to inform the cerebellum of ongoing cortical activity. In addition to this cortical input, the cerebellum receives information from the reticular formation, the inferior olive (a major nucleus in the medulla), the vestibular system of the brainstem, and directly from spinal levels via the unconscious proprioceptive pathways, especially the spinocerebellar tracts. Conscious proprioceptive pathways and the lateral spinothalamic tracts send collaterals to the reticular formation. Their information affects cerebellar input through this system. All this information is collected by the cerebellum and discharged – where? – not down to spinal levels, but *up* to the motor cortex, via the thalamus.

Conscious joint position and movement sensation reaches the post-central cortex from the posterior columns of the spinal cord via the thalamus. The reticular formation of the brainstem also discharges upward through the thalamus via diffusely projecting thalamic nuclei. Although projections from the reticular formation never reach the cortex, their activity certainly affects the final cortical discharge.

Projection to the cortex is an orderly process. The basal ganglia project from the *anterior* ventral thalamic nucleus to the *pre*motor cortex. The cerebellum projects from the ventrolateral thalamic nucleus immediately behind the anterior ventral, to the motor strip. Sensory information is passed from the *posterior* ventral nuclei to the *post*-motor (sensory) cortex. These three cortical regions are connected in turn with each other through short and long fibers that course just beneath the cortical mantle. Thus, a corticospinal discharge consists of highly controlled complex projections from large

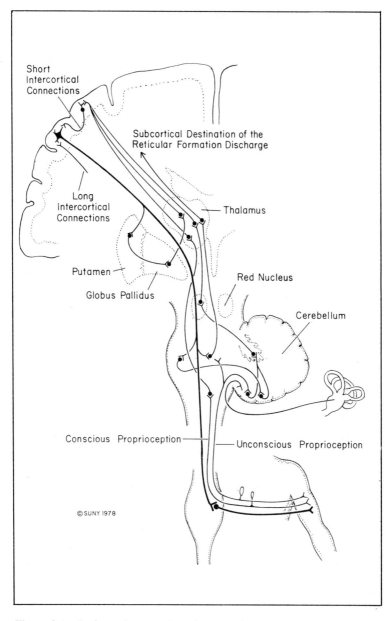

Figure 3-1. *Outline of neuronal connections that govern coordinated voluntary movement (see text).*

portions of the entire hemisphere, not of a simple message from a few Betz cells on the motor strip to a few anterior horn cells in the spinal cord.

When information finally arrives at spinal levels, it produces complex selective *activation* of certain anterior horn cell nuclei and simultaneous selective *inhibition* of others. The pattern of activation and inhibition shifts constantly and allows the individual to enter a boxing match, to play a sonata on the piano, or to do something simple like alternately slapping the palm and dorsum of his hand on his knee, or moving his fingers from his nose to a target. Medical students learn that tests of gait, rapid gross and fine alternating movements, and accuracy of finger-to-nose movements are "cerebellar tests." This chapter will make it clear that they are not. They examine the function of the entire nervous system, and the clinician must assemble evidence about *how* motor tasks are misperformed in order to determine the location of the disorder.

Watch the normal subject slap his hand rapidly on his knee, alternating palm and dorsum. Most of the movement occurs at the elbow; little in the fingers, wrist, and shoulder. The entire trunk is immobilized, and the opposite upper extremity takes no part in the movements at all. Early abnormalities, even of this simple coordinated movement, include flopping of the elbow due to poor fixation of the shoulder joint, and loss of smooth rhythmicity. If he is tapping a finger to his thumb, the taps become irregular and movement is no longer limited to the fingers, but spreads to wrist and elbow. Even extremities on the opposite side of the body show evidence of disinhibition by spread of reflexes or by associated abnormal movements. These abnormal new movements appear in spastic paresis, in ridigity, in cerebellar dyssynergia. Similar abnormalities occur in sensory loss and in disease of the anterior horn cells.

Fortunately for the clinician, lesions in each part of the nervous system produce distinct complaints and physical findings. The *way* patients mis-perform rapid skilled movements differs if the location of the lesion is different, but this distinction is a difficult nuance to transmit on paper. Other physical findings are more definite. Pyramidal tract lesions produce spasticity, hyperactive deep tendon reflexes, and pathological reflexes. Lesions of the basal ganglia produce complex abnormalities of movement, posture, and tone. Lesions of the cerebellum produce abnormal synergy of movements and decreased resting muscle tone with no alteration in resting posture. Patients with abnormalities of *conscious* proprioception complain of their sensory loss, but the system is invisible until it is tested specifically. There is no direct test for malfunction in the reticular formation or unconscious proprioceptive pathways.

Let us now examine the clinical abnormalities which result from malfunction in each of these brain systems, remembering always that tests of *coordinated activity* are not "cerebellar tests" or "pyramidal tests" but tests of the nervous system. The clinician must determine the significance of each abnormal finding through examination and cogitation.

SPASTIC PARESIS AND FLACCID WEAKNESS (THE "MOTOR SYSTEM")

In loose clinical parlance, we call it the "motor system." When we do, we are actually referring to the final pathways of the entire nervous system as it produces coordinated movements: the corticospinal system and the motor units. A motor unit consists of the anterior horn cell in the spinal cord, its axon, and all the individual muscle fibers innervated by that anterior horn cell. In the quadriceps femoris muscle, a motor unit may contain several hundred individual muscle fibers; in the extraocular muscles, a motor unit contains fewer than ten.

While the words "paresis" and "weakness" are often used as synonyms, they are not. *Paresis* means *spastic corticospinal* tract dysfunction with incomplete paralysis. (If the paralysis were complete, we would speak of —plegia.) *Weakness* implies *flaccid* dysfunction of portions of the *motor unit.* Thus, we speak of hemiparesis, quadriparesis, paraparesis, monoparesis; but we speak of weakness of the biceps or deltoid muscles, and we confuse ourselves by speaking about "weakness" of grip. Actually, paresis, weakness, and most of the other conditions that interfere with coordinated movement decrease the power of grip, but only those which damage the motor units produce actual weakness of the muscles of grip.

Spastic paresis and flaccid weakness divide the anatomical control of movement into two distinct parts that may easily be differentiated by the clinician at the bedside. The clear distinction in language not only helps the clinician to communicate more effectively with his colleagues but also helps him to remember the basic anatomy of the nervous system. In paresis, there is disorganization of complex cordinated functions, so grip is markedly diminished, but muscles used in the production of grip can generate considerably more power individually. In weakness, where the motor unit is deficient but central coordination is intact, muscle power is diminished equally during coordinated grip or individual muscle contractions. This is the critical *clinical* distinction between weakness and paresis of grip.

Ask the patient who has had a mild stroke, but still has some use of the hand, to squeeze your fingers. He is unable to hold on to the fingers and you easily escape. Now, ask him to hook his flexed fingers into your flexed fingers and pull. In this test of uncoordinated power, he fares much better and may have nearly normal strength.

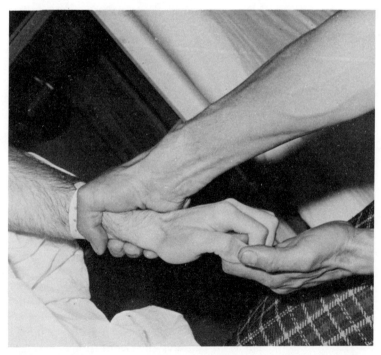

Figure 3-2. *Examiner and patient testing raw muscle power in finger flexors.*

Now repeat this test with a patient who has muscular dystrophy, polymyositis, myasthenia gravis, Guillain-Barré syndrome, or primary muscular atrophy, each of which represents disease in the motor unit, producing weakness. This patient's grip may be just as weak as the stroke patient's, but when he flexes his fingers into a hook and pulls against the examiner's flexed fingers, his muscular weakness is proportional to the weakness of grip.

This single test is a fundamental part of the functional examination of the upper extremity, because it clearly distinguishes between the two major portions of the motor system. Unfortunately, there is no similar test for the lower extremities. Naturally, the test may not be used if there is total paralysis, but under that circumstance, the anatomical question rarely arises.

Spastic Paresis

If loss of muscle power is not the primary defect in paresis, what is? We may think of paresis as the result of *incoordinated* muscle power. The normal selective inhibition of nervous system structures that produces finely tuned reciprocal activation and inhibition of spinal cord nuclei has been lost, and coordinated activities like grip, writing, and buttoning are deficient out of proportion to the power that may be directed to individual muscles on demand. Patients with paresis complain of "stiffness" and increasing fatigue with small amounts of exertion. A spastic leg suddenly "gives way" under him, and he falls. He recognizes the fall as the result of poor support, not of poor balance, and he remembers that the leg failed him. Patients with cerebellar disease complain of imbalance, and those with rigid Parkinson's disease do not know why they fall. As paresis increases, there is less and less coordinated muscle power and total paralysis eventually occurs.

Spontaneous clonus occurs with chronic spasticity, and spontaneous flexion reflexes appear in the form of sudden jerks of the leg, which seem to be activated as the patient is falling asleep at night, but may also occur during the day. If they are frequent and severe, they become exquisitely painful.

The motor incoordination of paresis is clearly visible during the examination. As the patients walks, his paretic arm does not swing normally at his side, because the normal rhythmic changes in muscle tone are no longer present. Rapid gross alternating movements are slowed and awkward, because the usual reciprocal action of antagonist muscles is lost. Rapid fine alternating movements are slowed, and muscles lose their smooth rhythmicity for the same reason. During the examination of these functions, new movements appear in more proximal joints that normally remain fixed because of coordinated *inhibition* of movement!

In addition to these abnormalities of coordinated movement, which are to some extent shared by all patients with lesions of the nervous system, the paretic patient develops specific findings related to his paresis:

1) Babinski's sign is the only absolute diagnostic abnormality for corticospinal dysfunction. But even in its absence, there is evidence of disinhibition of deep tendon reflexes with resultant hyperreflexia and spread of the response to muscles not normally involved.

2) The crossed adductor reflex is a perfect example of the spread of excitation during hyperreflexia. It is not necessarily a pathological reflex, but if it is asymmetrical or very active, it is abnormal. The crossed adductor response is elicited by tapping the knee on one side in the form of a normal knee jerk. This not only results in a snappy knee jerk, but if there is spasticity on the opposite side also, adductor muscles on the opposite side contract as well, producing adduction and internal rotation of the opposite lower extremity. This crossed adductor response results from disinhibition of reflex connections. The connections are always there, but the response is not normally seen because it is suppressed.

3)Trömner's sign, too, displays abnormal spread of excitation. Like the crossed adductor reflex, it is not necessarily abnormal, but if it is asymmetrical or very active, it indicates abnormal hyperreflexia. To demonstrate Trömner's sign, the examiner forcibly and suddenly extends the patient's middle finger with a snap of his wrist and a sharp slap of his middle finger against the patient's. Normally, this might mimic a deep tendon reflex and produce contraction in the flexor muscles of the patient's middle finger. If hyperreflexia is present, the thumb and other fingers flex as well (See p. 351).

4) Lastly, the distribution of paretic symptoms on the body follows the anatomy of the long motor tracts in the central nervous system. Lesions along the corticospinal system produce standard syndromes which may be used in the accurate localization of disease.

Localizing Significance of Paretic Syndromes

Hemiparesis

Pure hemiparesis almost always signifies disease above the midbrain – in the brain itself. If the face is paretic on the same side as the arm and leg, this establishes the localization in the brain, because corticobulbar fibers, which cross to control the opposite side of the face, leave the corticospinal system at the level of the midbrain. The lesion must be above this point if it is to involve both the face and extremities on the same side.

Hemiparesis does not always originate in the brain, because strictly unilateral lesions of the brainstem and upper spinal cord can paralyze one side of the body only; but in reality, lesions that cause strictly unilateral pathology are rarely found in such small structures as the brainstem and spinal cord. Consequently, with the exception of ischemic stroke, which may affect only one or the other side of the brainstem or spinal cord, diseases in these locations usually produce asymmetrical *quadri*paresis.

Crossed Hemiparesis

If a cranial nerve is paralyzed on one side, and the arms and legs are paralyzed on the opposite side, the syndrome is called crossed hemiparesis, and the lesion can occur *only* in the brainstem. The paralyzed cranial nerve defines the segmental level of the lesion within the brainstem: oculomotor nerve, midbrain; trigeminal nerve, upper pons; facial nerve, lower pons; tongue or vocal cord, medulla.

Quadriparesis

Many diseases cause quadriparesis. Arteriosclerotic vascular disease is a disseminated illness, although the individual stroke is not. Multiple sclerosis, infections, metastatic tumors, and a host of other conditions produce *bilateral* symptomatology, while others, like most primary brain tumors, produce essentially *unilateral* symptoms. The importance of quadriparesis is that it documents the presence of disease on *both sides* of the central nervous system. We have shown that a *single* lesion of the spinal cord or brainstem usually produces quadriparesis, but it is different in the brain, where lesions causing quadriparesis are almost always *multifocal* or *diffuse*,

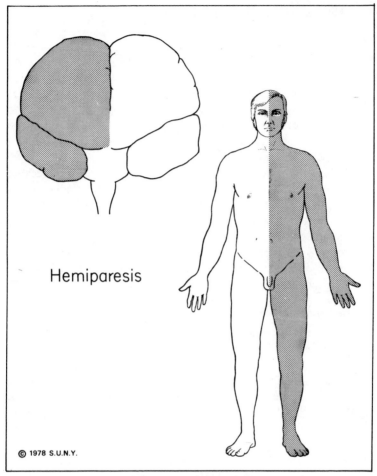

Hemiparesis

© 1978 S.U.N.Y.

Figure 3-3. *Hemiparesis.*

and this fact determines which diagnostic possibilities are likely to be accurate.

A search for quadriparesis is of vital importance to the diagnostic process. While it is proper to document the Babinski's sign and hyperactive reflexes on the left when a patient complains of *left*-sided paralysis, it is crucial to determine whether or not the reflexes and motor function on the *right* are normal, because the localization and the eventual diagnosis may turn on that point.

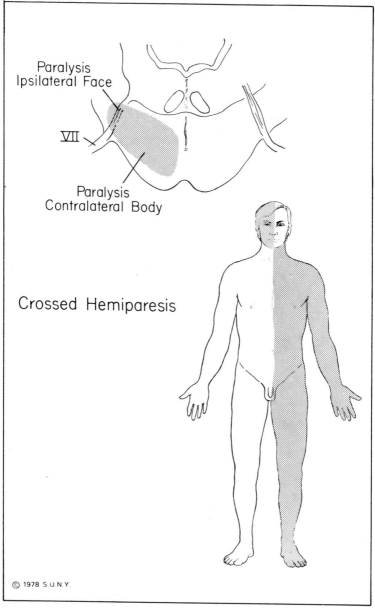

Paralysis
Ipsilateral Face

VII

Paralysis
Contralateral Body

Crossed Hemiparesis

Figure 3-4. *Crossed hemiparesis. A cranial nerve on one side and hemiparesis on the opposite side of the body.*

Paraparesis

Normal head and arms with spastic paresis in the legs is called paraparesis. Paraparesis occurs only from lesions situated between T2 and L2 in the spinal cord. Lesions above this level involve the hands and arms and produce quadriparesis. Lesions below L2 directly affect lumbar spinal neurons and cause weakness, not paresis, of the lower extremities and flaccid bowel and bladder. All forms of pathologic process may be encountered in the paraparetic patient.

The clinician may encounter a patient with double monoparesis in the lower extremities, which may be caused by a parasagittal lesion in the brain. This condition bears a superficial resemblance to spinal paraparesis and is easily misdiagnosed. Usually, however, in double monoparesis, the arms display some hyperreflexia, or there are seizures, dementia, or clouding of consciousness, indicating that the brain is involved. The sensory loss in double monoparesis is not sharply segmental, as it usually is in spinal parapesis. If the clinician recognizes atypical features in a patient who is ostensibly paraparetic and thinks about the possibility of a parasagittal lesion causing the syndrome, he will not be fooled.

Monoparesis

Small lesions situated in the cortex cause paresis in the hand, the foot, or the face, not complete hemiparesis. The anatomical reason for monoparesis is obvious as shown in Figure 3-6. Monoparesis is usually caused by metastatic cancer or a small ischemic stroke. Parasagittal meningioma causes unilateral or bilateral monoparesis of the foot.

Monoparesis is usually diagnosed on the basis of the examination not fitting the prediction the clinician may have made after he listened to the history. For example, the patient complained of progressive weakness of the hand or foot. The clinician was thinking about spinal cord or nerve, expecting signs of weakness. Instead, when he examines the patient, he finds a *paretic* limb with *increased* deep tendon reflexes. If the monoparesis is in the hand, there is markedly decreased power in the grip. But when the patient is asked to flex his fingers into a hook and pull against the physician's flexed fingers, there is surprisingly good strength.

Careful examination of the face and of the other extremity on the same side usually reveals slight hyperreflexia, or a minor droop

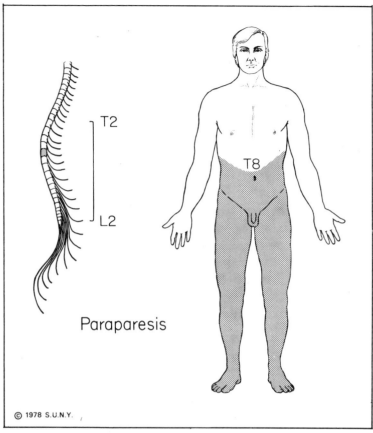

Figure 3-5. *Paraparesis. Lesions distributed between T2-L2.*

of the upper lip, which indicates that monoparesis is really only a special case of hemiparesis with emphasis on one part of the anatomy.

Flaccid Weakness

Disease of the motor unit causes a loss of muscle power. If anterior horn cells or their axons die, fewer motor units are available to move the joint. If there is muscle disease or myasthenia gravis, motor units that do operate are less effective. In each case, the firing

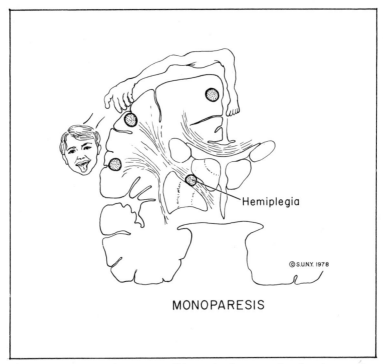

Hemiplegia

© S.U.N.Y. 1978

MONOPARESIS

Figure 3-6. *Monoparesis. A small lesion in the cortex involves innervation only to one limb or to the face, while a lesion of the same size in the internal capsule produces total hemiplegia.*

pattern of motor units is well coordinated by central nervous system activity, so it is to be expected that patients with flaccid weakness would usually display relatively well preserved coordinated movements when compared to the patient with paresis; and this is the case. For instance, the myasthenic patient in crisis, who can barely lift her hand, is still able to write legibly if someone holds the message board for her, and the author knows of one man with slowly progressive muscular dystrophy who works as a certified public accountant, keeping meticulous books by hand despite severe muscular weakness. These patients would be unable to perform in this manner if they suffered from paresis instead of weakness.

There are many associated findings in weakness, and these differ according to the portion of the motor unit affected. The electromyogram and nerve conduction velocity provide electrodiagnostic distinctions between diseases in various portions of the motor unit. These have been discussed in Chapter 2 (p. 33). Fasciculations, atrophy, and weakness are the clinical hallmarks of anterior horn cell disease. Peripheral nerve disease frequently causes atrophy, sensory loss, and may even produce fasciculations. Atrophy is not prominent if the disease process is at the myoneural junctions or in the muscles themselves, although people with chronic progressive muscular dystrophy do eventually develop significant wasting. In most patients, the anatomical distribution of flaccid weakness drastically limits the choice of possible diagnoses, so it behooves the clinician to develop expertise in the testing of muscle power and then to think carefully about the anatomical implications of the abnormalities he has discovered.

Localizing Significance of Focal or Generalized Flaccid Weakness

Focal Flaccid Weakness

Focal flaccid weakness is the most accurate localizing neurological sign. If a small nucleus of motor neurons at the C8-T1 level of the spinal cord, whose innervation is specific to the first dorsal interosseous muscle is affected, this will produce focal weakness, wasting, and fasciculations that are visible on the examination. The precise distribution of muscle involvement reflects the distribution of anterior horn cell damage in the spinal cord and defines the segmental level of the focal lesion. In the same manner, a lesion in the cervical, or the lumbosacral plexus, or in any other peripheral nerve, results in focal paralysis and wasting of muscles, plus sensory loss, in the distribution of that nerve distal to the lesion. If the upper extremity exhibits focal wasting and weakness, while the lower extremities display paresis, the lesion is in the spinal axis and indicates the need for myelography. If there is weakness in the arms but the lower extremities are normal, the lesion may be more distal; in the brachial plexus, shoulder, or even in the muscles themselves.

Generalized Flaccid Weakness

If focal flaccid weakness is the most localizing sign from the nervous system, generalized flaccid weakness is just the opposite, but despite the generalized nature of *symptoms*, diffuse motor unit disease has a very limited number of *causes*. If the clinician can discover which portion of the motor unit is affected, his diagnosis is almost established.

Thus, disseminated anterior horn cell disease usually means amyotrophic lateral sclerosis (or poliomyelitis). *Acute* disseminated peripheral nerve disease means Guillain-Barré syndrome (or porphyria or lupus erythematosus). *Chronic* peripheral neuropathy is a distinct disseminated peripheral nerve syndrome with many causes, that should never be mistaken for Guillain-Barré syndrome. Disease at the myoneural junction usually means myasthenia gravis, although the myasthenic syndrome must be considered, and, if home canning again becomes common, botulism may again be a diagnostic alternative. Finally, disseminated weakness due to muscle disease is caused by the inflammatory myopathies (polymyositis and its relatives) and by the muscular dystrophies.

The distribution of weakness differs somewhat in each disease process. Amyotrophic lateral sclerosis usually begins in one segmental region and spreads gradually to other levels but always displays its segmental emphasis. Guillain-Barré syndrome also may begin with local weakness but usually spreads rapidly during a few days or weeks to involve many other levels. Guillain-Barré syndrome is also usually associated with bilateral facial weakness, while peripheral neuropathy develops slowly and never affects the face. Myasthenia gravis and the myopathies produce more severe weakness in proximal limb and trunk muscles, and leave distal muscles more nearly intact.

In order to formulate a localizing diagnosis, the clinician should first make a general statement to himself about the type and distribution of motor disability. Is there paresis? Is it hemiparesis? Quadriparesis? What segmental level is affected – brain, brainstem, or spinal cord? Or, if there is weakness, is the origin in the anterior horn cells or some other part of the motor unit? Answers to these initial questions provide the clinician with a great deal of diagnostic information, which may be amplified by the sensory examination and the details of the motor examination.

LOSS OF CONSCIOUS PROPRIOCEPTION

The sensations of joint position and of joint motion are important sensory functions in the control of voluntary movement. The spinocerebellar tracts do not reach consciousness and are not available for testing, except by exclusion, but conscious proprioception may be tested. Conditions that destroy large fibers in the dorsal roots or the posterior columns in the spinal cord cause loss of conscious joint position sense. Fibers destined for the posterior columns enter the dorsal roots and do not synapse. They travel directly up the dorsal columns of the spinal cord, without crossing, until they reach the medulla where they finally synapse in the gracile and cuneate nuclei. Second-order neurons cross to the other side on their way to the thalamus and eventually to the cortex, where the information finally reaches consciousness. Somehow, information reaching the parietal cortex on both sides is turned into language and returns to the examiner in the form of a verbal response to his tests. If parts of this pathway are destroyed at any point, the patient's verbal response will be inaccurate. Position sense testing has the advantage that it provides objective information, because the clinician already knows whether he moved the joint "up" or "down."

The anatomy of conscious proprioception is identical to the anatomy of paresis, except that in each portion of the central nervous system, the two functions travel in distinct parts of the neuraxis. This fact may be used to provide even more detailed information about the extent of a lesion at any particular level. Because they parallel each other in the nervous system, the standard forms of hemiparesis are mirrored by similar forms of proprioceptive loss. Hemihypesthesia, crossed hemihypesthesia, and sensory levels along the neuraxis display the same anatomical distribution as the paretic syndromes. If there is dorsal root disease, loss of conscious proprioception (and pinprick) occurs in segmental distributions.

All sensory functions converge on the brain, so isolated proprioceptive loss does not occur from lesions at that level. Some brain lesions produce aphasia or directly affect connections to speech centers, occasionally making it difficult to interpret the meaning of verbal responses. Sensory pathways in the brainstem are all carried in the medial lemniscus, so crossed hemianesthesia syndromes affect perception of pain *and* proprioception equally.

At spinal levels, lesions may affect conscious proprioception and pain sensation individually, because these tracts travel in separate fascicles on opposite sides of the spinal cord. Lesions of the spinothalamic tract affect perception of pinprick. This tract is formed of second-order fibers which receive information near the segmental level of entry and cross immediately to the other side. They are on their way directly to the thalamus where they, too, will synapse. Thalamocortical fibers eventually bring this information to consciousness.

Because proprioceptive fibers do not cross in the spinal cord, but pain and temperature perception does, a lesion confined to the right side of the spinal cord produces loss of conscious proprioception on the right, below the level of the lesion, and loss of pinprick sensation on the left below the level of the lesion. This is called "dissociated" sensory loss. If the pyramidal tract is involved as well, there will be paresis on the right.

Classically, tabes dorsalis was the most common diagnosis in patients with loss of conscious proprioception, but this form of syphilis is not common now. Loss of conscious position sense in modern neurologic practice is most frequently caused by multiple sclerosis, cervical spondylosis, spinal cord tumors, early stages of Guillain-Barré syndrome (occasionally), and rarely by subacute combined degeneration of the spinal cord due to pernicious anemia. The patient complains of staggering gait, especially in the dark, and of sensations of unsteadiness. He watches the ground carefully as he walks, because visual cues help to substitute for lost proprioception. He complains of "numbness" in the affected limbs, but if the deficit is limited to a loss of conscious proprioception, testing reveals normal pain and light touch perception, so the "numbness" is not immediately explained. Occasionally, a patient with loss of position sense discovers his disability when he bumps his head on the sink as he stands in the morning, eyes closed, washing his face! Momentary loss of visual cues allowed him to bend down horizontally without knowing it. Romberg's test is based on exactly this phenomenon. The patient is able to stand with eyes open. But if there is loss of position sense, he falls, *without perceiving the change in posture* when he closes his eyes. Closing the eyes produces unsteadiness in normal people. Patients with spasticity, cerebellar ataxia, Parkinsonism, and many other conditions may fall when they close their eyes, but in those conditions, the patient *knows* he is falling because conscious proprioception is intact.

In the upper extremities, "numbness" due to proprioceptive loss may produce complaints of clumsiness and dropping things like cigarettes or pencils. Such things are held effortlessly and without special regard in the hands of normal people, but if there is loss of proprioception or light touch, small things fall out of the hands when the patient forgets to think about holding on to them. Incidentally, this is different from the dropping done by many hysterical patients, who drop small things *as they pick them up*. Patients with weakness drop heavy things like milk pails and large frying pans, or they complain that they cannot pick them up in the first place.

Techniques for Testing Conscious Proprioception

To test position sense in the foot the examiner braces his own hand against his body or the examination table while the patient lies supine, eyes closed. The clinician grasps the great toe on its *sides* and moves it "up" and "down" in a large arc so the patient learns the correct responses. Once the clinician is certain the patient understands his task, the arc is reduced so each quick movement is progressively smaller. Most adults can detect 1 to 2 mm of motion, and can report accurately on its direction. Old people are usually less sensitive to small movements of the toe. The examiner's fingers are usually more finely tuned to producing movement than the subject's toes are to detecting it, so the examiner usually can move the toe so little that the direction or even the movements are not detected. If the threshold is asymmetrical on the two sides, or if the motion is not detected with a 4 mm or greater motion, this probably represents a defect in conscious proprioception.

This is not the case in the hand. Fingers have delicate innervation, and there is usually no threshold for movement of the fingers. Even when the examiner immobilizes the middle phalanx of the finger with one hand, and makes the smallest possible movements of the distal phalanx with his other hand, the motion and direction are always easy for normal people to detect. The patient with a threshold on one side only, or the patient who does not detect movement of a millimeter or two in the distal phalanx, is displaying loss of position sense in that finger. Patients with loss of proprioception that appears minor during this examination may complain bitterly about clumsiness in the hand, even without associated neurological disability in other systems, because this examination technique, fine as it may be, is still grossly inaccurate compared to the detailed information needed for normal hand function.

The hand is innervated by several spinal segments. This allows for detection of small segmental lesions through position sense testing. The examiner may also be able to identify the site of a lesion in the posterior columns by establishing a sensory *level* to position sense in much the same manner as he tests with a pin. Test position sense in the thumb (C6), middle finger (C7), and little finger (C8). Multiple sclerosis frequently produces small lesions in the dorsal root entry zone, with complaints of "numbness" and "clumsiness," which are actually caused by segmental loss of conscious proprioception. Multiple sclerosis also produces small lesions in the dorsal columns, with sensory levels to position sense testing.

Loss of position sense on the skin of the trunk occurs regularly in patients with spinal cord disease. I do not know whether this represents the same anatomical system as joint position sense, but many patients with numerous sensory lesions due to multiple sclerosis for instance, cannot clearly detect a change of pinprick sensation across a sensory level on the trunk. This is where the crisp "up" and "down" answers at higher levels become valuable, as they suddenly deteriorate when the skin is moved at lower levels. This technique provides accurate results only if the skin *above* the test site is immobilized with the other hand. Otherwise, large areas of skin move with each test movement, and the patient may be responding to skin movement far above the sensory level.

DISEASE OF BASAL GANGLIA
AND ABNORMAL VOLUNTARY MOVEMENT

Disorders of the basal ganglia produce complex and varying abnormalities of voluntary movements and posture, but each disorder produces its own pathologic findings. Basal ganglion disease also interferes with the normal performance of rapid gross and fine alternating movements, finger to nose testing, gait, writing, and buttoning. These will be discussed in a separate chapter on the Movement Disorders (See 141ff.).

CEREBELLAR DYSSYNERGIA

Cerebellar anatomy is so arranged that the midline cerebellar cortex attends primarily to trunk and lower extremity function so that lesions of the vermis produce ataxia of gait and truncal ataxia.

The cerebellar hemispheres are placed lateral to the vermis and are primarily concerned with function of the upper extremities. Lesions of the hemispheres produce dyssynergia of the upper extremity on the same side. "Dyssynergia" is a more accurate term than "action tremor" for the disorganization of movements in cerebellar disease, because these abnormalities may be thought of as exaggerations of the dyssynergy present in normal people. The movements and postures of normal people are always accompanied by small inaccuracies of coordination, which are constantly corrected as they appear. The reader who doubts this should attempt to draw a straight line without a ruler and watch his own normal "dyssynergia." In cerebellar disease, synergy is progressively exaggerated when the patient attempts to move or to maintain static posture against gravity. The patient with cerebellar disease has difficulty buttoning, typing, and writing which is out of proportion to the amount of obvious dyssynergia. This characteristic helps the clinician to distinguish the condition from essential tremor.

There is no defect of posture at complete rest in cerebellar disease. In early cerebellar disease, there is no change in resting muscle tone, but as disability progresses, hypotonia appears and deep tendon reflexes may be diminished in accordance with diminution of muscle tone. There are also changes in the cadence of speech. The plunging cadence of normally coordinated language gives way to syllabic speech in which each syllable is spoken at about the same rate as every other syllable. In some cases, the cadence is completely disorganized, and the patient can barely make himself understood. Jerk nystagmus is another characteristic of cerebellar disease, and there are forms of nystagmus that are said to be specific for cerebellar disease. Unfortunately, jerk nystagmus rarely provides localizing information as accurate as the rest of the neurological examination or the CT or nuclear brain scans.

The reader knows now that the "cerebellar tests" he learned about in school do not test only the cerebellum. Rather, they examine the entire coordinated function of the nervous system. The best way to detect cerebellar disease is to establish that other systems are not abnormal by specific examination of the motor system, conscious proprioception, and by thinking about the specific diseases of the basal ganglia and deciding that they are not present. Failing this, the presence of dyssynergia that "looks like cerebellar dyssynergia," hypotonia, nystagmus, or alteration in the cadence of speech leads the clinician to the conclusion that the cerebellum is also involved.

ESSENTIAL TREMOR

Patients with essential tremor have no discoverable pathologic etiology for their tremor. Essential tremor, too, may be considered an accentuation of the essential tremor shared by all normal people. If it is mild, the easiest way to demonstrate such tremor in the office is to place an 8" x 11" sheet of writing paper over the outstretched hand and fingers. This procedure magnifies normal tremor and allows easy evaluation of the severity and symmetry of abnormal tremor.

It is frequently difficult to distinguish essential tremor from the tremor of Parkinsonism, and from cerebellar dyssynergia, because patients with essential tremor may exhibit features of either of these. Usually, essential tremor occurs solely during activity, but occasional patients have tremor at rest. Usually, essential tremor is rapid and regular, but occasionally it is slower and may be irregular, resembling dyssynergia. Elderly patients with essential tremor frequently develop tremor of the head and voice early in the illness, which may be mistaken for cerebellar degeneration or Parkinson's disease.

It is important to remember that patients with essential tremor do not have a detectable pathologic cause for their tremor, so even careful neurological examination fails to disclose associated pathological findings. Muscle tone is normal, reflexes and gait are unchanged, and coordinated movement of the upper extremities is disorganized only to the extent of the tremor itself. Despite significant tremor, these patients can usually button and tie and write.

If the physician is still concerned about the diagnosis of essential tremor and wondering whether his patient might have cerebellar disease or Parkinsonism, he may be reminded that essential tremor is rarely a disabling disease, because the incoordination is proportional to the degree of tremor. On the other hand, Parkinsonism and diseases that cause cerebellar dyssynergia are progressive and, eventually usually fatal. Therefore, the patient who has had tremor for five years or more, before he finally comes to the physician, and who is not disabled by his tremor, most likely has essential tremor. This is especially true if the rest of the neurological examination is normal. Lastly, patients with essential tremor have frequently discovered that alcohol, even in small doses, quiets the tremor. This is not a characteristic of any other tremulous condition.

There are two distinct types of essential tremor: "senile tremor" and "familial tremor." Senile tremor has nothing to do with the patient's mentation. If the clinician uses this term, he needs to reassure his patient on that point. The tremor is so named because it begins in older people; always after 50, nearly always after 60. Senile tremor frequently begins as head-shaking and spreads later to the hands, but the order may be reversed. It is almost never disabling. Patients come to the physician because of embarrassment or because they worry that people will think they have been drinking. The patient with senile tremor may respond well to propranolol (Inderal®) or, if necessary, to thalamotomy, but may decide not to treat his tremor at all, because he finds adequate consolation in the reassurance that the tremor does not represent a crippling disease, like Parkinsonism.

Familial tremor is transmitted as an autosomal dominant gene. The tremor usually begins before age 30, frequently before age 20. It is gradually progressive during life, but is rarely disabling. Patients with familial tremor almost always have a family history of tremor which is readily available to the physician. If a patient with familial tremor does develop significant disability from his condition, despite propranolol therapy, he may become an excellent candidate for thalamotomy.

Medicinal tratment for essential tremor is limited to propranolol. Most patients begin to respond at doses of 40-80 mg per day, but occasionally patients need much higher doses in the range of 160-200 mg per day. If these large doses do not stop the tremor, and if the patient is experiencing significant disability or embarrassment from his familial tremor, he should consider thalamotomy. The procedure is delicate, but in experienced hands, thalamotomy carries low risks, and the younger person with no progressive brain disease who has a condition eminently responsive to thalamotomy, should have the benefit of this treatment.

VERTIGO

Vertigo is not identical to dizziness or lightheadedness. The vertiginous patient feels a *sense of motion,* either of himself, or of objects around him. The motion need not be spinning. The heaving of the bed during intoxication or fever is an equally vertiginous sensation. Vertigo may cause staggering if it is severe. Even with mild vertigo, the patient has a sense that he might stagger if he is not careful.

The Anatomy of Vertigo

The anatomy of vertigo is the anatomy of the vestibular system. The labyrinth, the vestibular portion of the eighth nerve, vestibular nuclei in the lower pons, and their connections in the cerebellum are the sites of lesions that usually cause vertigo. Cervical spinal cord and even brain lesions may produce vertigo, but these are uncommon. The reader quickly realizes that true vertigo is a localizing symptom of a sort, because its primary anatomical location is in the posterior fossa or the petrous bone. "Dizziness" or "lightheadedness" are not localizing complaints, unless the complaint means that the patient was actually sensing motion.

Peripheral Vertigo vs Central Vertigo

The site of the lesion is the most constant determinant of the severity of vertiginous symptoms. If vertigo originates in the membranous labyrinth of the inner ear, it is more likely to be severe, acute, and disabling, and to be associated with autonomic symptoms like nausea, vomiting, pallor, and cold, sweaty skin. Vertigo originating within the central nervous system is likely to be more chronic, less disabling, and unassociated with autonomic symptoms, but accompanied by localizing abnormalities, which are found during the neurological examination.

An exception to this rule is vertigo due to ischemic stroke or transient ischemic attacks in the brainstem, because these conditions are associated with acute disabling vertigo and may be accompanied by nausea, vomiting, and autonomic symptoms. Even so, the associated symptoms and signs of nervous system disease allow the clinician to formulate an accurate localizing diagnosis.

Peripheral Vertigo

Acute labyrinthitis and Ménière's disease provide an excellent forum for the discussion of peripheral vertigo. The patient is suddenly struck with knock-down vertigo, repeated vomiting, pale sweaty skin, intolerance to any movement of the head, tinnitus, and, if the condition is severe, deafness in one or both ears. Examination may disclose rotatory nystagmus, which may be more severe in one position, indicating altered function in the macule or the saccule as well as the semicircular canals. There are no other neurological abnormalities. Ménière's disease recurs in irregular fashion over many years. Acute labyrinthitis is a self-limited disease of days' or weeks' duration. Treatment of acute labyrinthitis is directed to relieving some of the vertiginous feelings. Medications like dimenhydrinate (Dramamine®) and sedation help the patient to get over the worst of his attacks. Ménière's disease is best referred to an otolaryngologist for long-term treatment if deafness progresses, or if the patient does not respond adequately to diuretics and antiemetics.

Central Vertigo

Vertigo of central origin is usually much less severe. The patient may not even complain of vertigo until he is asked about sensations of movement. He may then recount continuous feelings that his body or the world are moving. Usually, other symptoms such as paralysis and incoordination are much more disabling than the vertigo itself. Disease of the vestibular system universally produces jerk nystagmus, but nystagmus associated with central vertigo is usually vertical or horizontal, while peripheral causes of vertigo more frequently produce rotational nystagmus.

By itself, vertigo is not a symptom that provides a great deal of localizing information to the clinician, apart from the differential between peripheral and central causes. Neurological diseases associated with vertigo invariably present the clinician with other signs and symptoms of more importance than the vertiginous sensations themselves. Treatment of the vertiginous patient is directed primarily at the disease process unless the patient has acute labyrinthitis. In this case, vertigo is the prime symptom; the disease is partially relieved by medication and is self-limited.

CHAPTER 4

Evaluation of Visual Loss

INTRODUCTION

Visual complaints are of two types: The first concerns loss of vision itself; the second concerns defective control of eye movements. In the next two chapters, we shall consider these complaints and their diagnostic significance. Visual loss is critically important to patients. It also can form the basis for the physician's anatomical considerations concerning his patient's disease.

ANATOMY OF THE VISUAL
AND GAZE CONTROL SYSTEMS

The visual system is constructed with great economy and simplicity. Visual fibers which originate in the *superior* portions of the retina course through the optic chiasm and optic tract to the lateral geniculate body where they synapse; the second order fibers then travel through *superior* portions of the visual radiations to the *superior* lip of the visual cortex. Those fibers which originate in the *inferior* half of the retina eventually course through the *inferior* portions of the visual radiations which pass through the temporal lobe and end in the *inferior* lip of the visual cortex.

Likewise, visual fibers which originate on the *left* half of *each* retina course toward the *left* optic tract where they terminate in the left lateral geniculate body and synapse, finally bringing their information to the left visual cortex, and vice-versa. The optic chiasm provides a crossing point for decussating fibers.

The only confusing part of the visual system originates from the pupil. Because of the pupil, the retinal image is reversed, so the left side of the retina looks only at the right half of visual space and the

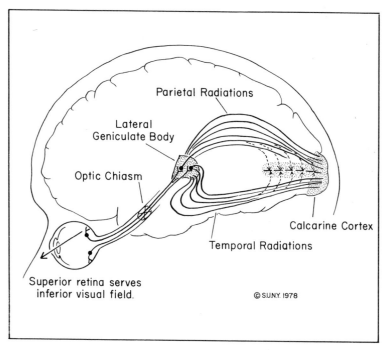

Figure 4-1. *Schematic outline of the visual system from a lateral projection.*

top half of each retina "looks down." The reader who keeps the simplicity of the fiber systems firmly in mind should be able to deal with crossed retinal images with little difficulty.

The brain functions in such a manner that the left hemisphere receives visual and somatic sensation from the right and produces movement on the right, providing in a single hemisphere the capability for instant perception and response to one half of the external world. A provocative article by Suttie,[6] written over 50 years ago, first introduced the author to the problem of decussation. In his article, Suttie emphasized that the "newer" parts of the nervous system all display a crossed function, while the "older" parts – the cerebellum, reticular formation, autonomic nervous system, anterior horn cells – do not. He suggested that the pyramidal tracts are

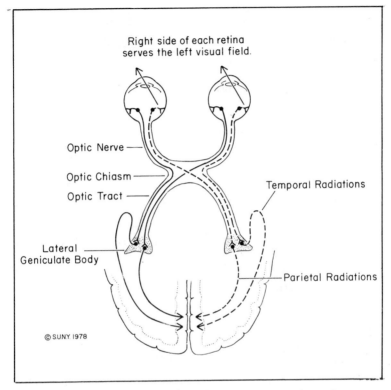

Right side of each retina
serves the left visual field.

Optic Nerve

Optic Chiasm

Optic Tract

Temporal Radiations

Lateral
Geniculate Body

Parietal Radiations

© SUNY 1978

Figure 4-2. *Schematic outline of the visual system from above.*

crossed because they represent the response of the "new" nervous system to its developing crossed visual capacities.

The human visual system is constructed to provide exquisitely detailed information from the central five degrees of the visual fields which are served by the macula. It also provides largely subliminal monitoring of the rest of the visual fields. With a minimum of conscious effort, the individual can avoid stationary objects near his path, and evade or take direct notice of moving objects that intrude from the periphery. If a peripherally perceived object is threatening or interesting, it is brought into central vision for closer inspection. This is preprogramed by the visual association cortex through connections with the frontal eye fields. The brainstem reticular formation governs the individual oculomotor nuclei and moves both eyes conjugately toward the object in a single, coordinated saccade.

Once an object is caught in central vision, the occipital cortex initiates smooth following movements to keep it in the central visual field. If the object moves too rapidly for the smooth pursuit mechanism, the frontal cortex generates a series of rapid saccades as needed, to maintain fixation.

The *visual*-ocular controls are augmented by *vestibulo*-ocular reflexes, which are discussed in the chapter on coma (pp. 164-165). The vestibular system keeps the extraocular muscles, cerebellum, and spinal cord informed about head and neck movements and about the static position of the head in space. This information may be converted directly into eye movements or coordinated with cortical mechanisms for accurate maintenance of ocular fixation, despite rapid movements of the individual and his object of fixation.

Not surprisingly, such a finely tuned system produces seriously disabling symptoms with a minimum of dysfunction. This is especially true of damage to central visual fields and of defective control of individual eye movements. We shall examine first the complaints and findings related to central and peripheral visual field defects and proceed in the next chapter to a consideration of extraocular muscle control. The reader who is interested in more detailed information about neurology of the visual and oculomotor systems and diseases which affect them, will find Cogan's *Neurology of the Visual System*[1] and Gay et al.'s *Eye Movement Disorders*[3] highly informative.

VISUAL COMPLAINTS AND THEIR SIGNIFICANCE

Loss of Central Vision

Patients are aware of even minimal central visual loss.
"It's blurred."
"Like a film in front of my eye."
"I can't read fine print."
"I can't see from my right eye."
"I'm blind!"
Loss of visual acuity brings the patient to his doctor immediately, and he always knows which eye is affected. Examination for loss of central vision centers first on the fact that visual acuity, and most

of color vision depend upon intact function of the central five degrees of macular vision.

Potts et al[5] showed that a macular lesion that affected only 0.4% of the Rhesus monkey retina, destroyed up to 25% of all the fibers of the optic nerve. Most central scotomata are not confined strictly to the macula, so the reader can see that the function of the optic nerve may be thought of as being highly representative of central visual fields. This helps to explain why optic nerve disease produces central scotoma with such regularity.

The funduscopic examination is of vital importance in many cases because it can rule out ocular causes for visual loss. Cataract, displaced lens, vitreous hemorrhage, retinal detachments, retinal artery or vein thrombosis are all easily visualized and diagnosed during the ophthalmoscopic examination. More subtle changes like macular degeneration are visible, but are difficult to see without a slit lamp.

Usually, optic atrophy is easily diagnosed because the nerve becomes whiter. Kestenbaum's rule is a valuable sign of optic atrophy. Normally, nine to 10 tiny vessels cross the temporal half of the optic disc. Ninety-five percent of the normal population has more than eight of these. If the examiner is practiced in the examination and can find only seven or fewer small vessels on the lateral surface of the disc, it is atrophic.[7]

The standard visual acuity chart is read with glasses on because we need to assess the best corrected vision. Most patients read downward and stop at their line of best vision. Some stop one line before they arrive at best vision, so all should be encouraged to read further toward the small print. Normally, patients do not read further than one line beyond their initial stopping point, but hysterical patients frequently stop at the big "E" or a line or two below it; then with forcible friendly encouragement, they may be able to read right down to 20/50 or better. Thus, the response to encouragement is an important diagnostic point.

Once the best visual acuity is established, confrontation central visual fields are easily performed. The patient covers one eye with a card and looks at the examiner's pupil: his left to the examiner's right. Then, a ballpoint pen tip or a red match tip or, best, a red-headed pin 2-3 mm in diameter, inserted into a pencil eraser or into a special holder, is brought directly between the pupils of the participants.

Red is the color of choice because it is the color first affected in early central visual loss. The first abnormality is that the object does not look as red in the abnormal eye as it does on the normal side. With more deficit, this desaturation of the red color may be perceived when compared to more peripheral portions of the same eye. Normally, we notice a desaturation of red color when the object is moved into the peripheral portion of the visual field, a fact the reader can document for himself with any red object at hand. Hold a red object in front of your fixation point and, without moving the eyeball, move the object in any direction away from the central five degrees of vision. It becomes "less red," and may even take on a brownish cast as it moves into more and more peripheral portions of the visual field. If central visual loss progresses, all red perception may be lost from central vision, and visual acuity drops precipitously. Eventually, the object disappears completely from central vision. This is called a central scotoma.

Once he has determined the *severity* of central visual loss, the examiner may investigate its *size* by confrontation visual fields, always keeping the test object on a vertical plane directly midway between the patient and himself. Patient, with one of his eyes covered, and clinician continue to look at each other. The patient's left pupil looks at the clinician's right, and vice versa. The initial maneuver involves identification of the patient's blind spot. The clinician finds his own, about 15° lateral to the direction of gaze, and moves his test object along the corridor of his blind spot until the patient loses the test object in his own blind spot. The relative size of the two blind spots may be assessed. Assuming the examiner's is normal, an enlargement of the patient's blind spot becomes evident if he does not see the object reappear as soon as the examiner does. Next, central and other peripheral fields are examined in the same manner.

Examination of central and peripheral visual fields by confrontation is exquisitely exact, because the clinician has complete control of the situation at all times. Unlike the tangent screen and perimetry testing, the clinician is instantly aware if the patient looks away, and he judges the extent of visual loss against his own normal visual field. This method of testing is also very easy. It does not require any special equipment and may be performed as an integral part of the rest of the examination.

Accurate assessment of severity and size of a central scotoma is of tremendous help to patient and clinician as they follow the progress of treatment over time. With precise information, the clinician may detect definite improvement when it occurs and mention it before the patient is really aware of it, or, if necessary, he can document that the process continues to worsen. In either case, patient and clinician may be in possession of the facts rather than being confined by ignorance.

The major problem with confrontation testing is not accuracy, but reproducibility over long periods of time. Confrontation testing may be used for diagnosis and for short-term follow up, but if the clinician is following an abnormal visual field over a period of years to detect the return of a tumor or other progressive disease, he cannot remember the exact outlines and should refer the patient to an ophthalmologist for reproducible visual field testing with perimeter or tangent screen.

Examination of visual acuity and even confrontation visual fields are subjective tests of retinal and optic nerve function. The afferent pupil, described by Marcus Gunn, is an objective test which documents absolutely that the eye is not functioning normally. The test is based on the fact that pupillary size is largely determined by the total amount of light coming into both eyes together. When extra light is shined into one eye, both pupils constrict to the same degree. When only one eye goes blind, both pupils remain symmetrical.

In Figure 4-3, (p. 77), imagine that lesion #1 is causing blindness in the right eye. A light flashed into that eye would produce no pupillary constriction on either side, but a light flashed into the left eye constricts both pupils equally. To observe the phenomenon of the afferent pupil, a light is shined first into the left eye, and the pupils are observed as they constrict. Then the light is instantly switched to the right eye, and the right pupil is seen to *dilate against the light,* because the stimulus to constriction which had come from the left eye is gone and is not replaced by light shining into the blind right eye. When the light is switched to the left again, the left pupil is seen to constrict dramatically when the light arrives.

The afferent pupil may be observed in the presence of vitreous hemorrhage, retinal or optic nerve disease anterior to the chiasm. Lesions behind the chiasm do not produce this finding. In patients with minimal loss of visual acuity, there is a bare gesture of pupillary noncompliance, but if there is significant loss of visual acuity and if the light is switched back and forth several times to "warm up the pupillary reactions," it is easy to see. The afferent pupil is diagnostic of abnormal function in an extremely limited portion of the patient's anatomy.

The afferent pupil does not occur with amblyopic eyes, with poor visual acuity due to congenital nystagmus or albinism, or in bilateral and equal optic atrophy. Of course, there is no abnormality of pupillary function in hysteria. The hysterical patient, who is significantly "blind" in one eye, may be accurately diagnosed as hysterical when pupillary reactions are normal. Surprisingly, the afferent pupil does not occur with cataract. The reason for this may be appreciated by the reader if he takes a moonlight walk on a cloudy night. The intense light and shadow normally present on a clear night are absent, but moonlight penetrates the sky's "cataract" quite well. In similar fashion, light penetrates a cataract to a normal retina and optic nerve, so the pupillary response to light is normal even though there is no clear image.

In temperate regions of the United States, multiple sclerosis is the most common cause of central visual loss. Optic neuritis may occur independently of multiple sclerosis, either spontaneously as a reaction to infection or, as with tobacco-alcohol amblyopia, due to nutritional deficiency or toxicity. Ischemic optic neuropathy produces sudden visual loss, frequently of an inferior portion of the visual field, in one or both eyes. There is a high incidence of diabetes and hypertension in these usually elderly patients. Ophthalmoscopic examination discloses an acutely swollen disc, frequently with flame hemorrhages and arteriolar narrowing. No effective treatment is available. Temporal arteritis frequently causes sudden total blindness in one eye, but blindness may also appear as a sector defect, and the funduscopic examination mimics ischemic optic neuropathy, so the syndrome of sudden unilateral visual loss, especially in an older person, suggests giant cell arteritis and strongly indicates prompt evaluation for this diagnosis.

Retinal diseases, such as macular degeneration or retinal detachment, may also produce central visual loss, but the cadence of these diseases is different from that of optic neuritis. Orbital tumors and inflammatory disease may also present as progressive loss of visual acuity and central scotoma. The complete list is very long. The clinician must first decide the anatomical location of the lesion, draw conclusions about its nature from the history and the rest of the examination, and then pursue the diagnosis with laboratory and radiographic examinations.

Loss of Peripheral Vision

"Hemianopsia" means loss of vision in one half of the visual field. "Homonymous hemianopsia" means that both eyes have lost vision to the left or the right. "Heteronymous" means that one eye has lost vision to the left, while the other has lost vision to the right. "Congruous" visual field losses occupy identical meridians of vision in an homonymous field. "Incongruous" visual field defects are homonymous but do not have the same shape and size. The most congruous visual field defects occur from lesions in the visual cortex. Theoretically, lesions of the optic tract should produce highly incongruous visual field defects, but in practice, direct lesions of the optic tract produce complete homonymous hemianopsia, because the optic tract is small and usually is completely destroyed by the lesion. "Quadrantanopsia" means that part of an hemianoptic field is destroyed. Lesions of the temporal radiations produce homonymous *superior* quadrantanopsia. Lesions of the parietal radiations produce homonymous *inferior* quadrantanopsia.

"I can't see from my right eye." (Right homonymous hemianopsia on exam.)

"I have half vision."

"I have trouble reading."

"Blurred vision."

Or no complaint at all.

Some patients with hemianopsia, or even with total loss of vision do not know it. These are special cases, in which the lesion is in the visual association cortex. Their disability will not be discovered unless the clinician routinely examines visual fields. Such patients, whose visual loss has not been discovered, are often thought to be demented, hysterical, or psychotic. An explanation for this phenomenon is not in the realm of this volume. There is a large literature concerning higher cortical function. The interested reader may find Geschwind's article on disconnexion syndromes illuminating.[4]

Some patients are not aware of hemianopsia until they have an automobile accident. Right homonymous hemianopsia causes drivers to sideswipe parked cars or to destroy mailboxes on the side of the road. Occasionally, such a person will run off the right side of the corner attempting to make a left turn. Drivers with left homonymous hemianopsia, if they are fortunate, recognize that they are driving in the middle of the road *before* their head-on collision.

The reading difficulties of hemianopsias are not caused by decreased visual acuity, because even a complete homonymous hemianopsia leaves half of each macula to function normally, and the visual acuity is normal. Patients with right homonymous hemianopsia have lost the peripheral portion of vision which allows the rest of us to follow a line of print across the page, and to make the accurate saccades required to bring the next word or words into central vision. If the patient can be made aware of the problem, he can keep his finger on the line and advance his eyes to the finger. This remains an unsatisfactory method for reading, even after practice.

Those with left homonymous hemianopsia read each line well, but they get lost when they attempt to find the beginning of the next line. This is easily remedied by the simple device of keeping a finger at the beginning of the line. Usually, hemianoptic patients do not understand precisely *why* they are having trouble, but a brief teaching session can help them to understand, and to make partial correction for their disability.

Cerebral Localization and Visual Field Defects

The visual system is a segmental function confined to the brain. Lesions of the brainstem and cerebellum cannot produce visual field defects. Additionally, because the visual system extends from the orbits all the way back to the occipital cortex, it forms a sort of "long tract" as it crosses the paths of cranial nerves III, IV, and VI, the pituitary region, motor and sensory systems to and from the body, and regions which govern complex functions like language. Knowledge of the characteristic visual field defects caused by lesions at various locations along the visual pathway, and of the relationships of other functions to the visual system, provides the clinician with very powerful diagnostic tools as he considers the history and physical findings. Figure 4-3 is designed to give the reader an outline of visual field defects and associated neurological abnormalities that accompany each lesion.

1) Lesions of the globe and orbit cause blindness in one eye only, frequently beginning with a central scotoma and complaints about loss of visual acuity. Constant pain, or pain on moving the

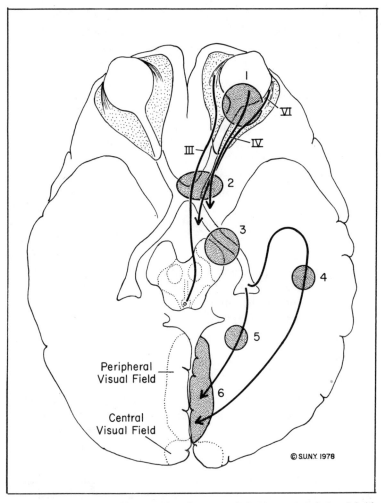

Figure 4-3. *Lesions of the visual pathways and their associated visual field defects. Each numbered lesion is discussed in the text.*

eye, are common. If there is an orbital mass, proptosis is evident and extraocular muscle palsies and pupillary paralysis are common. The discovery of an afferent pupil documents the presence of disease in this region.

2) Lesions around the optic chiasm do not produce highly pre-

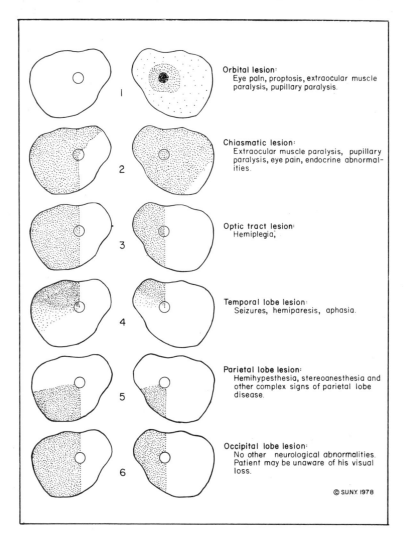

Orbital lesion:
  Eye pain, proptosis, extraocular muscle paralysis, pupillary paralysis.

Chiasmatic lesion:
  Extraocular muscle paralysis, pupillary paralysis, eye pain, endocrine abnormalities.

Optic tract lesion:
  Hemiplegia,

Temporal lobe lesion:
  Seizures, hemiparesis, aphasia.

Parietal lobe lesion:
  Hemihypesthesia, stereoanesthesia and other complex signs of parietal lobe disease.

Occipital lobe lesion:
  No other neurological abnormalities. Patient may be unaware of his visual loss.

© S.U.N.Y. 1978

dictable bitemporal hemianopsia because such lesions are usually discovered early in their course. In fact, many lesions of the region never have a chance to produce visual loss at all because they are discovered during an evaluation for endocrine or growth disorders, double vision, or headache. Symptomatology from the optic chiasm results from portions of an adjacent lesion which compromise the blood supply or press directly on the optic chiasm itself. Characteristically, chiasmatic lesions cause more loss of vision in one eye than the other because the effects of lesions on chasmatic function are not completely symmetrical. In the accompanying figure, the lesion is situated more to the right and has caused near-total blindness in the right eye. It affects crossing fibers from the left eye and has produced a left hemianopsia on that side, but it also affects the left optic nerve, with resultant loss of vision in the right superior field of vision on that side. The lesion we have depicted is causing far advanced visual loss. The hallmark of earlier chiasmatic lesions is a heteronymous visual field defect that affects one eye more than the other.

3) The optic tract is plastered closely to the cerebral peduncle. It is only a millimeter or two thick and about five millimeters wide, so a single small lesion in the area can cause total homonymous hemianopsia and hemiplegia. If the lesion extends a few millimeters into the substance of the midbrain from the cerebral peduncle, it causes total hemianesthesia as well, but without clouding of consciousness. The presence of devastating paralysis and hemianopsia without loss of consciousness leads the clinician to localize the lesion in the optic tract, because a lesion higher in the brain would have to destroy the hemisphere to produce the same findings. This would be accompanied by a significant mass effect, coma, and death.

4) and 5) Temporal and parietal visual radiations are distributed over a large expanse of the posterior hemisphere. Quadrantic visual field defects are common because few lesions are large enough to destroy the entire visual system in this region. The frequent incongruity of superior quadrantanopsia, caused by temporal lobe lesions, is emphasized in the figure. This probably occurs because tumors and acute vascular lesions are accompanied by a mass effect and damage the optic tract, which courses immediately adjacent to the medial temporal lobe. Surgical lesions of the temporal lobe do not produce incongruous visual field defects.[2]

Associated symptoms from temporal lobe lesions may consist of localizing seizures or, if there is a mass, it may cause hemiparesis by pressure on the adjacent motor system in the hemisphere. Aphasia occurs from both temporal and parietal lesions of the dominant hemisphere. Parietal lobe lesions cause simple sensory loss or loss of more complex functions related to language, which also are discussed in Geschwind's article.[4]

6) Homonymous hemianopsia with macular sparing has been a hallmark of occipital lobe disease, although there is no firm anatomical explanation. Additionally, this is the only part of the visual system which is not associated with other neurological functions, so occipital lobe lesions often produce homonymous hemianopsia with macular sparing, unaccompanied by any neurological abnormality except perhaps the mildest of sensory deficits.

Blood supply to the visual cortex on both sides usually originates from the basilar artery. Because of this, basilar artery disease frequently produces sudden onset of bilateral congruous hemianoptic defects, or total blindness, sparing only macular regions in some cases.

Lesions that cause visual field defects include all of the five pathological processes (see p. 3). Specific diagnostic considerations depend upon the cadence of the disease, the anatomical distribution of lesions revealed by the physical examination, and by the results of any laboratory examinations the clinician may perform.

Knowledge of the anatomy of visual loss simplifies the process of diagnosis and adds finesse to the clinician's capabilities. Treatment depends on the specific disease process discovered.

REFERENCES

1. Cogan, D.G.: *Neurology of the Visual System.* Charles C Thomas, Springfield, Ill., 1966.
2. Duke-Elder, S., Scott, G.I.: *System of Ophthalmology, Vol. XII Neuro-ophthalmology.* C.V. Mosby, St. Louis, 1971, pp. 426–427.
3. Gay, A.J., Newman, N.M., Keltner, J.L., Stroud, M.H., *Eye Movement Disorders*, C.V. Mosby, St. Louis, 1974.
4. Geschwind, N.: Disconnexion Syndromes in Animals and Man, II. Brain 88:585–644, 1965.
5. Potts, A.M., Hodges, D., Shelman, C.B., Fritz, K.J., Levy, N.S., Mangnall, Y.: Morphology of the Primate Optic Nerve III. Fiber Characteristics of the Foveal Outflow. Invest. Ophthalmol. 11:1004–1016, 1972.
6. Suttie, I.D.: A Theory of Decussation. J. Neurol. Psychopathol. 6:267–280, 1926.
7. Veith, N.W., Sacks, J.G.: Enumeration of Small Vessels on the Optic Discs in Normal Eyes. Am. J. Ophthalmol. 76:660–661, 1973.

CHAPTER 5

Evaluation of Abnormal Eye Movements

INTRODUCTION

This chapter outlines neural mechanisms for the control of eye movements, and discusses some of the common clinical syndromes associated with each part of the system. Accurate diagnosis of abnormal eye movements is complicated because the anatomy includes components from the brain, brainstem, peripheral nerves, and the eye muscles themselves. Furthermore, each anatomical area is affected by distinct disease processes. If he understands the anatomy of his patient's complaint, the clinician can reach a specific pathologic diagnosis without difficulty.

Figure 5-1 (p. 82) outlines the neural pathways for turning the eyes conjugately to the right. Since it represents a summary of most of this chapter, the reader is encouraged to refer to it as he reads. Remember that lesions at any point along the pathway interrupt all the functions below them, so a lesion in the supranuclear portions affects conjugate gaze. A lesion in the internuclear pathway affects only one eye, and causes diplopia and dysconjugate eye movements, but in a different manner from lesions of the nucleus or the nerve itself, which also cause diplopia and dysconjugate eye movements.

In addition to the distinctive symptomatology of individual portions of the oculomotor system, the pathways run near other neural functions. The discovery of associated neurological deficits also helps the clinician to determine the site and the extent of the pathologic process.

This chapter contains anatomical and functional terminology which may be new to the reader and needs definition before we begin.

Supranuclear refers to pathways from the cerebral cortex into the brainstem.

Internuclear refers to pathways coursing between the region of the abducens nucleus in the lower pons and the oculomotor nucleus in the midbrain, especially the medial longitudinal fasciculus (MLF).

Infranuclear are all the portions of a pathway which carry information outward from the nucleus. This includes the nerve, myoneural junction, and the muscles themselves.

Extortion is a rotational movement of the eyeball around the visual axis and is defined by the movement of the superior portion of the globe. When the observer sees the patient's right eyeball rotate counterclockwise, it is extorted. If the left eyeball rotates counterclockwise, it is *intorted.*

Oculomotor is the third nerve but also refers more generally to eye movements. I have tried to clarify this confusion in the text.

External ophthalmoplegia means paralysis of extraocular muscles. *Internal ophthalmoplegia* means paralysis of the pupil.

If the information in this chapter whets the reader's appetite, he may enjoy reading *Neurology of the Extraocular Muscles*[1] and *Eye Movement Disorders.*[2] Once he has mastered these volumes, he may plunge into the literature where he will find that the specialty of neuro-ophthalmology is a fascinating discipline.

PARALYSIS OF CONJUGATE LATERAL GAZE

Cortical Gaze Control

From frontal and occipital gaze control centers, the left side of the brain turns the eyes conjugately to the right. The frontal eye field initiates voluntary saccadic movements of the eyes ("Look to the right!"), while the occipital eye field initiates slower automatic pursuit movements ("Follow my finger!").

Ischemic stroke and cerebral hemorrhage are the most common causes for conjugate gaze paralysis because gaze paralysis from cerebral lesions only occurs immediately after acute lesions, disappears then, and can be revisualized only under special circumstances.

Brief malfunction of frontal or occipital cerebral gaze centers may be seen during head and eye turning seizures, when the eyes are (usually) deviated away from the side of the seizure focus; and dur-

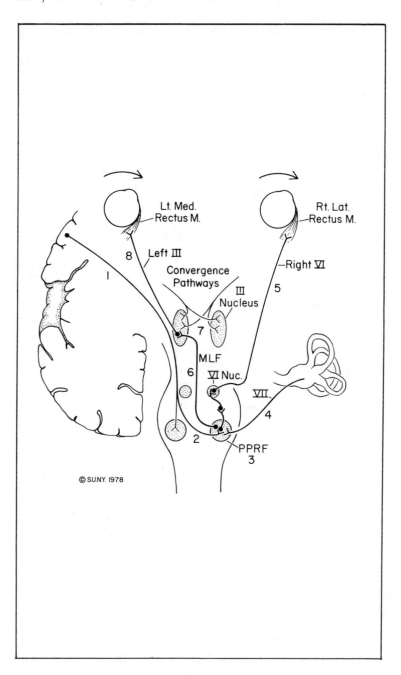

Figure 5-1. *Pathway for turning the eyes conjugately to the right. 1) Cortical control for conjugate lateral gaze originates in the frontal (voluntary) and occipital (automatic) eye fields. A lesion in these pathways produces temporary conjugate gaze paralysis. The eyes do not easily deviate away from the side of the lesion. 2) Supranuclear control is distributed bilaterally, but primarily to the opposite paramedian pontine reticular formation (PPRF). 3) The PPRF is the final determinant of conjugate lateral gaze. A lesion of the PPRF causes permanent paralysis of lateral gaze. The eyes cannot deviate toward the side of the lesion. The PPRF innervates individual motor nuclei via the internuclear connections. 4) Vestibular afferents also enter the pons and exert their influence on conjugate gaze. Lesions of the vestibular system cause vertigo and jerk nystagmus but do not cause paralysis of conjugate lateral gaze. 5) The internuclear pathway to the abducens nucleus is a two-neuron arc whose length is very short. It is almost never involved in disease and is not discussed. The right abducens nerve innervates the right lateral rectus muscle and turns the eye to the right. A lesion of this pathway causes right lateral rectus paralysis. 6) The medial longitudinal fasciculus (MLF) crosses the midline immediately and travels toward the opposite third nerve nucleus. A lesion of the MLF in its caudal portion causes a posterior internuclear ophthalmoplegia. 7) If the most rostral portion of the MLF is damaged, the pathway for ocular convergence is also involved. This pathway descends directly to the third nerve nucleus from cortical levels. A lesion involving the rostral MLF and convergence pathways is called anterior internuclear ophthalmoplegia (see text). 8) The left oculomotor nerve innervates the left medial rectus muscle and turns the eye to the right. A lesion of the oculomotor nerve causes paralysis of the medial rectus and other muscles innervated by that nerve. The pupil is unresponsive to light and is dilated because of parasympathetic paralysis with intact sympathetic innervation.*

ing the postictal period, when they may deviate toward the side of the seizure focus because of a Todd's paralysis of conjugate gaze.

A large ischemic stroke or a cerebral hemorrhage in the *frontal* lobe causes hemiplegia, clouding of consciousness or coma, as well as tonic deviation of the head and eyes toward the side of the lesion. When the patient regains consciousness, the gaze asymmetry disappears.

Gaze paralysis from lesions of the *occipital* eye field almost always occurs after an ischemic stroke in the distribution of the posterior cerebral artery. This small lesion does not cause unconsciousness, but there is invariably a dense homonymous hemianopsia. When occipital eye field cortex is involved, there is dramatic conjugate deviation of the eyes toward the side of the lesion. The hemianopsia is not the cause for the gaze paralysis, because lesions of other parts of the visual system produce dense homonymous hemianopsia without affecting conjugate gaze.

The patient with gaze paralysis due to an occipital lesion lies in bed, wide awake and responsive to questions, although he rarely initiates normal conversation. His head is deviated to some degree, but the eyes appear to be *forced* into far lateral gaze. Regardless of the examiner's position in the room, the eyes do not move to follow him. With considerable coaxing, the patient can bring his eyes out of the far lateral position, but when the examiner stops coaxing, they fall back immediately to their previous state, never having come fully to the midline. The patient may not volunteer that his vision is affected at all, because his language center may not be aware of the deficit. This is called Anton's syndrome.

If the eyes are deviated to the left, the lesion is on the left, and the patient has a right homonymous hemianopsia. The syndrome emphasizes the great power of the remaining occipital eye field in the initiation of the automatic conjugate lateral gaze when suddenly the balanced activity from the other side is lost. After a few days or a week, the powerful gaze deviation lessens and finally disappears. Hemianopsia is almost always permanent, once it is present, regardless of the cause or site of the lesion.

Pontine Gaze Control

Paralysis of conjugate gaze caused by a pontine lesion was first described by Foville in 1858, at a time when the French physicians were thrashing out the basic questions of clinical neuroanatomy. They were fairly certain that the left side of the brain always controlled the right side of the body, and they were beginning to recognize that apparent exceptions to the rule actually represented brainstem disease. Foville likened the action of the pontine gaze control center to a man driving a team of horses. The pontine gaze control center takes the reins guiding both eyes to one side in its one hand and produces conjugate eye movements while each nerve moves the muscles of one eye only.

The author has translated Foville's article and ten others which first described the classic brainstem syndromes that are frequently encountered.[6] Together they illustrate some aspects of the 19th century's developing understanding of clinical neuroanatomy and the difficulties encountered in establishing even the basic facts of anatomy without the firm concepts we now take for granted, like the neuron, the synapse, and decussation.

Gaze paralysis from a pontine lesion usually develops after an ischemic stroke, just as it does in the brain. At one time, neurologists referred to the "conjugate gaze center" of the pons, but such a "center" has not been found. Instead, it appears that one section of the paramedian pontine reticular formation (PPRF) is concerned with conjugate eye movements. Figure 5-1 indicates that cerebral gaze control from frontal and occipital eye fields and the vestibular apparatus innervate the PPRF. Each side of the PPRF receives impulses from *both* sides of the brain, and this accounts for the transient nature of cerebral gaze paralysis, but gaze paralysis due to a lesion in the PPRF is permanent because the PPRF is the end of the pathway governing conjugate gaze, and each PPRF deviates the eyes conjugately *only* toward its own side of the body.

The neurological examination easily distinguishes between cerebral and pontine lesions. If the lesion is in the brain, the eyes are deviated away from the hemiparesis, toward the side of the lesion. If the lesion is in the pons, the eyes are deviated toward the hemiparetic side, away from the side of the lesion, and usually there is paralysis of the face and tongue on the same side as the lesion.

Vestibulo-ocular reflexes are discussed in the chapter on the evaluation of the comatose patient (pp. 164-165). Diseases of the vestibular system cause conjugate jerk nystagmus, but in the conscious patient, there is no gaze paralysis. Nonetheless, because of its powerful physiological influence on conjugate gaze and its contributions to neurological symptoms, the vestibular system is included in Figure 5-1.

DYSCONJUGATE EYE MOVEMENTS

Actions of the Individual Extraocular Muscles

Normally, all 12 extraocular muscles, six in each orbit, act together to produce precise conjugate eye movements in all directions. If only one muscle is paralyzed, the paralysis may be identified by consideration of the direct actions of individual extraocular muscles. Students frequently give up in despair when they try to remember the actions of the individual extraocular muscles because they have tried to memorize the six cardinal directions of gaze for each eye, and have promptly forgotten them. The situation is greatly simplified if the student instead remembers a few cardinal facts of anatomy:

1) All eye muscles except the obliques are attached at the apex of the orbit, and their direction of action is toward the apex, regardless of the position of the globe. The resultant eye movements depend on the site of muscle attachment to the globe. The medial and lateral recti are attached to the medial and lateral sides of the globe and adduct and abduct the globe. The superior and inferior recti are attached to the top and bottom of the globe, and their action *depends upon the position of the globe in the orbit.*

2) The orbits are angled nearly 30° lateral to the forward angle of vision, and the direction of the superior and inferior recti parallels the axis of the orbit, so these two muscles have their most distinct function when the eye is abducted parallel to the axis of the orbit. Then, the superior rectus "looks up," and the inferior rectus "looks down." When the eye is adducted, the superior rectus intorts the globe, and the inferior rectus extorts it.

3) The oblique muscles have their bony attachment to the superior and inferior corners of the *anterior medial* wall of the orbit. Their direction of action is almost at right angles to the axis of the superior and inferior rectus muscles. The *inferior* oblique attaches to the inferior corner of the orbit and the inferior surface of the globe. The *superior* oblique, although it originates at the apex of the orbit, pulls through the trochlea on the superior orbital corner and attaches to the superior surface to the globe. These two muscles

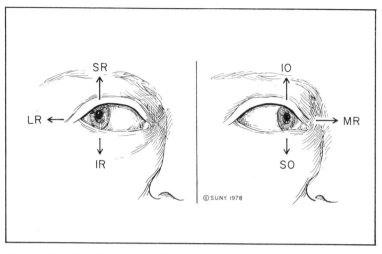

Figure 5-2. *This diagram emphasizes the primary functions of individual eye muscles. It stresses the fact that muscles which elevate and depress the axis of vision function most directly in the adducted or abducted position of the globe.*

have their most direct action when the globe is adducted toward their site of attachment. Then, the superior oblique "looks down," and the inferior oblique "looks up." When the eye is abducted, the superior oblique produces intortion, and the inferior oblique produces extortion of the globe.

There is no mystery to eye movements if these facts are kept in mind. However, diagnosis may be difficult if more than one muscle is paralyzed at a time. Involvement of the oculomotor nerve and its nucleus most commonly causes multiple muscle paralysis. A complete oculomotor nerve lesion causes paralysis of the medial, superior, and inferior recti and the inferior oblique. This leaves intact the functions of the superior oblique and lateral rectus muscles. Muscle tone in the lateral rectus abducts the eye. In abduction, the superior rectus depresses the visual axis and intorts the globe. The intortion is difficult to recognize, but the "down and out" position of the globe is characteristic of oculomotor nerve paralysis. If the pupillary pathway is destroyed, the pupil is dilated and unresponsive to light. The lid droops over the whole eye because of paralysis of the levator palpebrae superioris, and must be elevated to perform the examination.

Under normal conditions, the lateral rectus muscle, innervated by the abducens nerve, abducts the eye so strongly on command that sclera is not visible between the cornea and the outer canthus of the eye. If there is weakness of the lateral rectus muscle or incomplete sixth nerve paralysis, the eye may abduct beyond the midline but not enough to hide the sclera completely. Complete lesions of the abducens nerve produce complete paralysis of the lateral rectus muscle. This cannot be distinguished by examination alone from isolated paralysis of the lateral rectus muscle itself. In both nerve and muscle lesions, there is paralysis of abduction of the globe and double vision during attempted conjugate lateral gaze in that direction.

Isolated paralysis of the superior oblique muscle is unusual. It is discovered by asking the patient to adduct the globe and look down. Usually the clinician has discovered a third nerve paralysis and wonders whether the fourth nerve is also affected. Under these conditions, the eye does not adduct, and evaluation of intortion of the globe during attempted downward gaze may provide the answer. But accurate assessment of this function is difficult, and the clinician is likely to be dissatisfied with his answer. Fortunately, the diagnosis rarely depends on the results of this part of the examination.

Internuclear Ophthalmoplegia

Figure 5-1 illustrates the medial longitudinal fasciculus connecting the PPRF on one side of the lower pons to the third nerve complex on the opposite side of the midbrain. The MLF decussates in the lower pons immediately after it leaves the PPRF and travels closely beneath the floor of the fourth ventricle, only about a millimeter from the MLF on the opposite side. The MLF may be affected anywhere along its course by multiple sclerosis, ischemic stroke, brainstem hemorrhage, neoplasms of the brainstem and fourth ventricle, or acute infectious processes in the fourth ventricle.

The naming of MLF lesions is confused because there are two terminologies in the literature. The author has chosen the system most commonly used in this country. For the present, the reader need only be aware that there is another terminology in case he encounters it in his further reading.

A lesion of the MLF which occurs below the level of the third nerve nucleus produces a *posterior* internuclear ophthalmoplegia. This syndrome is recognized by an apparent paralysis of the medial rectus muscle during attempted conjugate lateral gaze. Further examination discloses that the medial rectus is not paralyzed at all, because there is no divergent strabismus on forward gaze, and the medial rectus functions normally during convergence movements. In addition to the paralytic component in the adducting eye, there is coarse nystagmus in the abducting eye, the significance of which has been widely debated. It seems probable now that the nystagmus represents spasmodic attempts to bring the adducting eye past the midline, through the use of convergence pathways.[5]

Anterior internuclear ophthalmoplegia even more closely resembles a nuclear medial rectus palsy, because there is apparent medial rectus paralysis during attempted lateral gaze *and* during attempted convergence. But again, there is no divergent strabismus on forward gaze, as would be expected if the medial rectus muscle were truly paralyzed. Figure 5-1 illustrates the pathways for convergence descending directly into the third nerve complex from occipital regions of the cortex. These are not affected except by lesions near the third nerve nucleus. Anterior internuclear ophthalmoplegia is much less common than posterior internuclear ophthalmoplegia, probably because of the great length of caudal portions of the MLF, which is several centimeters long, and because the lesion of anterior internuclear ophthalmoplegia quickly becomes a third nerve paralysis if it is only slightly enlarged.

Unilateral internuclear ophthalmoplegia is usually caused by ischemic stroke because the paramedian perforating arterioles from the basilar artery feed each side separately. If there is thrombosis of one of these, the MLF on that side may be destroyed without damage to its counterpart only a millimeter away but across the midline. Wernicke's encephalopathy may produce unilateral internuclear ophthalmoplegia for the same reason. Multiple sclerosis may produce predominantly unilateral symptoms, but bilateral dysfunction is usually evident if the clinician carefully investigates gaze in both directions.

Bilateral internuclear ophthalmoplegia is said to occur only in demyelinating diseases, especially multiple sclerosis. This seems to be a poor rule from the anatomical point of view, since brainstem glioma, tumors of the fourth ventricle, and other bilateral processes would seem to be likely causes for bilateral dysfunction of the MLF. However, in practice, the rule is usually vindicated, and it is a good one to remember—with reservations.

A *minimal* internuclear ophthalmoplegia may be diagnosed during the neurological screening examination, if the examiner asks his patient to follow his finger laterally and holds the eyes in the lateral position for a few moments. Nystagmus of the abducting eye becomes apparent under these conditions even though eye movements appeared conjugate. Weakness of adduction may be revealed if the examiner uses J. Lawton Smith's technique of stressing the medial rectus muscle by saccadic movements, using either the optokinetic tape or wider saccades between the examiner's two widely separated fingers.[3] As the patient looks back and forth between the two targets, the examiner may detect slowed adduction on one or both sides and thus establish his diagnosis of mild dysfunction in the MLF.

Discovery of mild bilateral internuclear ophthalmoplegia may be of central diagnostic importance to the patient whose symptoms suggest multiple sclerosis, but whose other neurological abnormalities are limited to spinal cord levels. Documentation of a minimal bilateral internuclear ophthalmoplegia establishes the dissemination of lesions above the foramen magnum, and may allow the diagnosis of multiple sclerosis to be made on clinical grounds (pp. 329-331).

Nuclear Ophthalmoplegia

Nuclear lesions may be diagnosed if associated signs also localize the lesion in the correct region of the brainstem. Nuclear abducens paralysis is often associated with facial paralysis on the same side and hemiparesis or hemihypesthesia on the opposite side of the body. Nuclear oculomotor paralysis on one side is also associated with contralateral hemiparesis or hemihypesthesia, and if the lesion affects the red nucleus as well, there may also be contralateral tremor.

The third nerve complex is distributed along the length of the midbrain, so lesions which leave the patient conscious usually do not affect the entire nucleus. Therefore, third nerve paralyses which do not involve all third nerve functions point to a nuclear lesion. The clinician must beware of "partial third nerve paralysis which spares the pupil," because myasthenia gravis may mimic many forms of external ophthalmoplegia. If the patient has extraocular muscle paralysis and the clinician is not absolutely certain of the cause, the edrophonium chloride (Tensilon®) test is an easy procedure and usually diagnostic if the patient has myasthenia gravis. It is embarrassing to hear later that the test was diagnostic in the office of some other physician!

While multiple sclerosis is a common cause of dysconjugate eye movements because it produces internuclear ophthalmoplegia, multiple sclerosis is not a common cause of nuclear paralysis, because this disease affects myelin around nerve fibers, not the nuclei themselves. If a patient has clearly documented nuclear paralysis, the clinician must consider many other diagnoses before multiple sclerosis.

Infranuclear Ophthalmoplegias

Oculomotor, Trochlear, and Abducens Nerve Paralyses

After the three oculomotor nerves leave the brainstem, they pass through the posterior fossa toward the cavernous sinus, where they join the first and second trigeminal divisions on their way to the orbit. They enter the orbit through the superior orbital fissure with the first trigeminal division and join the optic nerve and orbital contents before dividing: 1) to enter the globe for pupillary innervation, and 2) to innervate each of the extraocular muscles.

Isolated trochlear nerve paralysis is rare and will not be discussed here. Abducens paralysis occasionally occurs as an idiopathic and isolated complaint, much like Bell's palsy of the adjacent facial nerve. In such cases, it clears completely in a matter of several months. However, abducens paralysis may be a false localizing symptom of increased intracranial pressure from any cause, so double vision due to lateral rectus muscle weakness requires careful evaluation by the clinician. Because it may be a sign of disease elsewhere in the head, or an early sign of myasthenia gravis, a Tensilon test is indicated as part of the workup for abducens paralysis.

Oculomotor paralysis is the most frequent cause of neurogenic external ophthalmoplegia. It occurs especially frequently in relation to arterial aneurysms and diabetes mellitus. The oculomotor nerve travels in close association with the superior cerebellar, posterior cerebral, and posterior communicating arteries, and within the cavernous sinus it courses next to the carotid siphon. Aneurysms on these vessels may cause third nerve paralysis, which frequently, but not always, is associated with pain.

Because diabetic neuropathy also causes painful external ophthalmoplegia, the question of diagnosis is frequently unresolved if unilataral oculomotor paralysis occurs. Diabetic oculomotor paralysis spares the pupillary fibers more frequently than aneurysm, but this is not an absolutely reliable distinction. Myasthenic "oculomotor paralysis" *always* spares the pupil!

Angiography is usually relatively safe, while a ruptured aneurysm is potentially fatal. Surgical treatment for unruptured aneurysms may be highly successful and, for these reasons, nonmyasthenic oculomotor nerve paralysis is a strong indication for complete angiography unless there is clear evidence that the cause is unrelated to intracerebral aneurysm. Lesions of the cavernous sinus may involve all three oculomotor nerves and the first and second trigeminal divisions together. Once the oculomotor nerves have entered the orbit, they travel with the optic nerve, and lesions here cause ophthalmoplegia, blindness, and proptosis.

Neuromuscular Junction Disease

Diplopia is frequently the first complaint in myasthenia gravis, because the extraocular muscles require exquisite control for normal function, and any loss of control is immediately visible. Usually, when the myasthenic first complains of diplopia, careful examination also reveals ptosis or progressive drooping of the lid on sustained upward gaze. The general muscle examination reveals weakness or easy fatigability of other body muscles. A detailed discussion of myasthenia gravis is found in Chapter VI (pp. 124ff.).

The Tensilon® test may be disappointing in myasthenia, although Tensilon® usually produces some improvement in muscle strength. If the clinician does not note a diagnostic improvement after Tensilon®, a trial of pyridostigmine (Mestinon®) may produce progressive improvement over several days, although diplopia may never disappear completely. Pyridostigmine and the other treatments for myasthenia often produce incomplete restoration of muscle function all over the body. This may be hardly noticeable in the quadriceps, but if there are only a few degrees of strabismus, the patient may complain bitterly of disabling diplopia.

Extraocular muscles are not as severely involved in the myasthenic syndrome as in myasthenia gravis, but double vision is a prominent early symptom of botulism. Both of these conditions affect the myoneural junction, but in a different manner from myasthenia gravis.

Ocular Myopathies

Dysthyroid myopathy: This is not a neurological disease, but it must be exceedingly common because people with evident dysthyroid myopathy are often encountered at the grocery store, the theater, and the hospital lobby even by neurologists who don't treat the disease! J. Lawton Smith has emphasized that dysthyroid myopathy may occur when the patient is clinically euthyroid or even slightly hypothyroid.[4] He emphasizes the vital importance of performance of the thyroid suppression test, even if the T_3 is normal, because despite normal circulating thyroid hormone, the abnormal gland is not suppressed as it should be. In addition to the proptosis, congestion and swelling of the lids and conjunctivae, patients with dysthyroid myopathy develop fibrosis and shortening of specific muscles, especially the inferior, superior, or medial recti, with resultant diplopia. Smith recommends frequent eye exercises during each day in an attempt to stretch these muscles. He stresses the importance of corrective surgery for shortened muscles if specified medicinal treatment and exercises do not stop the process.

Progressive external ophthalmoplegia: One form of muscular dystrophy is strictly limited to the lids and extraocular muscles. The patient complains of slowly progressive ptosis and diplopia, with decreasing range of eye movements but no other neurological dysfunction. The disease is hereditary, but may be recessive, and there may be no family history. In about one fourth of cases, palate, bulbar muscles, and muscles of the face become involved, resulting in nasal speech, dysphagia, and loss of facial expressiveness. There is no treatment. If the diagnosis is suspected, it should not be accepted without the performance of a Tensilon® test, because myasthenia gravis is treatable and may superficially resemble progressive external ophthalmoplegia.

Ptosis

ˌTwo muscles elevate the upper lid: The levator palpebrae superioris, innervated by the third nerve, and Müller's muscle, innervated by the sympathetic divisions of the autonomic nervous system. Weakness of either muscle may produce ptosis, and each may easily be distinguished from the other.

The levator palpebrae superioris is striated muscle and forcibly lifts the lid as the eye looks up. Müller's muscle is smooth muscle and maintains lid tone according to activity in the sympathetic system. First, the patient with ptosis is asked to look up. If the lid elevates normally, the ptosis is of sympathetic origin. If the lid remains lowered despite attempts to look up, it is either of third nerve origin or hysterical.

The examiner may diagnose hysterical ptosis by watching the forehead. He must first establish that facial muscles are not weak by having the patient close his eyes and grimace. Then, the patient is asked to look up. The patient who is truly trying to look up wrinkles his forehead as he does so. The hysterical patient with "ptosis" or "upward gaze paralysis" does not.

Nystagmus

Nystagmus consists of visible alternating movements, which are usually involuntary, of one or both eyes. If nystagmus is binocular, the movements are usually conjugate. Two basically different kinds of nystagmus are distinguished on the basis of the physical examination and cause: pendular nystagmus and jerk nystagmus.

The movements of pendular nystagmus are equally brisk in both directions. This is in contrast to jerk nystagmus, which has a slow phase, caused by asymmetrical extraocular muscle tone, and a rapid corrective jerk, as the eyes regain their point of fixation with a saccade.

Pendular Nystagmus

Most patients with pendular nystagmus have decreased visual acuity, and know it. Congenital retinal disease, high myopia which was unrecognized in childhood, albinism, complete color blindness, and congential cataracts pose no diagnostic problem. Patients who become blind as adults may eventually develop pendular nystagmus.

Their diagnosis is also known when the nystagmus finally develops.

But occasionally, a person complains of headache or some other unrelated complaint, and the careful physician discovers pendular nystagmus in the course of his thorough neurological examination. This may be congenital nystagmus and, if it is, it must be recognized in order to spare the patient further diagnostic procedures. Congenital nystagmus is not associated with serious intracranial disease. Visual acuity is usually decreased, and the nystagmus itself has diagnostic characteristics:

1) Congenital nystagmus is pendular horizontal nystagmus on forward gaze and remains pendular and horizontal during upward and downward forward gaze. This characteristic is *the hallmark* of congenital nystagmus and does not occur in nystagmus due to serious intracranial disease.

2) As gaze is directed laterally, congenital nystagmus changes to jerk nystagmus in the direction of gaze. There is usually a "null point" at some position lateral to forward gaze where the directional component changes, and nystagmus is minimal.

3) Patients with congenital nystagmus do not complain of changing vision.

If the examination matches these three criteria, the diagnosis of congenital nystagmus is established and needs no further attention.

Occasionally, patients with serious intracranial disease develop unilateral or bilateral pendular nystagmus. This occurs most often in patients with multiple sclerosis and the patient is aware of other serious neurological disabilities.

Jerk Nystagmus

Jerk nystagmus is usually normal. Optokinetic nystagmus (railroad nystagmus) is the normal method used by the eyes to look at stationary objects as the individual moves past them. The normal response to vestibular caloric stimulation consists of jerk nystagmus, as the eyes are drawn toward the side of cold caloric stimulation by the activated vestibulo-ocular reflexes and jerk back repeatedly to the point of original fixation. Jerk nystagmus is named according to the direction of the rapid saccade.

End-point nystagmus must be recognized when it occurs, because it, too, is normal. When patients are asked to look far laterally and held there, the eye muscles fatigue and drift toward the midline, only to be jerked back on target. End-point nystagmus does *not* normally occur at 30° of lateral gaze, so the clinician who wishes to avoid being confused will take his patient *only* 30° laterally during his neurological screening examination. Then, if he sees nystagmus, he *knows* it is abnormal.

End-point nystagmus occurring at lesser angles of lateral gaze may be caused by muscle weakness. Myasthenia gravis causes slow coarse nystagmoid movements because the weakened extraocular muscles allow the eyes to drift toward a neutral position before the patient again reestablishes fixation.

Drug intoxications of many kinds produce nystagmus. Phenytoin is the most common cause of drug-induced nystagmus in neurological patients and produces vertical nystagmus first, followed, if intoxication increases, by nystagmus in all directions of gaze.

Serious neurological disease in the brainstem and cerebellum, and even in the spinal cord, optic chiasm, and the brain, may be associated with jerk nystagmus. Unfortunately, jerk nystagmus does not usually provide accurate localizing information, and those few patients with truly localizing nystagmus invariably have associated neurological findings, so the non-neurological clinician need not learn about them. Instead, he may rely on his standard neurological examination for localization, and recognize the presence of jerk nystagmus as an associated abnormality.

Hysteria

Complaints of double vision are common in nervous people, but the examination fails to disclose dysconjugate eye movements or pupillary abnormalities. The patient who complains of double vision in one eye is almost certainly hysterical unless he has dislocation of the lens or retinal detachment. Patients with a large iridectomy foramen may have monocular diplopia because, in effect, they have two pupils. All organic lesions which cause monocular diplopia are readily visible with the ophthalmoscope and need not cause confusion.

Convergence spasm occurs occasionally in hysterical patients. It appears superficially like bilateral abducens nerve paralysis, but is not accompanied by any evidence of intracranial disease. Pupillary constriction and spasm of accommodation also occur at the same time.

A Note on "Blurred Vision"

When the patient complains of "blurred vision," don't believe him – quiz him! The complaint of "blurred vision" may mean that he needs new glasses, or he has cataracts; central scotoma, visual field defect of any kind, double vision, or oscillopsia. The anatomical differential includes ophthalmic disease, disease of the retina, optic nerve, chiasm, brain, brainstem, cerebellum, peripheral nerves, myasthenia gravis, and primary muscle disease! "Blurred vision" is a dangerous complaint if it is not analyzed, but a rewarding one to the clinician who is alert, ferrets out its correct meaning, and finds the cause.

REFERENCES

1. Cogan, D.G.: *Neurology of the Ocular Muscles,* 2nd ed, Charles C Thomas, Springfield, Ill.,1956.
2. Gay, A.J., Newman, N.M., Keltner, J.L., Stroud, M.H.: *Eye Movement Disorders,* C.V. Mosby, St. Louis, 1974.
3. Smith, J.L., David, N.J.: Internuclear Ophthalmoplegia. Two New Clinical Signs. Neurology 14:307–309, 1964.
4. Smith, J.L.: in *Neuro-ophthalmology.* Symposium of the University of Miami and the Bascom Palmer Eye Institute. Smith, J.L., Ed. C.V. Mosby, St. Louis, 1972, pp. 1–10.
5. Stroud, M.H., Newman, N.M., Keltner, J.L., Gay, A.J.; Abducting Nystagmus in the Medial Longitudinal Fascicules (MLF) Syndrome—Internuclear Ophthalmoplegia (INO) Arch. Ophthalmol. 92:2–5, 1974.
6. Wolf, J.K., ed.: *The Classical Brainstem Syndromes*, Charles C Thomas, Springfield, Ill., 1971.

CHAPTER 6

Diseases of the Motor Unit

INTRODUCTION

The motor unit consists of an anterior horn cell in the spinal cord, its axon, the myoneural junctions, and the individual muscle fibers innervated by that anterior horn cell. All skeletal muscles are organized according to motor units, and diseases of the motor units may be classified according to that portion primarily affected.

Motor unit disease is the most difficult for the non-neurological clinician to diagnose because he is usually not familiar with the details of peripheral nervous system anatomy. Thus, when patients complain of generalized or focal weakness, the non-neurological clinician may be ill-equipped for the anatomical analysis of symptoms that make accurate diagnosis possible. I shall attempt to emphasize the clinical and anatomical characteristics of the various disease entities in this chapter and to provide details of some treatment plans. The clinician may find that the Medical Research Council's booklet *Aids to the Investigation of Peripheral Nerve Injuries*[19] is of great help in defining the relevant anatomical organization because it provides information about innervation by cutaneous and muscular nerves in upper and lower extremities and demonstrates how the power of each muscle may be examined.

Most patients with motor unit disease should be referred to a neurologist or to some other specialist with a particular interest or competence in the treatment of these diseases. With the exception of the chronic peripheral neuropathies and the focal entrapment neuropathies, many of these diseases are uncommon and at least potentially fatal. Some of them are eminently treatable. Those that are not, like amyotrophic lateral sclerosis, often can be made more bearable if the clinician has experience with aids to combat progres-

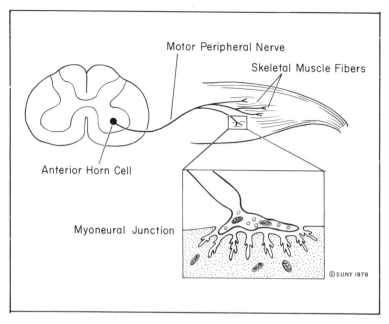

Figure 6-1. *The motor unit.*

sive disability and a humane interest in the emotional management of terminal illness.

AMYOTROPHIC LATERAL SCLEROSIS (ALS)

We still do not know the cause of ALS except that it is inherited as an autosomal dominant trait in about 5-10 percent of ALS patients. Even in these cases, the chemical pathogenesis is a mystery. Nearly 20 years ago, Russian workers claimed to have transmitted ALS from humans to Rhesus monkeys, but their work has been discredited. Discussion of the possible role of poliomyelitis virus in the causation of ALS has recently been rekindled by the report of Pertschuk et al,[21] who found evidence of poliomyelitis and measles antigen in jejunal biopsies of several ALS patients. Their work still awaits independent confirmation. Johnson[13] has recently reviewed evidence of the viral pathogenesis of ALS. There is preliminary evidence that certain of the HLA alleles may be related to the oc- curence of ALS, but researchers using different human populations are in disagreement about which alleles are significant.

Because we still have no cause, ALS is still classified as a "degenerative" disease. We shall see in a later chapter that the term "degenrative" is merely a mask for current ignorance (pp. 251); when future research reveals a chemical, toxic, or infectious patho- genesis, the term "degenerative" will be discarded in favor of a more accurate designation.

History and Physical Examination

Amyotrophic lateral sclerosis usually develops after age 35 and before age 70, with an average age of onset of about 60. It is a relentlessly progressive disease of lower motor neurons in the brain- stem and spinal cord and of "upper motor neurons" in the brain. Patients with amyotrophic lateral sclerosis develop disseminated weakness, wasting of muscle mass, and fasciculations from their an- terior horn cell disease, coupled with varying degrees of spasticity because of the progressive upper motor neuron deterioration. It is vitally important to remember that ALS patients *uniformly* have *normal* sensory examinations.

There are three clinical forms of ALS syndrome: 1) *Amyotrophic lateral sclerosis* itself is the most malignant of the three and consists of combined upper and lower motor neuron signs. Such patients usually die within three years of the onset of their dis- ease. 2) A diagnosis of *progressive muscular atrophy* is given to pa- tients whose disease clinically appears to be limited to the anterior horn cells. These patients may have a very prolonged clinical course of 10-15 years before death. Most of them eventually develop signs of spasticity before they die. 3) If no fasciculations or focal weakness are found and there is only asymmetrical spastic quadri- paresis without other specific cause, a diagnosis of *primary lateral sclerosis syndrome* may be entertained. The reader can understand that this is a much more treacherous diagnosis, since many diseases of the brain and spinal cord may produce progressive spasticity. However, there are patients who die with the syndrome of progres- sive spastic quadriparesis whose CNS shows the pathological changes of ALS syndrome with least emphasis on the anterior horn cells.

Although ALS is a chronic progressive disease with an insidious onset, patients with ALS may occasionally give a history that suggests a sudden onset. One farmer said his disease had begun last Tuesday morning. That was the day he could no longer lift his milk pail to carry it to the milk house. A lady with autosomal dominant ALS made her own diagnosis at a card party when she suddenly recognized that she could no longer hold her bridge hand. She looked, saw the atrophy, and knew. In both cases, atrophy was prominent in affected muscles, eloquent evidence of the chronic nature of the affliction.

Amyotrophic lateral sclerosis usually begins in a single muscle group such as hands, bulbar muscles (tongue and pharynx), or feet and legs. By the time a patient finally sees his doctor, there is evidence of wide dissemination over the body, but throughout the patient's remaining life, ALS maintains its regional preferences and even attacks certain muscle nuclei in a single limb more severely than others. The clinician who maintains a mental picture of his patient's illness may therefore develop an image of diffuse disease, mottled by patches of more severely affected motor nuclei. For instance, the left side may have more spasticity and more wasting and atrophy than the right, but the right biceps muscle is much more affected than the left, and grip on the left may be severely damaged far more than other general functions on that side. This "mottled" distribution of ALS may help to distinguish patients with this disease from those with cervical spondylosis because in spondylosis, neuron pools from one side of a given segment are affected to about the same degree.

Sometimes it is difficult to document spasticity in an ALS patient because weakness and areflexia caused by lower motor neuron diseases hide this sign. If hyperreflexia and spasticity are prominent early features, they may subside as the patient becomes more and more weakened, wasted, and areflexic.

Differential Diagnosis

One *hallmark* of ALS is the complete absence of sensory abnormalities. When a clinician thinks he has made a diagnosis of ALS, he should double check the sensory examination because other treatable diseases may mimic the spasticity and lower motor neuron signs, but if the patient also has damaged sensory pathways, they can be unmasked, investigated, and identified.

The distinction between cervical spondylosis and ALS may be especially difficult. Bony bars over the intervertebral spaces may project backwards, compressing the spinal cord against the fibrous ligaments of the posterior spinal canal, or the spur may embarrass the blood supply to the spinal cord in such a way that segmental anterior horn cells are damaged, begin to fire spontaneously, and produce fasciculations. As these anterior horn cells die, there is progressive focal weakness and wasting. This process is not always accompanied by radicular pain and limitation of neck motion. Most older people have evidence of cervical spondylosis on their neck x-rays, so plain spine films are not of great diagnostic assistance, and even the presence of a complete spinal block during myelography does not rule out the possibility of amyotrophic lateral sclerosis. In such a case, the clinical examination may disclose wasting and fasciculations of the tongue, even before there is dysarthria and dysphagia. Or there may be early wasting and fasciculations in the lower extremities. Electromyography can show that the fasciculations come from abnormal motor units and document the widespread nature of ALS if it is present. In patients who have only cervical spondylosis, motor units in the lower extremities are normal, and there is no disease in the tongue. Many patients with cervical spondylosis have a loss of position sense in the lower extremities or focal loss of light touch, pin, or position sense in the hands. This, too, helps to establish the diagnosis of cervical spondylosis with spinal cord compression.

Other diseases that occasionally mimic ALS are spinal cord tumors, syringomyelia, neurosyphilis, multiple sclerosis (primary lateral sclerosis syndrome), and progressive neuropathies. Their resemblance to ALS is usually only superficial, and the alert examiner immediately discovers physical evidence that rules out ALS and allows a specific and accurate diagnosis to be made.

Among the diseases that mimic ALS, foramen magnum meningioma is the most formidable because it is difficult to establish a diagnosis in this region of the neuraxis, and because symptoms of this tumor may exactly mimic bulbar amyotrophic lateral sclerosis. The patient with either ALS or foramen magnum meningioma develops dysarthria, asymmetrical fasciculations of the tongue, dysphagia, nasal speech, and quadriparesis in the limbs. If the patient with menigioma is lucky, he also has obvious sensory loss, which alerts the clinician to the presence of his curable lesion, but sensory loss does not universally occur in this condition.

The patient who ostensibly has bulbar ALS *must* have complete myelography to demonstrate unequivocally that the structures around 360° of the foramen magnum are normal. If the radiologist uses iodinated oil myelography, the procedure must be performed in the prone and supine positions, and the contrast agent must be carried into the posterior cranial fossa. This situation is a prime indication for the use of the new water-soluble contrast agent, metrizamide (Amipaque), especially in conjunction with the CT scanner, because this combination can demonstrate the area of cervical spinal cord, foramen magnum and posterior cranial fossa with unsurpassed clarity.

Without detailed investigation of the region indicated, the clinician cannot confidently tell his patient that there is no available treatment for his fatal disease. Usually, such investigation is indicated even for the patient with widely disseminated signs of ALS, because the procedure is usually safe, and the possible benefits, even though they are unusual, are immense.

Amytrophic lateral sclerosis syndrome may occasionally represent a remote effect of carcinoma, so some clinicians recommend a full cancer workup during the initial hospitalization, in addition to complete myelography.

Clinicians frequently mistake the wasting and weight loss of actual ALS for the systemic wasting of cancer. Remember that patients who complain of weight loss need to be examined for fasciculations, weakness, and spasticity *before* the chest x-ray and the entire metastatic cancer evaluation is performed. If fasciculations are infrequent, the clinician may have to examine single muscles for several minutes each to discover them. Once they are found, the electromyographer can determine whether they represent abnormal motor units and whether the abnormality is disseminated. If not, there is still time to order the x-ray studies, and cancer becomes a more likely diagnosis because ALS has been ruled out as a cause for the weight loss.

Management

The death of spinal cord and brain neurons cannot be delayed by treatment, but disability caused by shrinking numbers of active motor units may be delayed by physical therapy and exercise. Patients with gradually progressive ALS find that regular programs of muscle-strengthening exercises allow them actually to improve muscle power and to increase their stamina over long periods of time. Indeed, during middle stages of ALS, there are many months of apparent plateaued decline, the result of axons sprouting from still normal motor neurons and re-innervating orphaned muscle fibers, thereby maintaining contractility of the muscles themselves.

Patients should be advised to ignore muscles that already are nearly paralyzed and to concentrate on strengthening the muscles used in walking, lifting, and gripping. The exercise program should begin immediately and should continue for the rest of the illness. The goal is not to prolong life, but rather to delay disability as long as possible. Goldblatt has written a sensitive article about the treatment of ALS patients.[9] In the article, he discusses the failure of various medicinal treatments and the unscrupulous perpetration of ineffective treatments upon ALS patients. Goldblatt stresses practice with enunciation and speech training as well as physical fitness, and emphasizes the need of ALS patients and their families for psychological support as they observe the progress of the disease together and prepare for total disability and death. If patient, family, and physician cooperate to delay further disability as long as the patient is willing to fight, recognizing that there is still no cure and no magic, the impact of this terrible disease can be mitigated. A competent professional person can be an important support to a family's morale by his presence, by his accurate assessment of progress as it occurs, and by giving specific suggestions that help to combat disability.

An Aside on Quackery

In the neurological community, patients with ALS and MS are targets for the quack who offers them useless treatments for a high price. Most of these treatments are not especially dangerous, and families can sometimes afford the several thousand dollars they waste, but they cannot afford to waste their limited time together as a family and they especially cannot afford to waste their limited store of emotional strength and hope on a practitioner who is out to make his buck at their expense. Patients usually know it when they go to a quack, but they have decided they want to try it anyway. Friends send them articles from newspapers, and they wonder whether the treatment might really be the final breakthrough. Quackery has at least four major characteristics that may be recognized by physician and patient as they talk together about whether the patient will decide to go for treatment.

1) Quackery offers dramatic relief from chronic, disabling, frequently fatal diseases for which there is no effective medical therapy.

2) The treatment may be based on a shred of legitimate medical information, but there is no legitimate evidence that it is effective in the treatment of the disease. The announcement of this new therapy appears in the lay press before it does in the medical literature.

3) The quack is willing to treat without first establishing a diagnosis. Several of my MS and ALS patients went to an acupuncture clinic, where, as part of their initial evaluation, they were asked "What is your diagnosis?" They were then given a "complete physical examination" that included neither a neurological history nor neurological examination, nor a perusal of my chart, and they were treated with acupuncture for the disease I had diagnosed. It is patent quackery to claim to treat the pathogenic processes of ALS or MS in the central nervous system by sticking needles into a patient's earlobe, but to do this without first establishing that the diagnosis is correct simply compounds the offense.

4) The quack makes no effort to gather accurate data about the results of his new treatment. Instead, when confronted with the question by patients or by governmental agencies, he produces testimonials by patients whose diagnoses were not established in the first place. Even after money and time have been wasted by legitimate researchers to disprove his claims, the quack persists in his treatment and, in fact, continues his advertisements.

When your patient goes to a quack, do not dismiss him. Educate him beforehand about the characteristics of quackery, tell him it is all right to leave the quack if he decides to, and when he comes home, continue to care for him because he will need your help even more when this last hope has been dashed.

DISORDERS OF PERIPHERAL NERVES

Introduction

Symptomatology of peripheral nerve disease ranges from the simple localized numbness in, for example, a cut finger after nerve twigs are damaged, to total body paralysis and sensory loss during an attack of acute polyradiculitis. Systemic illnesses may produce peripheral nerve symptoms by direct immunological attack on nerve myelin protein, by altered metabolism of Schwann cells, by disease of the vasa nervorum, and by other unknown means. Metabolic disorders, like uremia and vitamin deficiencies, and infectious invasion of peripheral nerve structures, like herpes zoster and leprosy, also produce symptoms of peripheral nerve dysfunction. The number and kinds of peripheral nerve syndromes are bewildering, and there is treatment for only a few of the common neuropathies seen in this country.

There are two major categories of peripheral nerve disease that allow the clinician to begin to make his differential diagnosis. The first of these are the *generalized polyradiculoneuropathies*, including acute and chronic Guillain-Barré syndrome, chronic peripheral neuropathy and carcinomatous neuromyopathy. The second group consists of *mononeuritis syndromes* or *mononeuritis multiplex*. These include Bell's palsy (possibly), compression neuropathies, and peripheral nerve syndromes caused by some systemic diseases. These two categories do not distinguish absolutely between various illnesses as we shall see later, but the distinction allows the clinician to begin his differential diagnosis in a straightforward anatomical manner.

GENERALIZED POLYRADICULONEUROPATHIES

Acute Polyradiculitis (Guillain-Barré Syndrome)

Authors have had divergent views of acute polyradiculitis because of controversy that arose when Guillain, Barré, and Strohl described an ostensibly new disease in 1916. They clearly distinguished this syndrome from the one described by Landry more than 50 years previously because some of Landry's cases died and none of theirs did, and their cases developed paralysis more slowly than Landry's. Additionally, they were then in possession of the lumbar puncture, and they had discovered elevated CSF protein without an elevation of CSF cell count, something Landry could not have done, because the procedure of lumbar puncture had not then been developed. These turned out to be trivial distinctions without a difference, so Landry's paralysis and the syndrome of Guillain, Barré, and Strohl are now recognized as one disease.

Most patients with acute polyradiculitis give a history of previous infection, vaccination, or trauma during the past month, but this is not universal. Most patients with this syndrome develop progressive paralysis and sensory loss for an average of ten days to two weeks, but some progress rapidly to maximum paralysis in only a few days, while others have continuingly progressive disease for months and blend into a second syndrome of chronic relapsing polyradiculitis. If lumbar puncture is performed during the initial diagnostic workup, the protein may be normal, but during weeks 2-5 of the illness, it is almost universally elevated. Usually, there are no cells in the spinal fluid even though the protein is elevated. This discrepancy was important to early workers because it helped them to distinguish acute polyradiculitis from poliomyelitis and bacterial infections of the nervous system. Another helpful diagnostic characteristic of polyradiculitis is that paralysis is usually fairly symmetrical. Clinicians used this characteristic to distinguish polyradiculitis from the asymmetrical paralysis characteristically found in poliomyelitis. Usually, patients with acute polyradiculitis show no signs of current infection at the outset of their disease, but fever and leukocytosis have been reported, as has lymphocytic pleocytosis in the spinal fluid.

Radicular pains are a fairly constant complaint among acute polyradiculitis patients. These may begin before there is any paralysis or sensory loss. They are aching pains, not aggravated by any particular activity. Even gentle palpation of weakened muscles is painful. Pain continues throughout the disease and may, at times, be very severe. It is important to tell patients early that this will be a painful illness, although usually the pains are not unbearable, simply very annoying.

Pathogenesis

Despite discrepancies in the rapidity of evolution and in the specific clinical symptoms among different patients with acute polyradiculitis, there is a unifying pathology, first well described in 1949 by Haymaker and Kernohan in their classic paper.[10] The reader who is interested in a review of the historical controversy surrounding this disease is referred especially to that article.

More recently, Asbury et al[3] reviewed cases of acute polyradiculitis from the Massachusetts General Hospital and concluded that perivenular monocytic inflammation represents the initial pathologic anatomy. In older lesions, they found evidence of proliferating Schwann cells attempting to repair the damage, and they found secondary effects of damaged axons in the forms of Wallerian degeneration and demyelination of central nervous system tracts whose axons ascend directly from peripheral nerve cells. Asbury's case 19 is especially important, because this patient died of an unrelated disease 19 years after complete clinical recovery from an attack of acute polyradiculitis. He *still* had perivenular round cell infiltration in his peripheral nerves, indicating the constant activity of this syndrome despite clinical evidence that weakness and sensory loss had disappeared. Currently, it is felt that Guillain-Barré syndrome results from a direct immunological attack on the myelin protein of peripheral nerves, related perhaps to a misdirected immune response to previous infection.

Diagnosis

The clinician cannot easily detect perivenular monocytic inflammation, so he must make his diagnosis on clinical, not pathological, grounds. Characteristic neurologic syndromes recur and allow an accurate diagnosis to be made even though there are no pathognomonic physical findings. The most consistent of these is facial diplegia.

Unlike unilateral facial paralysis, bilateral facial weakness is not disfiguring and is discoverable only if the clinician really *looks* for it. Facial diplegia is so characteristic of acute polyradiculitis that it may occur with almost no other findings except some radicular pain or a decreased reflex. It is common for patients with acute polyradiculitis to have mild-to-moderate paralysis of arms and legs and total facial diplegia. In fact, acute facial diplegia without *any* other physical evidence for disseminated radicular disease probably represents acute polyradiculitis whose manifestations in the body are slight enough that they are not evident to the clinician. Exceptions to this rule are meningeal sarcoid, chronic meningitis, bilateral acoustic neuroma, or meningeal carcinomatosis, and each of these should be diagnosed by the distinctive history available in each case.

The diagnosis of facial diplegia is easy once the clinician suspects its presence. Ask the patient to close his eyes *tightly*. When normal people do this, they bury their eyelashes almost completely in their periorbital tissues. If there is facial weakness, the lashes are visible, or the eyes may not even close at all. If the eyes do close, attempt to open them by pulling upward on the upper lid with your thumb. Under normal conditions, it is impossible to open tightly shut eyes without a major effort on the part of the examiner. In patients with facial weakness, the lid is easily opened, exposing the globe. The reader should try these maneuvers on normal people in order to have experience with the normal range of eyelid strength, because this test establishes unilateral facial weakness in Bell's palsy, bilateral facial weakness in acute polyradiculitis, myasthenia gravis, and facial forms of muscular dystrophy. It is a beginning point for important diagnostic examinations throughout the rest of the body.

Other tests of peripheral facial weakness are less satisfactory because they do not have distinct end points. Ask the patient to look up and observe whether his forehead creases normally. Ask the patient to grimace and evaluate the effort needed to push his lips together. Ask the patient to wiggle his nostrils or to tense his platysma muscle. It is important to record these responses as part of the examination in order to determine whether there is improvement or deterioration at a subsequent examination, but these tests of facial strength are not as accurate as eyelid closure.

We have already mentioned that radicular pain and muscle tenderness are important diagnostic signs for acute polyradiculitis. These are present in nearly every patient with the disease and are demonstrated by squeezing muscles already affected by weakness.

Autonomic dysfunction is also evident in many patients with acute polyradiculitis. Tachycardia is frequent. Bladder involvement may result in urinary retention, and constipation is common.

Patients with facial diplegia, radicular and muscle pain, tachycardia, and definite signs of peripheral nerve involvement such as flaccid weakness, generalized areflexia, sensory loss, all developing over a period of days, are obvious candidates for a diagnosis of acute polyradiculitis. If the clinician then performs a lumbar puncture and finds elevation of CSF protein with few or no cells in the spinal fluid, his diagnosis is established.

Management

Because acute polyradiculitis may progress to total paralysis of the muscles of respiration and of swallowing, these two concerns are of primary importance to clinician and patient once the diagnosis is made. Patients do not die of this disease if respiratory paralysis is managed well and if they are not allowed to aspirate food into the lungs. All other considerations are of secondary importance until breathing and swallowing are under control.

When the patient is admitted to the hospital, the inhalation therapist should be in immediate attendance to establish a total forced vital capacity. The responsible clinicians, nurses, *and the patient* should all *know* what the vital capacity is, and this test must be repeated every few hours to determine whether the vital capacity is decreasing, and how fast weakness is progressing. It is important that patient and family understand the reasons for professional concern and that they know that endotracheal intubation or tracheotomy can easily be performed and can be life-saving. The patient must understand that the vital capacity values are of such overriding importance to him that he will be awakened at night and must give his best performance even though he is sleepy; hospital personnel should be reminded that the value is inaccurate in patients with facial diplegia unless special care is taken to prevent leaks around paralyzed lips. Far from provoking unnecessary anxiety, this kind of directed concern is comforting to the patient, because he knows that his needs will be met and that he is being actively protected from his disease.

The only immutable rule about tracheotomy or endotracheal intubation in acute polyradiculitis is that it should be done *before* it becomes an emergency. A good rule is that initial intubation should be strongly considered if the total vital capacity drops below 50 percent of the expected. If this occurs slowly during the first week of hospitalization, the clinician may continue extremely watchful waiting. If it occurs during a six-hour period, it should be performed immediately. Once the course of the disease is established, tracheotomy should be considered if it appears that respiratory paralysis will persist longer than 2 weeks.

Blood gases may be monitored. The new patient should have blood gases drawn before there is any respiratory insufficiency in order to determine what is normal for him. But a decision for tracheotomy or intubation should not wait until blood gases are already altered by his respiratory insufficiency. He could be dead before the results return from the laboratory. Intubation is so easy, so life-saving, and so commonly required that there is no reason to wait for terminal respiratory failure to proceed.

Dysphagia is a different problem, but its effects are related to the problems of respiratory paralysis. The patient whose total vital capacity is moderately diminished by weakness may choke to death suddenly if he aspirates food from a paralyzed pharynx and cannot cough normally. He can best monitor his own capacity to swallow and should be asked repeatedly to determine whether his swallowing is normal. If it becomes weakened, he must alert the staff immediately. Depending on the course of weakness elsewhere in the body, the physician may choose several days of intravenous feedings, the use of a nasogastric tube, or he may decide to go directly to endotracheal intubation or tracheotomy. Patients with nasogastric tube feedings are much safer with an inflated endotracheal cuff in place to prevent aspiration of stomach contents after feedings.

Once decisions have been made about life and death aspects of the initial management, other issues become important in their turn. If patients with acute polyradiculitis do not die of complications, they can expect to recover completely. This means that permanent joint contractures, bladder contractures and fibrosis, or bedsores, are intolerable and must be prevented at all cost. Pneumonia is a danger; malnutrition a possibility. Anxiety and panic are undesirable and unnecessary when the patient has severe generalized weakness.

Patients with acute polyradiculitis are fully awake and cognizant of their surroundings. They appreciate specific information about their progress. They need to know that special treatments may occur for the prevention of pneumonia, contractures, and so forth. Even children are able to tolerate painful physical therapy if they know it is being done as gently as possible, but thoroughly to insure them that they will be normal adults in a few years instead of permanent cripples because of joint contractures.

Specific Issues Need Attention

Physical Therapy: There is a myth among neurologists that patients with acute polyradiculitis should not be allowed too much activity until recovery is far advanced because they might have a relapse. Certainly no patient has ever had a relapse until he *has* begun to recover, but there is no controlled experiment that has tested the myth, and none will ever be done. Accordingly, the standard recommendation for these patients is that active physical therapy awaits excellent return of strength, and even *then* the staff will tend to hold them back.

Even during the acute hospitalization, *passive* physical therapy is important to prevent contractures. All joints should be manipulated through their full range of motion at least twice each day, including weekends. Foot rests are placed to prevent contractured drop feet, and hand rolls hold fingers and thumbs in apposition. Passive PT is frequently painful, and patients may need analgesics like acetaminophen or even codeine before range of motion treatments. Hot packs over painful joints may be applied 30 minutes before the therapist arrives, or passive range exercises may be performed in a Hubbard tank, even for patients with severe paralysis, providing there are enough personnel available to watch the respirator, the patient, and the joints.

The physician must be kind, but resolute, in his prescription of passive range of motion. Because it is painful, family members usually request periodically that it be modified or stopped. But the long-range goal of normal joint function must supersede the short-range goal of comfort! Usually, patients and families can understand this, but the principle needs to be reiterated during the illness.

Nursing care: Regular turning is the best prevention for decubitus ulcers and pneumonia. The Circle Electric Bed is especially well designed for caring for acute polyradiculitis patients, because they may be turned head down in the prone position to allow tracheal secretions to drain out in great quantities. Antiembolism stockings are a routine part of the care of any bedridden patient, and low-dose heparin treatment may prevent thrombophlebitis.

Psychological management: Accurate daily information about the progress of the disease is important, beginning on the day of admission. Television, radio, and talking books (p. 295) are available, and may even be used in an intensive care unit if the patient has earphones. Family visits are important, and family members may learn to provide some of the patient's care. A "talking board" with letters of the alphabet may be made. These allow him to spell out words and phrases. Even severely paralyzed patients can work out signals that allow them to communicate by using the talking board.

Bladder and bowel management: Chronic bladder flaccidity leads to poor bladder function later unless it is cared for properly. Catheter drainage may result in a scarred, contracted bladder, so patients with acute polyradiculitis recover best if the nursing staff learns the Credé maneuver to empty the bladder. This is facilitated in patients with this disease because the abdominal wall is also flaccid. The operator simply finds the dome of the bladder and massages it with increasing firmness, pushing the bladder down into the pelvis. Once urine starts to flow, pressure is continued until all the urine has been expelled. This maneuver is repeated every several hours, night and day. If a catheter is used, *tidal drainage* is vitally important.

Severely paralyzed patients may need regular enemas or manual disimpaction if other methods do not keep the bowels soft and regular. Nurses and patient should work together to establish a bowel regimen that works for him. Prune juice is still surprisingly effective in this day of chemical laxatives!

Steroids and ACTH: We do not have adequate information about the place of steroids or ACTH in the treatment of acute polyradiculitis. Certainly the literature does not support a claim for dramatic results from their use. Some studies have found a statistical difference in favor of steroids, others have not. One recent prospective double-blind evaluation of the use of ACTH came to the unlikely conclusion that treatment during the first 10 days of hospitalization reduced the time from onset to complete recovery without affecting the severity of paralysis during the acute phase of the disease or the duration of hospitalization.[23] Steroids are certainly of trifling importance when compared to proper care of respiration, swallowing, nursing care, physical therapy, bowel and bladder control, and the prevention of pneumonia.

From this discussion, it is evident that polyradiculitis is not a routine disease to be treated at home or even on the regular hospital ward. These patients should be referred for neurological care when the diagnosis is made, and the neurologist should plan to have a team of consultants to help with tracheotomy, management of the respirator, inhalation therapy, and treatment of infectious complications; and he must have a trained and competent nursing and physical therapy staff to manage the patient and his paraphernalia 24 hours a day.

Chronic Polyradiculitis

Asbury et al[3] and others have described patients with typical acute polyradiculitis who died years later with pathological evidence of continuing immunologic attack on peripheral nerve tissue despite complete clinical recovery. Presumably, the process of repair is adequate in most cases to mask the continuing immunological damage. However, in some cases this does not happen and symptoms continue to fluctuate for many months or years. Some of these cases actually represent the neuropathy of lupus erythematosus or porphyria. Others seem to represent a chronic form of idiopathic acute polyradiculitis syndrome, and some of these cases respond well to prednisone therapy. Such patients should be referred to a neurologist for care, preferably to one with special interest in peripheral nerve diseases.

Peripheral Neuropathy

Figure 6-2 shows the distribution of peripheral neuropathy, beginning in a stocking distribution on the feet. Peripheral neuropathy affects the most distal portions of nerves, and since feet are the farthest part of the body from the central nervous system, they are invariably affected first. If neuropathy becomes so severe that it extends above the knees, then the hands also begin to develop sensory loss in a "nylon stocking and glove distribution."

Hysterical numbness may affect hands and feet, but in this case, the numbness is usually a "bobby sox and gloves" distribution, uncharacteristic of any organic disease of peripheral nerves.

In this country, diabetes mellitus and alcoholism are the most common discoverable causes of peripheral neuropathy. Leprosy is the most common cause in some parts of the world, but American physicians are unlikely to have occasion to diagnose this disease.

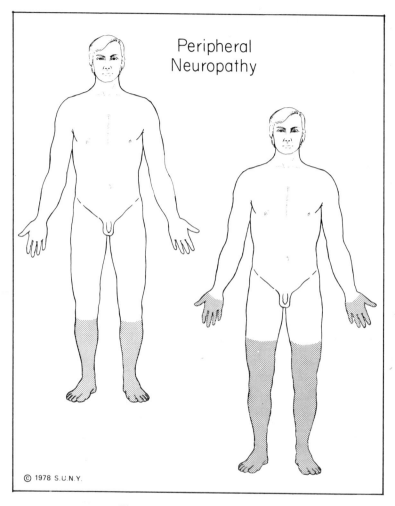

© 1978 S.U.N.Y.

Figure 6-2. *Peripheral neuropathy.*

Malnutrition occasionally causes neuropathy, especially thiamine or pyridoxine deficiency. Pernicious anemia is regularly associated with typical peripheral neuropathy as well as spinal cord degeneration. Industrial toxins have been implicated in the pathogenesis of peripheral neuropathies, but it is difficult to establish in any particular case that a specific toxin caused the trouble.

Some unusual neuropathies are heritable. The patient may have a family history of relatives with an abnormal gait. Usually, this is caused by Charcot-Marie-Tooth disease, but there are other less common heritable neuropathies.

The specific causes of neuropathy listed above account for most of the patients who eventually receive a specific diagnosis. The rest are left with no discoverable cause and no treatment. Occasionally, patients with neuropathy of many kinds develop severe burning pains in the extremities. These may be treated with phenytoin or even with carbamazepine to reduce the pain, even if this treatment does not stop the neuropathic process.

Carcinomatous Neuromyopathy and the Remote Effects of Cancer on the Nervous System

Even though a cancer is undetectable by careful radiographic and physical evaluation, and has not yet produced detectable metastases, it can nonetheless cause neurological dysfunction at all levels of the nervous system. The most common of these is carcinomatous neuromyopathy, but other remote effects of cancer include polymyositis-dermatomyositis (especially in older men), myasthenic syndrome (pp. 129-130), ALS syndrome, necrotizing myelopathy, Purkinje cell degeneration in the cerebellum, and encephalomyelitis syndromes in brain and brainstem. Because some cancers occur in association with immune deficiency states, they allow the direct invasion of the brain by organisms that are otherwise nonpathogenic. Herpes zoster and progressive multifocal leukoencephalopathy (pp. 123, 258-259) are two of these.

Therefore, patients who develop unexplained neurological syndromes may be candidates for evaluation directed to the discovery of a hidden cancer. Carcinoma of the lung is the most common cause of neuromyopathy, followed closely by breast cancer and various cancers of the gastrointestinal system.

RESTRICTED MONONEURITIDES

While the generalized polyradiculoneuropathies affect the peripheral nervous system diffusely, the mononeuritides are focal or multifocal manifestations of disease. They produce weakness and sensory loss in the specific distribution of affected nerves, and for this reason they are often more difficult for the non-neurological clinician to diagnose. The Medical Research Council's handbook is of special help in the diagnosis of these conditions.[19]

Bell's Palsy (Acute Peripheral Facial Paralysis)

Bell's palsy is a unilateral peripheral facial paralysis. Usually, the paralysis is preceded by pain in the ear or face, followed hours or a day later by weakness of the muscles of facial expression: the orbicularis oculi, the elevators of the forehead, the smile, the platysma. More than 90 percent of patients with Bell's palsy completely recover normal facial function. The remaining 10 percent have some residual synkinesis between smile and blink, or smile and tears, and some with residual paralysis or contracture. Even most of this 10 percent are not disfigured by their residua.

There has been little agreement about the pathogenesis of idiopathic Bell's palsy. In Wynn Parry's 25-year experience with acute peripheral facial paralysis,[25] 6 percent were caused by geniculate herpes zoster. These would be missed if the clinician did not search for herpetic vesicles in the external ear canal, where the facial nerve has its sole representation on the skin. Occasionally, a facial neuroma, acute mastoiditis, or some other disease in the skull causes the syndrome, but this leaves the majority of patients without a pathogenetic explanation.

One explanation has related Bell's palsy to an infectious process. Leibowitz[15] showed that Bell's palsy occurs in epidemics. Djupesland, et al[7] demonstrated, by careful sensory and electrical testing, that Bell's palsy is the most obvious manifestation of a more generalized cranial neuritis. Among 16 patients with Bell's palsy, they found only two who had no other cranial nerve involved. One patient had involvement of five cranial nerves. Additionally, there was evidence of acute or recent viral infection in many cases, although the authors were unable to isolate virus from any of their cases. Abramsky et al[1] found that lymphocytes from patients with both Bell's palsy and acute polyradiculitis were sensitized to peripheral nerve myelin basic protein P_1L, while lymphocytes from patients with several other diseases causing facial weakness were not.

During our discussion of acute polyradiculitis, we stated that patients with *bilateral* peripheral facial paralysis were probably only cases of acute polyradiculitis with restricted distribution. Now we find increasing evidence to link even *unilateral* peripheral facial neuritis with acute polyradiculitis. Unfortunately, Djupesland et al did not examine peripheral nerves of the rest of the body as well as the cranial nerves. If they had, they might have settled this important question.

The relationship of Bell's palsy to acute polyradiculitis and the frequency of facial paralysis during the usual course of acute polyradiculitis still fails to explain why the facial nerve is so sensitive to the inflammatory process. Perhaps the explanation has to do with the long course of the facial nerve within the bony facial canal, where only minimal edema or vasodilatation due to inflammation could produce a compression neuropathy. If this were the case, then surgical decompression of the facial canal might prevent those few cases of residual facial asymmetry that occur following Bell's palsy. This supposition has also sparked controversy.

The problem is that there is no way to distinguish the 2-5 percent of patients who will have disfiguring residual paralysis and synkinesis from the 90-95 percent of those who will recover completely. At one time, facial EMG and electrogustometry promised to establish the necessary distinction. Indeed, these examinations do distinguish among patients with partial or complete denervation.[14] All patients with partial or no denervation eventually return to completely normal facial function, but even patients with complete denervation have an excellent prognosis, because 73 percent of Langworth and Taverner's patients who had total denervation of the nerve were satisfied with the results of their eventual recovery.

Which patients require surgery? Those with complete denervation who will not recover completely. How can we identify them? We must wait until the nerve is completely denervated. But over half of these patients are satisfied with their recovery anyway, so is it justified to operate on the rest? Worse yet, once the nerve is completely denervated, is not the damage already done? In this case, perhaps surgery comes too late to help even those who might have had a bad result, and surgery adds to the expense of hospitalization, and the possible surgical complications of deafness and infection to the bad residual effects of Bell's palsy itself. The clinician whose patient has Bell's palsy might consider these problems and help his patient to avoid a surgical procedure unless better methods become available that can establish a poor prognosis early in the disease.

Steroid treatment also has a vogue. In theory, treatment with prednisone or ACTH would also reduce edema and inflammatory response in the facial canal. There are two prospective controlled studies that address this question. May et al[18] found no benefit from a 10-day high-dose tapered regimen of prednisone given immediately after diagnosis. Wolf et al[24] used a similar tapered-dosage regimen for 17 days. Their results indicate a possible decrease of crocodile tears (autonomic synkinesis) but no statistically significant difference in residual facial weakness.

Patients who develop an acute peripheral facial palsy *do* require consideration of the specific causes of their syndrome. If there are indications for special studies of the bony skull and mastoid region, these should be performed. Look into the ear canal to diagnose herpes zoster of the facial nerve. If the case appears to be an idiopathic Bell's palsy, the patient may be told that he has over a 90 percent chance of complete recovery, and most of the remaining 10 percent have no serious residua. There is no effective treatment, so clinician and patient simply must wait out the results. This is not a fatal disease. Under these circumstances, there is even question whether the slight risk of complications from a 10-day course of prednisone is warranted, and certainly, at the current state of the art, we have no means to identify in advance those patients who could really benefit from surgery.

Acute Brachial Neuritis

The patient with acute brachial neuritis develops unexplained severe pain in the shoulder, followed one or several days later by sensory loss and weakness in the upper extremity. Once paralysis appears, its distribution may be localized to one or more of the portions of the brachial plexus. There are no adequate studies addressing the treatment of this condition, but prednisone is usually prescribed in the hope that it might be of value. While recovery is usually incomplete, there is usually adequate return of function following the acute paralysis for the patient to return to normal living.

Compression Neuropathies

Carpal Tunnel Syndrome
Surprisingly, although median nerve paralysis was recognized in

the last century, its frequency was not appreciated, and surgical treatment did not become common until 1950. However, since that time there has been a steadily increasing stream of patients whose symptomatic compression of the median nerve as it passes through the carpal tunnel in the wrist is dramatically improved following surgical section of the transverse carpal ligament.

The symptoms are variable and frequently occur in both hands. The patient usually complains of numbness and weakness in the hands, and frequently there is pain in the wrist. But the pain may be centered more proximally. Patients frequently waken at night with pain in the forearm or arm and find they can relieve it by shaking their hand or sleeping with the hand draped over the edge of the bed. Occasionally, the sole complaint of pain may be in the neck, with numbness and weakness in the thumb and first two fingers, exactly mimicking the complaints of a soft cervical disc protrusion. In young people, a disc protrusion is usually not accompanied by abnormalities in the plain cervical spine films, and the diagnosis of carpal tunnel syndrome may not be made until cervical myelography reveals normal subarachnoid structures and the doctor reconsiders his original diagnosis.

In early cases, the examination may appear completely normal. Sensory loss is confined to the palmar surface of the thumb and first fingers and does not extend proximally from the wrist. If sensory loss is severe, the radial side of the ring finger may be less sensitive than the ulnar side. Weakness is best discovered in the opponens pollicis muscle, and atrophy appears in the thenar eminence. Other muscles innervated by the median nerve in the hand may also be weak.

The condition is being diagnosed earlier now, because physicians are aware of its frequency. Even if the patient has no physical findings, early compression of the median nerve may be detected by demonstration of prolonged latency during nerve conduction velocity measurements. Under these circumstances, surgery may be of immediate benefit.

Tardy Ulnar Palsy

As the ulnar nerve courses through the ulnar groove on the medial side of the elbow, it is exposed to repeated trauma, as everyone knows who has "struck his crazy bone." If the ulnar groove is anatomically shallower than normal, the situation is aggravated. People whose occupation requires prolonged sitting at a desk or table, and people who sit with constantly bent elbows may traumatize the nerve enough so that it becomes thickened, and nerve conduction velocity across the elbow is slowed. Palpation of the nerve in the ulnar groove may disclose its enlargement by comparison with the opposite side. The damage results in sensory loss over the little finger and half the ring finger but *only up to the wrist.* There is weakness of the opponens of the little finger, the abductor of the little finger, the interossei and the last two lumbricals.

Surgical or medicinal treatment is unsatisfactory, but patients can learn to live in such a way that they stop damaging their ulnar nerve. They may strap soft sponges to the elbow or perform some other maneuver that heightens their consciousness of that part of the anatomy, and then concentrate on living with elbows straight and without pressure on the ulnar groove. This usually allows a progressive diminution of symptoms over a period of months.

Acute Radial Nerve Paralysis

Entrapment neuropathies are more likely to occur in patients who have systemic diseases that tend to damage peripheral nerve tissues. In these conditions, pressure or repeated trauma that would be insignificant in normal people produces symptoms of focal nerve disease. Diabetes mellitus and alcoholism are the most common systemic illnesses that cause focal neuropathic symptoms as part of a generalized peripheral neuropathy.

Radial nerve palsy is a prime example of this, because it is nicknamed "Saturday night paralysis." The alcoholic whose nerves are already damaged comes home drunk, sleeps on his arm without moving, or falls asleep with his arm draped over the back of a chair. In the morning, his radial nerve has had hours of pressure ischemia and refuses to function. Normal people waken at night with momentary radial nerve palsy, but it disappears in a few moments when they turn over and sleep in a different position. Because of its great frequency under normal circumstances it is actually surprising that permanent paralysis is not more common.

Sensory loss is not as well defined in radial nerve palsy as in median and ulnar nerve paralysis, but the distribution of weakness is pathognomonic. Usually triceps strength is intact. The brachioradialis is paralyzed, and this produces an apparent weakness of the biceps muscle, confusing many examiners. Remember that brachioradialis and biceps act together to flex the elbow, so weakness of the brachioradialis causes weakness of elbow flexion even with normal biceps power. As the patient pulls, the examiner need only palpate the brachioradialis on the affected side to convince himself that it is paralyzed. Other paralyzed muscles include the supinator, wrist and finger extensors, and the extensors of the thumb.

Patients with radial nerve palsy should be questioned about exposure to lead, especially if the condition is bilateral. Under normal circumstances, recovery occurs in the next several months, and a cock-up wrist splint should be prescribed, which is available from the occupational therapy or orthotics service.

Other Compression Neuropathies

1) Peroneal palsy occurs when the common peroneal nerve is compressed as it courses over the head of the fibula. This is sometimes a complication of childbirth, of sitting with legs crossed, and of acute trauma. There is weakness of the anterior tibial, extensor hallucis longus, and peroneal muscles, producing a dropped foot and the danger of sprained ankle because the paralyzed peronei do not support it on the lateral side.

2) Meralgia paresthetica occurs if one of the femoral cutaneous nerves is compressed as it passes through the fascia lata on its way to the skin, or if it is compressed by a girdle or by carrying heavy boxes braced over it. There is nasty, irritative numbness in the distribution of the nerve, but no weakness because these are solely cutaneous nerves. Symptoms may recur throughout life. If they are extremely annoying, the patient may elect to have surgical enlargement of the fascial foramen.

3) Compression of individual roots at the level of the spinal neural foramen that may be related to herniated nucleus pulposas, tumors of bone or nerve, spondylosis, and many other processes also represent compression neuropathies. Diagnosis in each case depends upon an accurate clinical determination of the root that is involved, and radiographic proof of the offending lesion. Treatment depends upon the specific pathological process.

Mononeuritis Multiplex

Suddenly, with or without pain, conduction along a nerve trunk is interrupted at a specific site along its course. Later the same thing happens elsewhere in an asymmetrical repetitive pattern of multifocal disease. As one nerve regenerates, another is attacked. The physical findings depend upon which nerves are affected. This is mononeuritis multiplex, and it is caused by diabetes mellitus, polyarteritis nodosa and other connective tissue diseases, certain blood dyscrasias, sickle cell anemia, and other less common illnesses. Mononeuritis multiplex is not a common syndrome, but it is so distinctive that it cannot be misdiagnosed. Diabetic femoral neuropathy is one of the most common forms of mononeuritis multiplex. There is pain in the anterior thigh, followed hours or a few days later by paralysis of the whole anterior compartment of the thigh innervated by the femoral nerve. Recovery is very incomplete, and the incident may be repeated on the other side.

The cause of mononeuritis multiplex is probably related to disease of the tiny vasa nervorum. When they become occluded, the resultant "ischemic stroke" in the nerve produces mononeuritis. If the process is repeated in different nerves of the body, the result is mononeuritis multiplex.

Herpes Zoster

Herpesvirus lives with us during our lifetime after we have had the chickenpox. Usually, it appears to be a passive recipient of hospitality, but occasionally it may produce herpes zoster, "shingles." About six percent of acute peripheral facial paralyses are caused by herpes zoster. Zoster may occur in the distribution of any other nerve root as well.

The attack is heralded by a peculiar burning sensation that may begin near the dorsal root ganglion, posteriorly, and "grow" forward along the dermatome during several days. If there is a prominent skin eruption which displays the characteristic *grouped vescicles on an erythematous base*, the diagnosis is simple, but frequently there is only a slight rash that may be missed unless it is sought at the right time. The pain itself is characteristic enough to make the diagnosis because of its gradual spreading character, its intermittency during the day, and its strict limitation to one or several nerve root distributions. The skin over these distributions is tender to light touch, and there may be some loss of sensation in the affected area.

Older patients may develop permanent, postherpetic neuralgia of disabling severity. This may be relieved with phenytoin (Dilantin®) or with carbamazepine (Tegretol®) in most cases. In severe cases, a 10-day to 2-week course of chlorprothixene (Taractan®) therapy, 50 mg every six hours, may provide permanent relief, even after treatment is stopped.* If medicinal therapy does not stop the pain, the nerve root may be injected or sectioned, but this produces permanent sensory loss that may be almost as uncomfortable as the pain.

DISEASES OF THE MYONEURAL JUNCTION

Myasthenia Gravis

Introduction

The onset of myasthenia gravis is usually insidious. There is intermittent slurred speech or ptosis. Diplopia may occur occasionally during the day. Complaints of "fatigue" are common. The diagnosis may easily be missed at this stage. Every neurologist can recall his failures of diagnosis, and he is *certain* to recount his diagnostic triumphs.

For instance, a 20-year-old girl was about to be married when her smile changed. Her mother thought she looked unhappy. Apart from noting the unhappy smile, my examination was completely normal, and the family was greatly relieved that she was merely nervous about her wedding. The next week, when she was swimming with her fiancé, she nearly drowned because of the rapid development of generalized myasthenic weakness. She had to be pulled from the water! Of course, her "unhappy smile" had been the transverse smile of facial muscle weakness, which occurs primarily in myasthenia and the muscular dystrophies.

On the other hand, a colleague had followed a young man for several years because of intermittent diplopia. The symptom was always the same, and each time the patient came to see him the examination was completely normal. My colleague proposed the possible diagnosis of a small arteriovenous malformation in the midbrain. I happened to see the patient when he displayed weakness of multiple extraocular muscles in both eyes, normal pupillary responses, and an otherwise normal neurological examination. Tensilon "cured" him on the spot!

*Farber, G.A., Burks, J.W.: Chlorprothixene therapy for herpes zoster neuralgia. South. Med. J. 67:808-812, 1974.

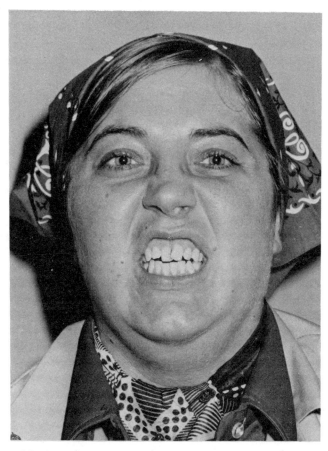

Figure 6-3. *Myasthenic patient smiling pleasantly at the photographer. The transverse smile is characteristic of facial muscular weakness in myasthenia and facial myopathies.*

Paralysis of jaw muscles is a common problem in myasthenia and may be the first complaint. I believe this is a pathognomonic sign for myasthenia gravis because no other disease, not even muscular dystrophy or amyotrophic lateral sclerosis, weakens the masseters, temporalis, and medial pterygoid muscles to the extent that they cannot even hold up the jaw against gravity. The complaint usually centers around trouble chewing and slurred speech, but as he

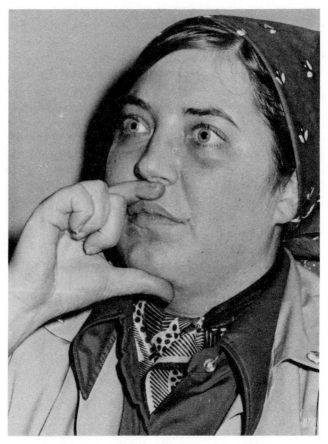

Figure 6-4. *Myasthenic patient with facial and jaw weakness. She props her lower jaw up and her upper lip down so she can speak clearly.*

gives his history, the patient with severe jaw weakness sits with his jaw propped up in his hand. Examination usually reveals generalized myasthenic weakness in the body and in muscles innervated by other cranial nerves.

In order always to make an accurate diagnosis when a patient complains of early symptoms of myasthenia, the clinician must keep in mind that strange symptoms, especially those that involve cranial nerve musculature, may be caused by this disease. Do not diagnosis myasthenia in every nervous person who complains of weakness. But if a person is concerned about his weakness, do not send him away as "nervous" without a Tensilon® test! Be aware that you will receive letters from colleagues, recounting their subsequent diagnostic successes among patients you have missed, and be charitable when you are able to return the favor!

Early Symptoms and Examination

Intermittent ptosis, double vision, slurred speech, slack jaw, trouble swallowing, transverse smile, and complaints of general "tiredness" are common early complaints. The tired myasthenic may lie down, but he is not sleepy. He simply has "no energy" to perform his work or to climb stairs. Workmen drop boards they are carrying and have trouble climbing onto the truck; housewives cannot carry the laundry from the basement; but still they all usually complain of "fatigue" not weakness.

Evaluation of muscle power is the most subjective part of the neurological examination. Each clinician must examine many people in order to establish for himself how strong normal people are by comparison to his own strength, depending upon their age and physical build. Otherwise, he will never be able to detect mild weakness and may even miss profound weakness when he does the examination.

The hallmark of myasthenia gravis consists of muscular weakness that improves with edrophonium chloride (Tensilon®) or pyridostigmine (Mestinon®). Most myasthenics display abnormal fatigability of muscles, and this is also a major diagnostic characteristic of the disease. The goal of the examination is to identify weakness in specific muscles and to demonstrate whether the strength of those muscles improves after intravenous edrophonium.

Begin with an examination of the lids and extraocular muscles. If there is diplopia, which of the 12 extraocular muscles are at fault? Is extraocular muscle weakness bilateral? Is pupillary activity truly normal? Unless the pupils are *completely normal*, the diplopia is probably *not* caused by myasthenia gravis because myasthenia affects *only* skeletal muscles.

Normally, the upper lid covers sclera above the cornea and part of the iris, but it does not cover any part of the pupil. As the myasthenic patient looks up, the lid may retract normally, but if he is held in upward gaze, the lid may begin to droop. When it droops to the edge of the pupil, it has become pathological. During this time, the examiner may assess how difficult it is for the patient to maintain upward gaze and whether rapid up and down eye movements at this time cause him increased weakness of the lid and the extraocular muscles.

Myasthenic diplopia may mimic central nervous system disease. Internuclear ophthalmoplegia (p. 88 ff.) also leaves the pupil intact and so may diabetic oculomotor nerve paralysis; and both cause diplopia. When myasthenia gravis causes the identical form of muscular weakness, the diagnosis may be established by a Tensilon® test, which is strongly indicated in all cases of diplopia unless there is definite evidence for another pathological process.

We have already discussed the procedure for testing facial weakness (p. 109). Bite strength may not be tested in patients with dentures, but patients who still have their own teeth can bite down on a tongue blade so hard that it cannot be pulled from the mouth, and the stick is destroyed as they bite down on it. In myasthenia, the tongue blade may be easily removed despite the patient's best effort. In myasthenia, the blade may only be dented by the teeth whereas normal people produce a splintered relic.

Body muscles are weaker proximally than distally in myasthenia and in the myopathies. Do not forget to examine neck flexors and extensors and muscles that flex and extend the back. In normal people, the biceps muscles are stronger than triceps. If the situation is reversed, the clinician may diagnose biceps weakness. Asymmetry of muscle power is important unless the patient is a tennis enthusiast, or has a profession that requires him to use one arm more than the other. In most cases, muscle power should be about the same on both sides. Clinicians must examine normals repeatedly in order to examine myasthenia patients adequately.

All diseases of the motor unit cause weakness, but only myasthenia gravis and the myasthenic syndrome (pp. 129-130) cause weakness that responds to edrophonium chloride. If the muscle examination discloses distinctly weakened muscles, a Tensilon® test may be used for diagnosis. Usually the examiner picks a series of five or six weakened muscles that can be examined rapidly and accurately. Then 1 cc (10 mg) of edrophonium is drawn into a syringe, and the needle is inserted into an antecubital vein. It is critically important to document that the needle is well into the vein, because even in myasthenia gravis there is no response to subcutaneous edrophonium. Two milligrams of edrophonium are injected initially, and the clinician waits at least 45 seconds to determine that the patient does not develop unusually severe muscarinic side effects, like abdominal cramps, nausea, salivation, vomiting. This almost never happens, but if it does, the test is terminated. If necessary, it may be repeated later with a prior dose of atropine.

After the 45-second waiting period, another 8 mg are injected, and the needle is removed. Within 30 seconds after the second injection, most patients develop muscarinic side effects. Tears come to the eyes. There is increased salivation and abdominal cramps begin. At this time, the clinician begins repeated examinations of his series of distinctly weakened muscles. The edrophonium effect reaches its peak in about two minutes, and effect may last in diminished degree for many hours.

If the edrophonium response is equivocal, the patient may be sent for electrical investigation of his myoneural junctions in the EMG laboratory, or he may be given a trial of pyridostigmine therapy. Frequently, when therapeutic doses of pyridostigmine are prescribed, the myasthenic whose response to edrophonium was equivocal develops increased muscle strength during the first several days of treatment.

Diagnostic Evaluation

Myasthenia gravis occurs in association with thymoma, hyperthyroidism, and connective tissue diseases like systemic lupus erythematosus. These associated conditions must be sought and ruled out before a diagnosis of idiopathic myastenia gravis is made. There are also families with hereditary myasthenia. Pregnancy may be the cause of first myasthenic symptoms, and the baby may have neonatal myasthenia for several months after delivery.

The myasthenic syndrome may mimic myasthenia gravis. This condition usually accompanies oat cell carcinoma of the lung, but it may occur in conjunction with other malignancies and even in otherwise apparently normal people.

The myasthenic syndrome causes weakness in extremities and trunk, more prominently than in cranial nerve musculature. The response to edrophonium is less dramatic than the usual myasthenic patient's response. Electromyography may disclose a neuromuscular block characterized by defective initial release of acetylcholine from the *pre*synaptic membrane. While the two myasthenias blend with each other in some cases, the electrical distinction is usually diagnostic.

Management

The management of myasthenia gravis is rewarding because there is nearly always something the clinician can recommend to make things better, even if it is only to stop medicinal treatment, perform a tracheotomy, and prescribe an intensive care unit and respirator for a period of time.

Education is the *key* to the management of myasthenia patients and every patient with a chronic disabling disease. The myasthenic who understands his disease, the proper use of his medications, and the workings of an intensive care unit can help immeasureably with his own management. Such a patient knows how to determine his "best dose," of pyridostigmine, and if the disease changes, he can change his dose effortlessly. Educated patients know when they are beginning to get into trouble, and they call for help before they have an emergency. Educated myasthenic patients can help to educate new myasthenics even better than their physicians can, and they can help each other to manage problems of chronic weakness as they arise.

There are three standard forms of treatment for myasthenia: 1) anticholinesterase medications, of which pyridostigmine (Mestinon®) is the most satisfactory; 2) prednisone and ACTH; and 3) thymectomy. Plasmapheresis is a fourth new treatment for severe myasthenic patients. This technique is not universally available, and its long-term effectiveness is unproven, although early reports suggest that plasma exchange may provide prolonged remission of symptoms, even among severely incapacitated patients.

Cholinesterase Inhibitors

Because it has fewer muscarinic side effects, and a somewhat smoother action than neostigmine, pyridostigmine (Mestinon®) is the cholinesterase inhibitor of choice. This medication binds cholinesterase, the enzyme that inactivates acetylcholine. Thus, pyridostigmine therapy provides more effective muscle contraction by prolonging the action of acetylcholine molecules at the myoneural junction. The effect of a single dose of pyridostigmine peaks at about two hours and lasts from three to six hours.

Once the diagnosis is established, the patient must learn how pyridostigmine affects *him*. This is best accomplished by giving an initial single dose of one tablet. The patient is instructed to observe his muscular strength and to note when strength begins to wane. The single dose may be repeated again six to eight hours later so that the patient develops a clear notion of its effects.

On the following day, the patient is instructed to wait until the effect of the first dose definitely begins to wear off and then to take a second tablet in an attempt to maintain more even control over the weakness. Since this procedure is usually carried out in the hospital, the physician's orders should specify that dosage timing is the patient's responsibility and cannot wait for the routine medication distributions. Over a period of days, the dosage interval may be established, and thereafter the interval doses may be increased ¼-½ tablet each time until there is no further increase in strength. Most patients need a dosage interval of 3-4 hours, and few benefit by more than three tablets at each dose.

During this educational period, the patient must learn about the side effects of pyridostigmine, because an overdose may cause extremely dangerous weakness that must be distinguished from myasthenic weakness or the patient may inadvertently paralyze himself, with fatal consequences. The most important characteristic of the weakness produced by pyridostigmine toxicity is that it usually appears within two hours after the most recent dose. If the patient limits his dosage interval to a period of three hours or longer, and if he is certain each time he takes pyridostigmine that the previous dose is beginning to wear off, he is unlikely to get into trouble. Also, it is definitely to his advantage to begin each day with mild, but definite myasthenic weakness. Most patients with mild or moderate myasthenia can do this by taking their last dose before they retire and abstaining from medication during the night.

Fasciculations in skeletal muscle are a major symptom of toxicity from pyridostigmine. Occasionally, it is possible to increase the patient's dose in the hospital to the point of fasciculations and mild weakness. If this is accomplished, he will never forget the sensation and the appearance of the fasciculations.

Muscarinic side effects of pyridostigmine affect smooth muscle and glands. Salivation, sweating, stomach cramps, diarrhea, nausea, and vomiting may be used by some patients as a sign of overdose if their muscarinic and nicotinic side effects happen to coincide. However, many myasthenic patients develop diarrhea before they have reached their optimal dose for skeletal muscle strength, and these patients find relief from cramps and diarrhea by the use of atropine tablets, 0.4-0.8 mg as needed.

Mestinon is available as doubly scored 60 mg tablets which may be broken accurately into halves or quarters. Scored Mestinon Timespan tablets, 180 mg, are also available. These produce a prolonged effect for about 10-12 hours. The use of Timespan tablets should be limited to a nighttime dose in patients who are so weak in the morning that they are in danger of suffocating or are unable to swallow a morning tablet without nighttime coverage. The Mestinon Timespan tablets should never be used as a daytime medication because the dosage cadence cannot be accurately controlled.

The goal of pyridostigmine therapy is admittedly optimistic: that the patient have completely normal muscle strength during each day. This is usually not possible for extraocular muscles because even the slightest dysfunction produces diplopia. The goal is frequently not even attainable with large skeletal muscle function, so when the goal is not approximated, additional treatment should be considered.

Prednisone - ACTH

Many myastheniologists prefer to institute prednisone therapy before thymectomy, especially in severely disabled myasthenic patients.[12,16,17] Daily or alternate-day high-dose prednisone therapy results in clinical remission of myasthenia in over 70 percent of patients. The remission reaches a peak in about three to five months after treatment begins; thereafter, the dose may be reduced drastically in some patients, and they are able to maintain a permanent remission. Some patients display an initial and temporary aggravation of myasthenic weakness, even with the use of prednisone on alternate-day schedules. They should be warned of this in advance so they may be prepared to come to the hospital temporarily for care during this period, if necessary.

If prednisone dosage can be reduced to very low levels, even chronic use is not hazardous, but patients who require chronic high-dose prednisone therapy to prevent generalized weakness or disabling diplopia should not be continued indefinitely on this regimen because of the serious side effects from this medication. These patients are clearly candidates of thymectomy.

The use of a short course of high-dose ACTH gel was popularized by Osserman. Patients whose myasthenia is worsening despite all available therapy frequently benefit from hospitalization in an intensive care unit, withdrawal of all anticholinesterase medication, tracheotomy or endotracheal intubation, and respirator care. Further improvement may be expected after a 10-day course of 100 units of ACTH gel, IM each day during that period. Several days after the last dose, anticholinesterase medications are reinstituted, and many patients are able to leave the intensive care unit greatly improved.

Thymectomy

There is general agreement that the thymus plays an important role in the etiology of myasthenia, and that thymectomy produces dramatic remission of myasthenic symptoms in some cases. At one time, it was thought that the best candidate for thymectomy was a young woman with no thymoma, whose generalized myasthenia gravis began less than two years before operation. Men, older people, patients with thymoma, and patients with long-standing myasthenia were less desirable candidates. More recently, several groups have advocated thymectomy for nearly all myasthenics, and they present evidence that all may have an equal chance for remission after surgery.[5,20]

When thymectomy was first performed for myasthenia gravis, it was done as a last resort for the treatment of severely ill patients. In those days, respirators were unsophisticated machines. Intensive care units did not function as they do now, and many of these patients died because their poor physical status compounded the usual complications of surgery. Initially, thymectomies were performed through a sternal splitting operation that further aggravated a patient's respiratory problems. Under those circumstances, it is surprising that thymectomy could gain any favor at all! More recently, a suprasternal approach has been devised. This does not involve major intervention in the chest and is almost without morbidity. This approach gained great favor until the revelation that thymus tissue may be scattered throughout the mediastinum. The surgeon may inadvertently miss unattached pieces of thymus because of poor visibility from the suprasternal approach, thus negating the results of his surgery.

Currently, thymectomy is recommended early in the treatment of myasthenia. If a patient is disabled on his best dose of pyridostigmine, or needs more than a minimal dose of prednisone for chronic maintenance, thymectomy is recommended immediately before the patient becomes seriously ill. There is a strong movement toward a return to sternal splitting operations because the surgeon can be more certain that he has removed the entire thymus. Most modern surgical candidates are in excellent physical condition, and postoperative care is greatly improved so the morbidity of even the more extensive surgery is minimized.[11]

"Never give up" is a central rule in the management of myasthenia. Thymectomized patients, especially those with many germinal centers in the thymus, may have to wait several years before their remission occurs. Even seriously ill myasthenic patients may recover strength in time. If prednisone does not help, perhaps a course of ACTH will. Given time and patience, things will usually get better. Myasthenia is a completely different disease from ALS or MS in this regard.

Pathogenesis

We have known for many years that the myoneural junction is the culprit in myasthenia, but for some time after the discovery that miniature endplate potentials in myasthenic muscles were abnormally small, the defect was thought to be inadequate packaging of acetylcholine in the *pre*-synaptic vescicles. In recent years, there is increasing evidence that myasthenia gravis is an autoimmune disease caused by an immune response to acetylcholine receptor protein in the motor end plate on the *post*-synaptic side of the junction. Recently, Andrew Engel et al[8] have demonstrated for the first time the presence of antireceptor protein IgG and components of complement on the motor endplate of myasthenic muscle. They postulate that worsening myasthenia results from the direct effects of the immune complexes on muscle endplate. The use of antithymocyte globulin, plasmapheresis, and immunosuppressive drug therapy in myasthenia result directly from these and other considerations of the immunological pathogenesis of the disease.[4,6,22] The reader may profit from further reading in a recent symposium on myasthenia gravis.[2] (See addendum, p 140.)

DISEASES OF MUSCLE

Introduction

One of the most exciting fields of research during the past 20 years relates to the ultrastructure and physiology of muscle. In the late 1950s we were still interested in the fact that actin and myosin reacted *in vitro* in the presence of ATP and magnesium ions. Currently, even high-school classes may be exposed to the detailed normal chemical anatomy of striated muscle and the chemical and anatomical processes of excitation-contraction coupling.

As the details of muscle anatomy and physiology became known, researchers also discovered new diseases related specifically to portions of that ultramicroscopic anatomy. Nemaline myopathy represents an aberrant growth of the Z-disc. Mitochondrial myopathies represent various malformations of that organelle. Central core disease results either from defective maturation of muscle or perhaps from defective innervation, but its electronmicroscopic pathology is highly specific. Various kinds of periodic paralysis had been recognized for many years and the relation of paralysis to serum potassium was known. But as the understanding of the function of muscle endoplasmic reticulum matured, it became obvious that the vacuolar change in this disease represents swollen endoplasmic reticulum, malfunctioning because of specific chemical abnormalities; and the paralysis occurred because under normal conditions, the endoplasmic reticulum is responsible for transmitting muscle cell membrane excitability into the depths of each muscle fiber. In periodic paralysis, it does not do this.

The literature concerning these developments is too voluminous to detail here, and the diseases are unusual enough that the clinician not specifically interested in muscle disease need only know of their existence. The reader who wishes to follow this literature should begin reading articles published between 1965 and 1970. He should look for the names of G.M. Shy, L.P. Rowland, A.G. Engel, and W.K. Engel. If he begins there, he will develop an understanding of basic muscle structure. Then he can pursue the literature forward and follow the developments that have occurred since that time.

We shall confine ourselves to the more common muscle diseases. These may be divided into two major categories: the hereditary muscular dystrophies and the acquired myopathies.

Hereditary Muscular Dystrophies

The various muscular dystrophies are inherited diseases, transmitted by autosomal recessive, autosomal dominant, and sex-linked genes. They may be classified into four major categories: 1) sex-linked muscular dystrophy (Duchenne's); 2) limb-girdle and facio-scapulo-humeral muscular dystrophy; 3) ocular and oculopharyngeal dystrophy; and 4) myotonic dystrophy.

Sex-Linked Muscular Dystrophy

Duchenne's muscular dystrophy is confined to boys because of its sex-linked nature. This is the most common form of muscular dystrophy and the most malignant. The child usually demonstrates weakness by the age of five and frequently much earlier. Physical examination characteristically discloses apparently hypertrophied calf muscles despite severe weakness. As the disease progresses, this pseudohypertrophy is replaced by gradually progressive atrophy. These boys usually do not survive past the age of 20. There is an unusual, but milder form of sex-linked muscular dystrophy with a life expectancy up to age 50, but these patients have prolonged severe disability.

The diagnosis of Duchenne's muscular dystrophy is usually straightforward. There is a family history of muscular dystrophy among the mother's male siblings and among cousins of affected children, offspring of the mother's sisters. Serum enzyme determinations reveal astronomical levels of skeletal muscle creatinine phosphokinase (CPK). Carrier females may be identified by modest elevations of CPK, so genetic counseling is available for the sisters of affected boys.

Limb-Girdle and Facio-Scapulo-Humeral Muscular Dystrophy

These are restricted muscular dystrophies limited either to proximal muscles of the trunk and extremities or to these areas and skeletal muscle of head and neck. The restricted muscular dystrophies are usually mild by comparison with Duchenne's muscular dystrophy, although they may cause severe chronic disability during a nearly normal life span. In some families, there is a strong autosomal dominant heredity. Other cases are apparently sporadic, probably representing an autosomal recessive characteristic.

The diagnosis is usually made in the twenties to thirties by complaints of muscular weakness. Weakness is confined to the proximal muscles, and close examination may reveal congenital absence of muscles of trunk or upper extremities. Serum CPK is usually elevated but may be nearly normal if the condition is only very slowly progressive.

Ocular and Oculopharyngeal Muscular Dystrophy

The extremely localized form of dystrophy causes progressive external ophthalmoplegia. It has been discussed briefly under the myopathic disease of eye muscles (p. 93). Some patients with progressive ocular muscular dystrophy also develop nasal speech and dysphagia due to progressive weakness of pharyngeal muscles. Ptosis is the most disturbing complaint and may be treated with upper lid crutches attached to the glasses or by surgery to shorten the upper lids.

Myotonic Muscular Dystrophy

This form of muscular dystrophy has attracted the most attention because myotonia and muscular weakness appear to be only two manifestations of a generalized metabolic defect affecting cells throughout the body. This is a multiorgan disease that produces early baldness, cataracts, testicular atrophy and mildly decreased fertility, dementia and cerebral atrophy, defects of intracardiac conduction with abnormal EKG and potentially fatal arrhythmias. Myotonic dystrophy is transmitted as an autosomal dominant trait. The expressivity is extremely variable. One member of the family may demonstrate dementia and cataracts only, with few distinctive dystrophic features, while another displays the entire syndrome.

The diagnosis is usually made at the bedside because of the characteristic facies, with high forehead due to frontal balding and atrophy of temporalis muscles, and a transverse smile; family pictures, if available, may demonstrate similar traits in close relatives. The muscle examination discloses characteristic percussion myotonia or effort myotonia. When the thenar eminence or other muscles of the body, including the tongue, are percussed lightly with the reflex hammer, there is prolonged contraction of the muscle, which only gradually subsides. Similarly, patients with this disease have difficulty opening their eyes after forcibly closing them, and they have trouble opening a tightly closed fist. During EMG, the characteristic "dive-bomber sound" of myotonia appears as the needle is inserted into resting muscle or is moved about within the muscle.

There is no treatment for any of the muscular dystrophies. Patients with severe myotonia may find some relief from quinine or quinidine preparations. The Muscular Dystrophy Association provides some financial help for diagnostic workup and provides wheelchair and other necessary appliances for dystrophic patients. For this reason, patients with muscular dystrophy of all kinds should be referred to the Muscular Dystrophy Association so they may receive these needed benefits free of charge.

Acquired Myopathies

– Dermatomyositis and polymyositis are the most important of the acquired inflammatory myopathies. Dermatomyositis is one of the connective tissue diseases related to scleroderma and systemic lupus erythematosus. Weakness and muscle tenderness appear rapidly or in subacute fashion and are accompanied by at least a fleeting rash. At times, the rash may be very prominent, but in other cases there may be so little rash that it is missed unless the clinician examines his patient carefully on several different occasions.

Polymyositis may actually represent the same disease in which the rash was never seen. However, polymyositis is also associated with numerous primary diseases. This is especially true of occult or already diagnosed cancer in elderly men. The diagnosis of polymyositis and dermatomyositis may be very difficult if muscle enzyme levels in the serum are not elevated and if the muscle biopsy fails to reveal typical inflammatory lesions. Patients with rapidly progressing weakness, and muscle tenderness, with or without a rash, are candidates for the diagnosis and should be referred to a clinician with special interest in muscle diseases, if possible. The weakness of polymyositis frequently responds to treatment with prednisone.

REFERENCES

1. Abramsky, O., Teitelbaum, C.W.D., Arnon, R.: Cellular Immune Response to Peripheral Nerve Basic Protein in Idiopathic Facial Par-

alysis (Bell's Palsy). J. Neurol. Sci. 26:13–20, 1975.

2. Ann. N.Y. Acad. Sci. Vol. 274, 1976.
3. Asbury, A.K., Arnason, B.G., Adams, R.D.: The Inflammatory Lesion in Idiopathic Polyneuritis. Its Role in Pathogenesis. Medicine 48:173–215, 1969.
4. Barnes, A.D.: The Use of Antithymocyte Globulin in Myasthenia Gravis. Postgrad. Med. J. 52 (Suppl. 5):110,111, 1976.
5. Buckingham, J.M., Howard, F.M., Jr., Bernatz, P.E., Payne, W.S., Harrison, E.G., Jr., O'Brien, P.C., Weiland, L.H.: The Value of Thymectomy in Myasthenia Gravis: A Computor-Assisted Matched Study. Ann. Surg. 184:453–457, 1976.
6. Dau, P.C., Lindstrom, J.M., Cassel, C.K., Denys, E.H., Shev, E.E., Spitler, L.E.: Plasmapheresis and Immunosuppressive Drug Therapy in Myasthenia Gravis. New Engl. J. Med. 297:1134–1140, 1977.
7. Djupesland, G., Degre, M., Stien, R., Skrede, S.: Acute Peripheral Facial Palsy. Part of Cranial Neuropathy? Arch. Otolaryngol. 103:641–644, 1977.
8. Engel, A.G., Lambert, E.H., Howard, F.M.: Immune Complexes (IgG and C3) at the Motor End-plate in Myasthenia Gravis. Ultrastructural and Light Microscopic Localization and Electrophysiologic Correlations. Mayo Clin. Proc. 52:267–280, 1977.
9. Goldblatt, D.: Treatment of Amyotrophic Lateral Sclerosis. Adv. Neurol. 17:265–283, 1977.
10. Haymaker, W., Kernohan, J.W.: The Landry-Guillain-Barré Syndrome. A Clinicopathologic Report of Fifty Fatal Cases and a Critique of the Literature. Medicine 28:59–141, 1949.
11. Jaretzki, A. III, Bethea, M., Wolff, M., Olarte, M.R., Lovelace, R.E., Penn, A.S., Rowland, L.: A Rational Approach to Total Thymectomy in the Treatment of Myasthenia Gravis. Ann. Thorac. Surg. 24:120–128, 1977.
12. Johns, T.R.: Treatment of Myasthenia Gravis: Long-Term Administration of Corticosteroids with Remarks on Thymectomy. Adv. Neurol. 17:99–122, 1977.
13. Johnson, T.R.: Virological Studies of Amyotropic Lateral Sclerosis: An Overview. In: *Amyotrophic Lateral Sclerosis. Recent Research Trends.* Andrews, J.M., Johnson, R.T., Brazier, M.A.B., (Eds.) Academic Press, New York, 1976, pp. 173–180.
14. Langworth, E.P., Taverner, D.: The prognosis of Facial Palsy. Brain 86:465–480, 1963.
15. Leibowitz, U.: Epidemic Incidence of Bell's Palsy. Brain 92:109–114, 1969.
16. Mann, J.D., Johns, T.R., Campa, J.F.: Long-Term Administration of Corticosteroids in Myasthenia Gravis. Neurology 26:729–740, 1976.

140 / PRACTICAL CLINICAL NEUROLOGY

17. Mann, J.D., Johns, T.R., Campa, J.F., Muller, W.H.: Long-Term Prednisone Followed by Thymectomy in Myasthenia Gravis. Ann. N.Y. Acad. Sci. 274:608–622, 1976.
18. May, M., Wette, R., Hardin, W.B., Sullivan, J.: The Use of Steroids in Bell's Palsy: A Prospective Controlled Study. Laryngoscope 86:1111–1122, 1976.
19. Medical Research Council War Memorandum No. 45. *Aids to the Investigation of Peripheral Nerve Injuries.* Her Majesty's Stationery Office, London 1943 (Reprinted 1976) Available at Medical Book-stores. (Price about $3.00)
20. Papatestas, A.E., Genkins, G., Horowitz, S.H., Kornfeld, P.: Thymectomy in Myasthenia Gravis: Pathologic, Clinical, and Electrophysiologic Correlations. Ann. N.Y. Acad. Sci. 274:555–573, 1976.
21. Pertschuk, L.P., Cook, A.W., Gupta, J.K., Broome, J.D., Vuletin, J.C., Kim, D.S., Brigati, D.J., Rainford, E.A., Nidsgorski, F.: Jejunal Immunopathology in Amyotrophic Lateral Sclerosis and Multiple Sclerosis. Identification of Viral Antigens by Immunofluorescence. Lancet I:1119–1125, 1977.
22. Pirofsky, B., Reid, R.H., Bardana, E.J., Baker, R.L.: Antithymoctye Antiserum Therapy in Myasthenia Gravis. Postgrad. Med. J. 52 (Suppl. 5): 112–116, 1976.
23. Swick, H.M., McQuillen, M.P.: The Use of Steroids in the Treatment of Idiopathic Polyneuritis. Neurology 26:205–212, 1976.
24. Wolf, S.M., Wagner, J.H., Jr., Davidson, S., Forsyth, A.: Treatment of Bell Palsy with Prednisone: A Prospective Randomized Study. Neurology 28:158–161, 1978.
25. Wynn Parry, C.B., King, P.F.: Results of Treatment in Peripheral Facial Paralysis. J. Laryngol. and Otol. 91:551–564, 1977.

ADDENDUM

While this book was in preparation for press, an important volume on myasthenia gravis recently came into print:

Dau, P.C. (Ed.): *Plasmapheresis and the Immunobiology of Myasthenia Gravis.* Houghton Mifflin, Boston, 1979.

The serious student should first refer to this text before proceeding with the other references in this chapter.

CHAPTER 7

The Movement Disorders

INTRODUCTION

Parkinsonism is the most frequently disabling of the movement disorders. Huntington's chorea is discussed among the untreatable adult dementias (pp. 212), but chorea and athetosis are also symptoms of other conditions which do respond to treatment. Dystonic postures and movements are a common part of the symptomatology of many diseases of the basal ganglia. Generalized dystonia musculorum deformans is rare, and the clinician may never see a case, but limited dystonia, in the form of spasmodic torticollis, blepharospasm, or dystonic writer's cramp, is not rare and is frequently thought by physicians to be of hysterical origin. This belief is no longer tenable. Hemiballism and Wilson's disease are rare, but because they are treatable, it is important to recognize them when they do appear. Most of the movement disorders begin insidiously, and because of this, they are frequently misdiagnosed in their early stages. However, each has a distinctive clinical history, symptomatology, or laboratory abnormalities. They share the presence of abnormal movements and postures at rest and during activity.

PARKINSON'S DISEASE

The three cardinal symptoms of Parkinsonism are tremor, rigidity, and hypokinesia. These may develop alone or in any combination, but as the disease progresses, all three are usually present, at least in some degree.

141

Parkinsonian Tremor

Parkinsonian tremor at rest is the most easily diagnosed of the three. It disappears momentarily as the patient moves, only to return shortly after he relaxes. Mild resting tremor is easily suppressed by the patient, so the clinician may need to make his observations surreptitiously as he takes the history or otherwise engages the patient. Parkinsonian tremor is a slow tremor, about 4 Hz. In mild cases, only a finger or a thumb may be involved. If several digits are involved, they may move individually, sometimes with a rotatory motion around the axis of the digit.

Parkinsonian symptoms are always bilateral, but they usually develop asymmetrically, so the patient may complain of trouble in only one extremity. However, because it is a bilateral affliction, the clinician can usually detect bilateral signs of Parkinsonism during the first interview. This is important because patients with focal brain pathology may develop some unilateral Parkinsonian features, but the presence of strictly unilateral abnormalities during the examination helps to distinguish these patients from those with true Parkinson's disease. When bilateral tremor develops without other Parkinsonian symptoms, it also raises the questions of essential tremor (pp. 62-63).

Parkinsonian Rigidity

Even mild rigidity interferes with buttoning, tying, writing, and other finely coordinated movements. Rigidity is the underlying explanation for the Parkinson patient's imbalance and gait disturbance. It is much more disabling than tremor. Parkinson patients are not severely disabled with even moderate tremor, unless it is accompanied by rigidity.

Rigidity is most easily detected by having the patient relax an upper extremity as much as possible, while the examiner flexes and extends it at the elbow. The elbow is fixed in place with one of the examiner's hands while his other moves the arm up and down in a linear motion. If the wrist is pronated and supinated at the same time, still maintaining the linear motion at the elbow, rigidity becomes even more evident. Minimal rigidity may be augmented by asking the patient to draw a large circle in the air with the opposite upper extremity, as the examiner continues his testing. In normal subjects, there is no change in resting tone during this maneuver, but when patients with rigidity or spasticity draw the circle, their resting muscle tone on the opposite side increases dramatically.

"*Cogwheeling*" becomes apparent during this procedure if the thumb of the stabilizing hand at the elbow is placed over the biceps tendon. As the examiner extends and flexes the elbow with the other hand, his thumb feels rapid small changes in biceps tendon tone; "br-r-r-r-t!" Even if there is no spontaneous tremor at rest, cogwheeling documents its subliminal presence because the sign represents tremor hidden behind rigidity. "Cogwheel rigidity" is said to be a sign of Parkinsonism. It actually represents *two of the three* cardinal signs of the illness, but the two components are distinct and different. Cogwheeling and rigidity also occur during flexion and extension of the lower extremities at the knee or hip, but they are more difficult to elicit because of the large bulk of the lower extremity.

Parkinsonian Hypokinesia

Families occasionally bring an early Parkinson patient to the physician for symptoms which represent hypokinesia.

"Old age is creeping up on Dad during these last few months. He has slowed down a lot. It takes him forever to get shaved and dressed in the morning, and he dawdles over meals. He does not answer immediately when we speak to him, and when he does, he talks so slowly and softly that we do not hear him well. We wonder if his mind is affected. If he smiles during a conversation, the smile gets "stuck" and stays there after the laughter has died. When he does get up and go somewhere, he frequently stands for a moment before he starts to walk, and sometimes stops, and simply stands, as he is going around the corner. When we get out of the car, we have to speak to him, or he might just sit there."

Hypokinesia is exasperating to the family, but the physician may easily miss it in his office. The patient is so quiet that he becomes unnoticed as conversation flows around him. Because of his silence, he may easily be considered demented. In order not to be fooled, the clinician must become aware of movement in his office; how he and family members change their tone of voice and facial expression, how brief is a smile, how often they gesture and move in their chairs, or turn their heads as conversation moves about in the room. Then he can compare these things to similar activity in his patient. Once hypokinesia is recognized as a symptom, it becomes overwhelmingly obvious during the rest of the interview.

When the patient answers direct questions, his answers are to the point, and he is evidently not demented, but when he gets up to enter the examining room he may get "stuck" and simply stand motionless next to his chair, or in front of the examining table.

The examination itself is abnormal too. Hypokinesia is universally accompanied by at least the beginnings of rigidity, and there may also be tremor. If tremor is already present, the diagnosis is easy, but do not miss the patient whose chief symptom is hypokinesia, because this is a crippling complaint. He may respond well to treatment and postpone his eventual disability for several years.

Associated Symptoms

Other Parkinsonian symptoms relate to rigidity and hypokinesia or they may reflect dystonic characteristics of Parkinsonism.

Imbalance

Parkinsonian imbalance is dangerous, because it leads to bad falls and broken hips. The imbalance is probably caused by rigidity. Normal people constantly and rapidly correct minor imprecisions of standing posture, but the patient with rigid Parkinsonism cannot do this. Consequently, he may fall without warning while standing at the sink or walking around the house. By the time his muscles have made the small corrections necessary to adjust to the first postural inaccuracy, he is already well on his way to the floor. Unlike the spastic patient who remembers that his leg "gave way" under him, the Parkinson patient usually cannot say why he fell.

Festinate Gait

Festination is related to Parkinsonian imbalance. When he festinates, the Parkinson patient walks forward or backward, sometimes with increasing speed until he runs into a wall or falls. The physician may discover the earliest sign of approaching festination by asking the patient to stand, feet together, eyes closed. Then the examiner tries to knock him off balance with sharp, unpredictable pushes, forward or backward. Normal subjects stand firm during surprisingly sharp pushes. The trunk sways, but they recover without taking a step. Under the same circumstances, the Parkinson patient takes one or several steps backward or forward before stopping. If he is more severely affected, he may begin uncontrollable festination, and fall into the examiner's arms. Early warning of festination in the Parkinson examination is an important sign, because festination is dangerous. It may be prevented by prompt treatment, which can save the patient from a broken hip.

March à Petits Pas

Several kinds of Parkinsonian gait result in small steps. The usual rigid gait consists of short, shuffling steps. If hypokinesia is prominent, the shuffle may be interrupted by prolonged stops, as though the patient were "stuck" in place. The more dramatic *march à petits pas* is less common. It occurs when the patient begins to walk. He moves forward, not necessarily out of balance, with tiny rapid steps. If he is fortunate, these elongate in a moment into a Parkinsonian shuffle or a fairly normal gait. Some patients never escape from this form of *march à petits pas* without outside help: "Stop! – Now lift your right leg and take a big step!" This command may allow him to take the first step, and move out. One would think a Parkinson patient could learn to tell himself; "Lift your right leg," but the author has been unable to teach a patient to do this, even with help from the family. Somehow, the process of cortical learning fails to connect with this gait.

Lying Down vs. Standing Up

Parkinson patients display a dramatic disparity between fairly well-preserved ability to move about erect and vast immobility in bed. Many Parkinsonians complain they cannot turn over or even move in bed without help. Yet, once they stand up, they may walk with ease. When they start levodopa treatment, they frequently report that the first sign of improvement was a return of the ability to roll over in bed.

Blepharospasm

Blepharospasm is an involuntary closure of the eyelids, with inability to open them by the usual means. Blepharospasm is occasionally the initial complaint in an otherwise healthy person, who later develops clear symptoms of Parkinson's disease. In the author's experience, this dystonic symptom has always been misdiagnosed as hysterical, despite the absence of any prior history of nervous disposition. Parkinsonian blepharospasm has characteristic features which distinguish it from hysteria. Despite the severe disability of being essentially blind, Parkinson patients with blepharospasm frequently carry on, while hysterical patients use relatively mild symptoms to explain why they stopped various life activities. The Parkinson patient quickly learns that he can open his eyes, at least momentarily, if he pulls downward on the lower lid of one or both eyes, or does some other related maneuver. Usually the orbicularis oculi is not in spasm as it is in the normal subject who tries forcibly to close his eyes. Instead, the lids are shut, but the eyebrows are in the neutral or slightly elevated position.

Unfortunately, anti-Parkinson medications offer little help with blepharospasm. Tarsal splints, which attach to the glasses and hold the lids open mechanically, are uncomfortable and only occasionally effective.

Etiologies of Parkinsonian Syndromes

There are numerous causes for Parkinsonian syndromes. After the world pandemic of influenza in the years following 1918, there was a large outbreak of Parkinsonism, and for years thereafter, most patients who developed Parkinsonism were "postencephalitic." Parkinsonism may also develop after other forms of viral encephalitis, after carbon monoxide poisoning, and as a result of chronic manganese intoxication. Parkinsonian rigidity is extraordinarily common among patients who take phenothiazines for psychiatric disability.

Parkinson's disease, without an evident antecedent, is considered to be a "degenerative disease," which means that we do not yet know what causes it. Parkinsonism may be inherited as an autosomal recessive genetic trait, but in hereditary cases, there is a spastic component to the illness as well.

Shy-Drager Syndrome (Idiopathic Orthostatic Hypotension)

In 1960, Shy and Drager[11] reported cases of disseminated neurological disease with Parkinsonian features, orthostatic hypotension, fasciculations and wasting in muscles, loss of sweating, flaccid bladder, and atrophy of the iris. This syndrome was thought to be rare, but centers which see large numbers of Parkinson patients regularly discover cases of Shy-Drager syndrome. They are usually misdiagnosed initially because of one or another of the symptoms which may appear first.

For instance, patients with Shy-Drager syndrome may develop bladder atony early in the course of their disease. In this case, men go to urologists for a prostatectomy, while women have pelvic sling repairs from their gynecologist.

On the other hand, patients with idiopathic orthostatic hypotension may be treated initially with fludrocortisone acetate (Florinef®) for this complaint until bladder or Parkinsonian symptoms appear.

Shy-Drager patients whose first symptoms are tremor and rigidity may later develop fainting spells when they stand up. In this case, the orthostatic hypotension may initially be blamed on levodopa therapy. If a Parkinsonian patient develops flaccid bladder, orthostatic fainting, or unusual symptoms suggestive of amyotrophic lateral sclerosis, examine him for the other features of the Shy-Drager syndrome.

This is a terrible disease because the course is protracted and relentlessly progressive. Symptoms may be controlled for a time by the use of levodopa for Parkinsonian symptoms, Urecholine for the bladder paralysis, and fludrocortisone for the orthostatic hypotension, but the syndrome leads ultimately to total disability and death, unaccompanied by dementia, which might be a blessing, under the circumstances.

"Arteriosclerotic" Parkinsonism

The concept of "arteriosclerotic Parkinsonism" is similar to the concept of "arteriosclerotic dementia," an easy explanation, but inadequate as a proper diagnosis. Patients with multiple, tiny lacunar strokes due to hypertensive arteriolar disease do develop shuffling gait, flexion posture, dysarthria, and dysphagia, but they also have spasticity, pseudobulbar emotionality, and they *do not shake.* This condition is easily distinguished from classic Parkinson's disease, and the term should be abandoned in favor of an accurate one such as "lacunar state" or "multiple small strokes."

Onset and Course of Parkinsonism

We generally consider that Parkinsonism is a disease of the elderly. Unfortunately, this is not universally true. Symptoms may begin as young as the thirties. When Parkinsonism begins in early life, the clinican must be certain he is not actually seeing a case of Wilson's disease (p. 157). Serum ceruloplasmin and urine copper excretion studies can help rule out this possibility.

Parkinsonism is a relentlessly progressive disabling disease. Sometimes progression is slow, and the patient appears to be stable over many years, but in other cases progression is rapid, and the patient becomes disabled and then bedridden in a few years. Despite the advent of levodopa, Parkinson's disease remains progressive. Initial treatment with levodopa, sometimes appears miraculous and may even completely erase the symptoms for a while, but the disease continues to progress beneath the calm exterior. Symptoms will eventually return, despite continuing treatment, unless the patient dies from some other cause. It seems that levodopa gives the patient a five- or six-year handicap on his disease, but he must not count on levodopa alone to provide him with a permanent cure.

Treatment of Parkinsonism

Levodopa and Carbidopa-Levodopa Preparations

The availability of levodopa for general use in Parkinson's disease has changed the face of treatment. Medications like trihexyphenidyl (Artane®) and benztropine (Cogentin®) are nearly completely ineffective by comparison to levodopa, and should no longer be used in Parkinsonism, except for patients who cannot tolerate, or do not respond, to levodopa.

Levodopa is one of the few medications whose clinical use resulted from an understanding of the biochemistry of the brain. Biochemical analyses indicated early that there was abnormal dopamine metabolism in Parkinsonism. Shortly thereafter, studies on experimental animals revealed a dopaminergic nigrostriatal pathway. Lesions of this pathway resulted in death of neurons in the substantia nigra, marked depletion of dopamine in the striatum (caudate nucleus and putamen) on the same side of the brain and a movement disorder on the opposite side of the animal's body. Replacement therapy with levodopa relieves the movement disorder and replenishes striatal dopamine.

The effectiveness of levodopa in Parkinson's disease relies on its ability to enter the striatum and be transformed into dopamine by striatal dopa-decarboxylase. As dopamine, it activates dopamin-ergic synapses. In most cases, there is considerable relief of Parkin-sonian symptoms; occasionally complete remission is produced. Some patients do not respond to levodopa and others actually be-come worse on the medication. Recently, autopsy studies on Par-kinson brains have revealed depletion of striatal dopamine and of striatal dopa-decarboxylase.[7] It may be that the group which does not respond to this medication consists of patients who are unable to transform exogenous levodopa to dopamine. Some may actually have progressive supranuclear bulbar palsy (p. 211) that was mis-diagnosed as Parkinsonism. Increasing understanding of striatal biochemistry may provide more specific anti-Parkinson drugs.

Levodopa may be prescribed alone as 250 mg or 500 mg cap-sules or tablets. It is also available in a 1:10 ratio by weight combi-nation of carbidopa and levodopa called Sinemet®, which is available as 10/100 (carbidopa 10 mg/levodopa 100 mg) and 25/250 (carbidopa 25 mg/levodopa 250 mg) scored tablets. Carbi-dopa inhibits dopa-decarboxylase activity in non-neural tissues of the body, permitting a larger fraction of ingested levodopa to reach the brain. Sinemet causes fewer gastrointestinal side effects than levodopa alone, but as patients reach therapeutic doses of Sinemet®, dystonic side effects are more common than with levodopa. Be-cause of the presence of carbidopa, patients on Sinemet® use about 1/4 the total dose of levodopa at therapeutic dosage levels.

Strategy for Treatment with Levodopa

Strategy for the use of levodopa or Sinemet® depends first upon the fact that patients continue to experience a growing relief of symptoms as they increase their dose, but when toxic side effects ap-pear, these become more uncomfortable than the disease. There-fore, the proper dose of levodopa in either form is *just less* than the dose which causes side effects. There is no definite milligram amount. The patient must discover his "best dose" himself by in-creasing the dosage gradually to the point of first side effects, and then returning immediately to the preceding dosage level. **Note:** If levodopa is prescribed according to this schedule, 100 percent of pa-tients will have at least transient side effects!

A second part of the strategy of long-term management with levodopa derives from the fact that a patient's "best dose" may change from time to time. This is especially true during the first months of treatment, perhaps because they do not push to proper levels during the initial program or possibly because of a real change in dosage requirements. Whatever the reason, patients need to test periodically to determine that they really are on their best dose by increasing the dose one or two tablets a day. If side effects again develop, the previous dose is established as correct. On the other hand, side effects may develop on a dose previously established as correct, and patients must be prepared to decrease the dosage level accordingly.

Levodopa is prescribed initially at low dosage levels and increased gradually over a period of six to 12 weeks to toxicity. There is no need to push this medication rapidly in a disease as chronic as Parkinsonism. Indeed, it is important to *avoid* side effects at low dosage levels, because their presence may make it difficult for the patient to establish his proper dose with accuracy, and it may also make him uncomfortable about the medication altogether. Because some patients do not respond immediately to levodopa preparations, they should plan to remain on "their best dose" for several months before concluding that the medication is ineffective for them.

Prescribe plain levodopa at a starting dose of 250 mg three or four times each day. At five- to seven-day intervals, this dose is increased by 500 mg per day. Patients taking levodopa usually arrive at their proper dose when they are taking 2-5 grams per day.

Prescribe Sinemet® at 50 mg (one half of a 10/100 tablet) three times each day. This may be increased every four to seven days by 100 mg per day. Patients taking Sinemet® usually arrive at their best dose when they are taking 500-1500 mg per day.

Patients who cannot tolerate plain levodopa because of nausea and vomiting may do well on Sinemet®. Patients who develop intractable dystonic movements on Sinemet® may be more comfortable on levodopa. Both preparations offer about the same degree of anti-Parkinsonian activity if the patient arrives at a comparable dose.

Caution: If the physician prescribes levodopa alone, he must warn his patient against concomitant use of therapeutic vitamin tablets containing 5 mg of pyridoxine. This vitamin is part of the co-enzyme for dopa-decarboxylase, which transforms levodopa to dopamine.

Dopa-decarboxylase is present in non-neural tissues of the body as well as in the brain, and the availability of large amounts of pyridoxine allows rapid transformation of levodopa to dopamine in the non-neural tissues, completely negating its neurological action because the medication never reaches the brain. Because of the presence of carbidopa, an inhibitor of non-neural dopa-decarboxylase, patients taking Sinemet® need not be concerned about pyridoxine.

Caution: If the physician discovers that a patient taking plain levodopa is also taking therapeutic vitamins without his prior knowledge, this helps to explain why the patient was a "dopa failure," but the physician must not simply stop the vitamins! He must recommend first that levodopa be stopped for a day – then the vitamin preparation. Several days later levodopa may be restarted at standard starting doses and built up toward a proper dosage level as though the patient had never been treated. If the patient simply stops the vitamins and continues large doses of levodopa, he will have a severe toxic reaction.

Caution: Because Sinemet® contains carbidopa, an inhibitor of dopa-decarboxylase, it may not be prescribed with large doses of levodopa. If the physician wishes to switch his patient from levodopa to Sinemet®, the patient should take his last dose of plain levodopa in the afternoon, none during the night, and begin Sinemet® the following morning on a dosage schedule that provides about one fifth the dose of levodopa that he was taking previously. This will probably be an inadequate dose of Sinemet® because the usual dose of Sinemet® is about one fourth the dose of plain levodopa. It is easier for the patient to have a mild relapse of Parkinsonism, and then reach for his proper dose of Sinemet®, as described above, than it is for him to develop sudden toxic side effects as he changes preparations.

Patient Education

Levodopa in its various forms requires intense patient education as treatment begins. Patients and families need to discuss treatment strategy with their physician in order to understand how to define a "best dose" and how to reach it. During treatment, they need to be reminded about the recurrent need to establish that they are still taking their proper dose of levodopa. If they call, wondering whether the patient is toxic, they may cut back the dose sharply for a day and then begin again at a lower dosage level. If the patient does not improve, or if he is worse, they have their answer, and may return to the previous dose, or investigate a higher dosage level to determine whether his symptoms actually represented too *small* a dose. In any case, the answer is *their answer,* not the physician's. *They* must balance therapeutic effectness against known side effects to achieve their optimum, in light of their patient's total living conditions.

Lastly, they must be educated to the fact that they are in possession of a powerful anti-Parkinson agent, not a miracle. Levodopa has been universally disappointing to Parkinson patients, even when they were much improved by it. The lay and professional press has hailed levodopa as a miraculous treatment, and even small failure is a disappointment. Trihexyphenidyl, at least, had the dubious advantage that no one expected much from it, and patients were happy with any improvement. Now, they need to accept levodopa for what it is – not a cure, very imperfect, merely an excellent medication.

Side Effects of Levodopa Preparations

When levodopa was first used as an experimental drug, it was considered dangerous because it caused severe orthostatic hypotension. This unwarranted concern is still present in the medical and lay community. It may be that orthostatic hypotension was caused by the rapid dosage increases required by in-patient experimental protocols. Perhaps, instead, it occurred in unrecognized cases of Shy-Drager syndrome. In any case, levodopa is an extremely safe medication if it is used sensibly, and side effects are usually dose-related and not life-threatening.

If the dose is increased gradually as outlined above, the first side effect of plain levodopa is usually nausea. This occurs during the 30-60 minutes following a dose and lasts less than an hour. If the dose is increased beyond this point, the patient begins to vomit in a similar time sequence. Some patients taking plain levodopa, and many patients on Sinemet® develop uncontrollable dystonic grimacing and tongue movements, or dystonic movements in the hands and lower extemities. These side effects are strictly dose-related and disappear promptly when the dose is reduced.

Some patients develop nocturnal confusion or even an organic psychosis on levodopa. This, too, is dose-related and subsides promptly when the dose is decreased. Patients with dementia frequently cannot tolerate enough levodopa to reduce Parkinsonism because of psychotic side effects, and for this reason, levodopa should be prescribed in smaller initial doses, and increased more slowly for such patients. The physician must warn the families of a demented Parkinson patient that psychosis may occur and that he may not be able to tolerate the medication. There are many other reported side effects to levodopa. These, however, are uncommon. Most reported side effects of acute toxicity are strictly dose-related and carry no hazard if the medication is decreased.

Long-term side effects are the most troublesome because they first appear after the patient has taken his medication for several years, with good control of symptoms and few side effects. Dystonic facial and extremity movements become prominent and distressing. Worse yet, there are sudden fluctuations in Parkinson symptoms. These have been called the "on-off" effect. The patient suddenly finds himself immobile ("off") and must wait until this phase passes before he can continue his activities. As the "off" phase passes, he may have a period of fairly normal activity, or may pass directly into a toxic, dystonic state! The on-off effect is dose-related. It disappears to completely "off" as the patient reduces the dose and develops returning Parkinsonism. At this point, the patient must choose between two bad alternatives—"on-off" with some "on," or largely "off." These late side effects herald the return of Parkinsonism despite the best treatment available. They should warn the clinician to start thinking about other modes of treatment which might still be available to his patients.

Contraindications to the Use of Levodopa

Levodopa has been reported to aggravate narrow angle glaucoma and to increase the growth of malignant melanoma. Patients with these two conditions should not use levodopa in any form. Patients taking monoamine oxidase inhibitors, apart from carbidopa, must stop these before they start levodopa. Methyldopa (Aldomet®) markedly potentiates the effect of levodopa in the same manner as carbidopa, and should not be used concomitantly with levodopa preparations. Dementia is not a direct contraindication to the use of levodopa but usually results in organic psychosis before the medication becomes effective as an anti-Parkinson agent.

Bromocriptine

In 1974, Calne and co-workers[1] treated Parkinson patients with 2-bromo-alpha ergocriptine (bromocriptine), a molecule known to stimulate dopamine-sensitive receptors. Numerous publications have appeared since then, testifying to the effectiveness of bromocriptine in the treatment of Parkinson's disease.[2,6,9,12] Long-term experimental treatment trials are now underway in patients. Bromocriptine has theoretical advantages over levodopa, because it has a direct action on dopamine receptors without a requirement for biotransformation in the striatum.

Side effects of bromocriptine are similar to those of levodopa. The "on-off" effect may be reduced in frequency but not in severity,[8] and gastrointestinal distress is lessened. However, patients develop confusional states, aggressive behavior, and prolonged hallucinations which may last several *weeks* after bromocriptine has stopped.[9]

Bromocriptine may become a substitute for levodopa, but even if it does not, it represents the first of a new generation of anti-Parkinson agents, whose goal is more specificity against the symptoms of the disease, fewer side effects, and fewer active metabolites to confuse body metabolism.

Thalamotomy

Destruction of certain thalamic nuclei, or of the globus pallidus or substantia nigra, either by freezing, injection of alcohol, or extirpation, relieves Parkinsonian symptoms on the opposite side of the body. When levodopa was first introduced, many severe Parkinson patients had already had thalamotomy on one or both sides, and they derived additional benefit from levodopa therapy. Patients whose Parkinsonism was less severe, and those who have developed Parkinson's disease in the intervening years, have usually improved enough without levodopa therapy that they have not needed thalamotomy. Indeed, for a number of years, this procedure became a vanishing operation, and there were even predictions that it would no longer be of value because levoopa prevented progression of Parkinsonism. In the recent past, patients on levodopa have confirmed the progressive nature of their disease, and they have begun to fail despite the best levodopa therapy. These people are again being referred for thalamotomy.

Thalamotomy is especially effective for the patient with asymmetrical Parkinsonism, in whom tremor is the primary component. However, each patient must be evaluated by an experienced neurosurgeon before a determination can be made.

CHOREA-ATHETOSIS

Huntington's chorea and the clinical diagnosis of choreiform movements are discussed in the section on untreatable dementias (p. 212). But several other types of chorea-athetosis occur which are not accompanied by progressive dementia.

Sydenham's Chorea

Onset of restlessness and inattention in school may bring a child to a physician as a behavior problem. On other occasions, the movement disorder itself is recognized as an abnormal event. Sydenham's chorea is related primarily to rheumatic fever, and may eventually be accompanied by rheumatic heart disease. For this reason, once it is diagnosed, the child should take prophylactic penicillin to prevent further attacks. The chorea itself may be treated with bedrest and either phenothiazine or haloperidol. Girls who have Sydenham's chorea may develop chorea gravidarum later in life.

Chorea Due to Focal Brain Lesions and Metabolic Disease

Acute hemichorea may develop after ischemic stroke in the caudate nucleus. Systemic disease, like lupus erythematosus or hyperthyroidism, is occasionally accompanied by choreiform movements. Tardive dyskinesia, the movement disorder associated with long-term use of many different phenothiazine preparations, is characterized by dystonic movements of face and neck with accompanying choreiform motions. Metastatic tumor may cause hemichorea or bilateral chorea. Treatment is directed to the original pathologic process.

Children below the age of 10 or 12 years of age normally display irregular small choreiform movements as they sit, eyes closed, arms outstretched. These should not be confused with pathological choreiform states. Instead, they represent the normal function of an immature nervous system.

DYSTONIA

Dystonia refers to complex involuntary movements and postures which may form part of the symptomatology of previous head trauma, cerebral palsy, and Parkinsonism, or may be due to the side effects of therapy with such chemically diverse medications as levodopa and phenothiazines. Dystonia musculorum deformans is a specific heritable disease which may be transmitted as an autosomal dominant or autosomal recessive trait. Expressivity of the dystonia genes is extremely variable. Onset may occur in early childhood with a malignant course leading to disability and early death, or it may occur later in life as localized and very slowly progressive dystonia.

Zeman has outlined the history of dystonia as a symptom, a disease, and as a bone of nosological contention.[13] For many years, dystonia was considered to represent an hysterical reaction, because there are no recognizable central nervous system lesions, and because the movements are so complex that they resemble voluntary or hysterical movements. Additionally, even severely disabled dystonic patients fail to show pathological reflexes or sensory loss, and it was difficult to give such patients an organic diagnosis without firm neurological abnormalities. It is now accepted, at least by most of the neurological world, that dystonic symptoms, including dystonia musculorum deformans, spasmodic torticollis, blepharospasm, and even dystonic writer's cramp, are manifestations of an organic, not psychiatric, dysfunction.[10]

Medical treatment of dystonic syndromes is usually unrewarding. Beneficial results have been reported and refuted from levodopa, haloperidol, and carbamazepine. The most effective treatment for disabling dystonic symptoms is thalamotomy.[3,4,5] The adult with distressing dystonia and the child with generalized dystonia must be evaluated for thalamotomy if they do not respond to medicinal therapy, because thalamotomy has produced long-term improvements where other treatment has failed.

The clinician who is confronted with a case of dystonia would be wise to refer that patient immediately for neurological consultation. Should medicinal management not provide adequate relief, he should plan for a referral to a neurosurgical center with experience in the treatment of dystonia. Do not consign the dystonic patient to his home or to psychiatric care on the basis of an unfounded belief in a psychiatric etiology!

HEMIBALLISM

Hemiballism consists of irregular wild flinging movements of upper or lower extremities. It is different from tremors because of the extreme irregularity of the movements, and because of their violent swinging character. Ballistic movements may become so severe that the patient is exhausted by them or may even break a bone as he hits things with the arm. Ballism may occur in a limb which is completely paralyzed for voluntary movements. The causative lesion is usually an ischemic stroke in the upper midbrain tegmentum or the subthalamic region. At one time, it was thought that the responsible lesion universally occupied the subthalamic nucleus of Luys. This is not so, but the lesion usually does involve that nucleus or its afferrent or efferrent pathways.

Treatment of hemiballism is thalamotomy, which may be dramatically successful. There is no effective medicinal therapy.

WILSON'S DISEASE

Wilson's disease may appear in a young child as an episode of acute or chronic hepatitis and result in death in a few months. At older ages of onset, symptoms from the central nervous system, including personality change, tremor, dystonic movements, and dysarthria, become more prominent, and liver symptoms are less obvious. The young person who develops the onset of liver and central nervous system involvement, or the young person suspected of having "Parkinsonism," is a suspect for Wilson's disease. The diagnosis is usually made quite simply by taking a serum ceruloplasmin test. Ceruloplasmin is markedly decreased, and urinary copper excretion is markedly increased in this disease. The Kayser-Fleischer ring on the cornea is pathognomonic of the disease, but it may be confused with arcus senilis unless the ring is examined under a slit lamp by an experienced examiner.

Wilson's disease is treatable with penicillamine, but the clinician who makes this diagnosis should not attempt to treat such a patient without help from a neurological consultant, preferably one with experience in the treatment of this disease.

REFERENCES

1. Calne, D.B., Teychenne, P.F., Claveria, L.E., Eastman, R., Greenacre, J.K.: Bromocriptine in Parkinsonism. Brit. Med. J. 4: 442–444, 1974.
2. Calne, D.B., Williams, A.C., Neophytides, A., Plotkin, C., Nutt, J.G., Teychenne, P.F.: Long-Term Treatment of Parkinsonism with Bromocriptine. Lancet II:735–738, 1978.
3. Cooper, I.S.: Dystonia Reversal by Operation on Basal Ganglia. Neurology 7:132–145, 1962.
4. Cooper, I.S.: Effect of Thalamic Lesions Upon Torticollis. N. Engl. J. Med. 270:967–972, 1964.
5. Cooper, I.S.: 20-Year Followup Study of the Neurosurgical Treatment of Dystonia Musculorum Deformans. In: *Advances in Neurology* Vol. 14, *Dystonia*, Eldridge, R., Fahn, S. (Eds.) Raven Press, New York, 1976, pp. 423–447.
6. Godwin-Austen, R.B., Smith, N.J.: Comparison of the Effects of Bromocriptine and Levodopa in Parkinson's Disease. J. Neurol. Neurosurg. Psychiatr. 40:479–482, 1977.
7. Lloyd, K.G., Davidson, L., Hornykiewicz, O.: The Neurochemistry of Parkinson's Disease: Effect of L-DOPA Therapy. J. Pharmacol. Exp. Therap. 195:453–464, 1975.
8. Kartzinel, R., Calne, D.B.: Studies with Bromocriptine Part 1. "On-off" Phenomena. Neurology 26:508–510, 1976.
9. Kartzinel, R., Shoulson, I., Calne, D.B.: Studies with Bromocriptine Part II. Double-Blind Comparison with Levodopa in Parkinsonism. Neurology 26:511–513, 1976.
10. Marsden, C.D.: The Problem of Adult-Onset Idiopathic Torsion Dystonia and Other Isolated Dyskinesias in Adult Life (Including Blepharospasm, Oromandibular Dystonia, Dystonic Writer's Cramp, and Torticollis or Axial Dystonia). In: *Advances in Neurology* Vol. 14, *Dystonia*, Eldridge, R., Fahn, S. (Eds.) Raven Press, New York, 1976, pp. 259–276.
11. Shy, G.M., Drager, G.A.: A Neurological Syndrome Associated with Orthostatic Hypotension. Arch. Neurol. 2:511–527, 1960.
12. Teychenne, P.F., Kartzinel, R., Perlow, M., Pfeiffer, R., Calne, D.B.: Clinical Studies with Bromocriptine in Idiopathic Parkinsonism. Tr. Amer. Neurol. Assn. 101:302–304, 1976.
13. Zeman, W.: Dystonia: An Overview. In: *Advances in Neurology* Vol. 14, *Dystonia*, Eldridge, R., Fahn, S. (Eds.) Raven Press, New York, 1976, pp. 91–102.

CHAPTER 8

Evaluation of the Comatose Patient

INTRODUCTION

Two complementary but distinct methods of examination for the comatose patient are presented in this chapter. The first, which I have called the "coma examination," is directed toward an evaluation of the depth of coma and allows the examiner to distinguish rapidly between patients whose coma is caused by mass lesions above the tentorium and those whose coma is of metabolic etiology. The second, which I have called the "neurological examination in coma," outlines techniques for examining the comatose patient to localize the site of the lesion that caused his coma. This examination has the same goal as any other neurological examination, but the techniques are different because the patient is comatose. There are detailed lists of the structural and metabolic causes of coma which may be found in other medical texts. These are not reproduced in this volume.

THE COMA EXAMINATION

Stupor, somnolence, coma, deep coma – these are some of the imprecise terms used to describe patients with various degrees of unconsciousness. The terms lack precision because they are based on general observations of the patient rather than on anatomical considerations derived from specific physical findings. The coma examination consists of observations of four specific variables, which evaluate function in four anatomical systems of the brain. The examination may be performed in less than three minutes, and at the end of that time, the examiner may make accurate statements about the depth of coma, whether it is possibly reversible, and the probable cause. By repeating the examination of these four variables from time to time, he may assess the results of treatment. The four variables are:

1) Motor response to deep pain.
2) Pattern of respiration.
3) Pupillary size and reactivity to light.
4) Vestibulo-ocular reflexes.

An understanding of the functional anatomy involved in each of these four aspects of the examination is important, so we shall discuss them individually before we show how they may be used in a clinical examination.

1) Motor Response to Deep Pain

Neurophysiologists have distinguished between decorticate and decerebrate postures in animals with experimental brain lesions. These represent reflex postures, organized at lower nervous system levels, which appear only when the lower levels are released from higher control.

If large portions of the cerebral cortex and subcortical white matter are removed, but the diencephalon (basal ganglia, thalamus, hypothalamus) remains intact, the animal is said to be decorticate and develops a stereotyped posture. In man, the decorticate posture consists of flexion of the upper extremity, usually across the chest, and extension of the lower extremity. This posture is best observed as a response to deep pain, and is characteristic of early phases of coma.

To produce increasingly intense deep pain, the examiner places the tip of his thumb under the ridge of the patient's eyebrow and presses with increasing firmness over the bone. The normal subject's response is to raise the hand to remove the offending thumb. The earliest change toward decorticate posturing is an incomplete gesture, the hand coming to the general vicinity of the face or eye, but not effectively removing the thumb. In the completely decorticate posture, the hand reaches only to the level of the chest.

If the entire brain of an experimental animal is separated from the brainstem by section of the neuraxis at the midbrain level, the animal is said to be decerebrate. The human decerebrate posture consists of extension of the lower extremity as mentioned above, but the upper extremity response is even less appropriate, because now it *extends* down the patient's side in response to painful stimulation over the eye, usually with an internal rotation at the shoulder and wrist.

If the brainstem of the experimental animal is sectioned at lower pontine levels, all reflex postures are destroyed, resulting in flaccid quadriplegia, As human coma deepens from midbrain levels, decerebrate responses become weaker and disappear shortly before death.

This means that most comatose patients exhibit specific responses to painful stimulation during most of their coma. The clinical question is *how* they respond, and what that response means in terms of pathologic anatomy. Patients with coma of metabolic origin are exceptions to this rule. Some metabolic toxins, such as general anesthetics and alcohol, affect brainstem structures early, and produce loss of brainstem reflex postures in response to pain, while other brain and brainstem reflexes are preserved.

"No response to pain" is frequently recorded incorrectly on in-patient charts. This deprives the doctor and his patient of vitally important diagnostic information. The statement frequently reflects the examiner's inadequate method of stimulation. Pinching the skin or slapping the face produces superficial pain, which is not an adequate stimulus. Responses to painful stimulation may be evaluated only after *deep pain* of adequate *intensity* and *duration* have been applied.

2) Patterns of Respiration

Cerebral respiratory centers exert inhibitory control over pontine respiratory centers. Left to themselves, the pontine centers produce rapid hyperventilation, but the higher centers prevent this and, through their inhibitory function, maintain accurate control over blood CO_2 and oxygen tensions.

The earliest change in respiratory pattern occurs if a minimal dysfunction of higher inhibitory centers develops for any reason. Under this circumstance, the pontine centers escape periodically and produce transient hyperventilation, thus lowering the blood CO_2 tension. When the CO_2 tension falls enough, the sluggish cerebral center again exerts itself to inhibit pontine hyperventilation, and respirations are shut off temporarily only to repeat the cycle again in a few moments. This kind of cyclic respiration is seen in normal elderly people during sleep, in patients with delayed circuation times, and in early coma. It is called Cheyne-Stokes respiration.

Cheyne-Stokes breathing is frequently thought of as a "bad sign," but the reader can see that it is actually one of the earliest abnormalities in respiratory pattern. It is a "bad sign" only because it presages deeper levels of coma if accurate diagnosis and effective treatment are not immediately available.

In the decerebrate animal, whose neuraxis has been sectioned at the midbrain level, all cerebral control over pontine respiratory centers is removed. Released from cerebral inhibitory influences, the pontine centers produce uninterrupted hyperventilation. In man, this is a breathing pattern characteristic of deep coma; once it is heard, it can never be forgotten. If the patient is lying on his back, the observer hears loud, apparently labored, rapid snoring respirations which intrude on other noises in the hospital, even through closed doors. This respiratory pattern is called central neurogenic hyperventilation. It is distinguished from acidotic hyperventilation by the great depth of acidotic breathing and the terminal flaring of the rib cage at the depth of each expiration as the acidotic patient attempts to squeeze every possible bit of air from the lungs. Central neurogenic hyperventilation is merely rapid, not deep.

If neurological dysfunction deteriorates even more, pontine hyperventilation begins to fail, and breathing subsides, resembling normal respirations for a time. Then, occasionally, one can observe breathing which is arrested at the top of inspiration, so-called apneustic breathing. As the level of coma deepens even further, this organization is also lost, and only irregular brief gasps remain until death.

3) Pupillary Size and Reactivity to Light

Pupillary size is determined by the combined effects of sympathetic and parasympathetic tone. The parasympathetic outflow originates in the oculomotor complex in the midbrain and travels to the eye with the third nerve, constricting the pupil. If the parasympathetic pathway is destroyed, the pupil dilates because the sympathetics are acting alone.

Sympathetic tone originates in the hypothalamus and travels

downward through the brainstem to cervical spinal cord level, C8-T1, where it leaves the central nervous system to travel with the cervical sympathetic plexus around the internal carotid artery, finally entering the orbit with the ophthalmic artery. Activity in the sympathetic system dilates the pupil. Damage to the pathway anywhere along its tortuous route causes pupillary constriction because the parasympathetic system is acting alone.

When light hits the retina, nerve impulses travel through the optic nerve and into the optic tract, where they leave the visual system and go to the parasympathetic neurons of the oculomotor complex in the midbrain. The resultant parasympathetic discharge through the third nerve constricts the pupils bilaterally. Destruction of midbrain structures destroys parasympathetic tone and light response simultaneously. Because midbrain disease usually also destroys sympathetic pupillary pathways traveling through the area, lesions here are associated with mid-position pupils, which are unresponsive to light because influences from both autonomic pathways are absent.

Question: Using knowledge of the anatomy, can the reader predict the pupillary size and reactivity in the patient whose lesion is in the pons, not the midbrain?

Answer: Destructive lesions in the pons destroy only the sympathetic pupillary pathways and do not affect parasympathetic tone nor light response. Therefore, the pupils are pinpoint sized, but still respond promptly to light. These pupillary findings, coupled with flaccid quadriplegia, are diagnostic of acute pontine disease.

In human coma, there is no change in pupillary size and reactivity if only the cortex and subcortical white matter are involved. But if the hypothalamic outflow is compromised, the pupils become smaller, still retaining their light responsiveness. Such small reactive pupils are characteristic of early stages of coma due to mass lesions above the tentorium, probably because the hypothalamus is very sensitive to edema or pressure changes. Eventually, as midbrain structures become involved, small but reactive pupils change to small but unreactive pupils. This transition is of clinical importance because it is one sign that there is dysfunction in the vital midbrain region. Once this area is actually destroyed, coma is irreversible. As both sympathetic and parasympathetic systems fail in midbrain destruction, the pupils dilate to midposition, but never again regain their responsiveness to light. In preterminal coma, when all brainstem and body reflexes have disappeared, the pupils become fully dilated – perhaps because the constrictor muscle of the pupil also becomes flaccid, perhaps because of an agonal release of norepinephrine.

4) Vestibulo-Ocular Reflexes

To perform the doll's head eye movement maneuver, the examiner turns the patient's head forcibly to one side. When this is done, reflex connections in the brainstem attempt to turn the eyes toward the opposite direction, thus helping the individual to maintain fixation on an original object of interest. This reflex originates in the semicircular canals, where movement of endolymph signals the head movement to the vestibular portion of the eighth nerve. This information is distributed to the pontine paramedian reticular formation (PPRF), which controls conjugate eye movements, and the eyes move in response to these stimuli.

Cold water caloric stimulation is performed by placing the head in the proper position and instilling iced water in the external auditory canal. This cools the otic capsule, produces currents in the horizontal semicircular canal, and results in strong stimulation of the same reflex system without head turning.

These reflex connections are confined to the brainstem, but they are controlled by cortical activity during normal wakefulness. In the *normal subject,* rapid head turning produces a brief gesture of contralateral eye movement, but the subject quickly re-fixes the eyes on some object in front of him, so the observer finds *nearly absent* doll's head eye movements. Cold caloric stimulation is uncomfortable for the normal subject because of the sense of motion it produces, but the wakeful subject maintains constant fixation, despite the tendency to eye deviation, by producing rapid corrective saccades in the opposite direction called jerk nystagmus.

Like the rest of the functions discussed in this chapter, the vestibulo-ocular reflexes are amenable to analysis in terms of levels of anatomical dysfunction. Has the reader already thought ahead of the text to predict the first functional change when there is loss of cortical inhibition in early coma? This releases the vestibulo-ocular reflexes from cortical inhibition and produces *hyper*-active doll's head eye movements. Nystagmus disappears during cold caloric stimulation, and the eyes deviate conjugately toward the side of iced water instillation.

As the level of neurological dysfunction descends, midbrain structures, including the oculomotor complex, are damaged, and, for the first time, the response of extraocular muscles to forcible head turning and to cold caloric stimulation is dysconjugate because of defective medial rectus muscle function. At this point, the doll's head eye movements begin to be suppressed, but vigorous cold caloric stimulation still produces definite abduction of the ipsilateral eye, even though the opposite eye no longer adducts.

As pontine levels of dysfunction and death approach, the entire vestibulo-ocular reflex is destroyed, and neither turning of the head nor cold water in the ear produces eye movement.

The response to cold caloric stimulation is a critically important diagnostic event during the coma examination. If there is nystagmus, *the patient is awake*: hysterical, malingering, or perhaps in a catatonic stupor, *but not comatose*. If the eyes deviate toward the side of testing, the patient is comatose. If there is no response at all, he probably has wax in the external ear canal, is near death, or is in a metabolic coma.

Note on the Performance of Cold Water Stimulation

Strangely, wax in the ear canal is a most common cause of absent response to cold water caloric stimulation. The first part of the procedure *must* consist of an examination of the canals and removal of excess wax.

The horizontal semicircular canal is most accessible and is situated so that it becomes vertical when the patient's head is tilted 30° forward from the supine. One or two pillows under the head does this perfectly. A bath towel is placed under the ear to keep the bedsheets clean, and a 30-cc syringe is fitted with about two inches of thin rubber tubing to be inserted partially into the ear canal. Then, 20-30 ml of iced water is instilled slowly into the ear canal while the eyes are held open. The response usually begins in 20-30 seconds and lasts about a minute. After the effect has been observed and has passed off, the procedure may be repeated in the other ear.

This kind of cold water caloric stimulation is different from caloric testing done in the otolaryngology clinic. During the coma examination, the clinician is not interested in a finely graded evaluation of labyrinthine function. He wants to know whether the brainstem reflexes are functioning. For this reason, during the coma examination he should use **enough** *iced* water to be certain he has seen the response he seeks.

Rostro-Caudal Brainstem Dysfunction with Supratentorial Mass Lesions

In their germinal article, McNealy and Plum[1] brought clinical correlation of these four variables to the bedside. They examined a series of comatose patients with mass lesions above the tentorium. In many cases, the process was irreversible, and they followed the progress of coma to death. Their findings have been verified repeatedly by the neurological community. This single article gives the clinician a rapid, reproducible coma examination, which allows an accurate determination of the depth of coma in a few minutes.

McNealy and Plum found that each of the four variables deteriorated in an orderly, rostro-caudal manner as we have described above and, more importantly, that there was *concomitant deterioration of all four variables*. Note in Table 8-1 that at any given examination, all four variables are found at a given "level" of neurological dysfunction, so that the depth of coma may be named by the group of functions that were most recently destroyed – early and late diencephalic coma, midbrain coma, pontine coma. Naturally, there are asymmetrical aspects to the examination of each case, but hemiplegia does not affect the analysis nor any of the four variables except the motor response to pain.

Variable Brain Dysfunction in Metabolic Coma

There is no orderliness about the progression of metabolic coma as there is in coma due to supratentorial mass lesions. Plum and Posner's volume, *The Diagnosis of Stupor and Coma*,[2] has become a standard text and is highly recommended to the reader. Here we learn that *metabolic causes of coma* produce *highly variable* responses during the coma examination. This is to be expected, of course. Structural disease and the associated edema and hemorrhage impinge directly upon anatomical structures and destroy them, but alcohol, drugs, diabetic acidosis, liver disease, hypothermia and the like are associated with metabolic toxicity which affects different neuron pools in different fashions. So we might have

TABLE 8-1

Orderly Rostro-Caudal Progression of Dysfunction in Coma Due to Supratentorial Mass Lesion

Anatomical Stage	Response to Pain	Respiratory Pattern	Pupil Examination: Light	Size	Vestibulo-Ocular Reflex	Prognosis
Early diencephalic (Wakeful, dull)	Almost normal	Normal	Reactive	● ● 4 mm	Normal	
(Stuporous)	Incomplete; Decorticate	Cheyne-Stokes	Reactive		Hyperactive	Reversible Stages of Coma
Late diencephalic (Comatose)	Decorticate	Cheyne-Stokes	Reactive	● ● 3 mm		
		Central neurogenic hyperventilation (CNH)	Reactive		Hyperactive	
Early Midbrain (Deep coma)	Decerebrate	CNH	Reactive	● ● 2 mm	Hypoactive	Usually Irreversible Coma
Late Midbrain	Decerebrate	CNH	Unreactive		Dysconjugate: (Medial rectus paralysis)	

(Continued)

TABLE 8-1 (Continued)

Anatomical Stage	Response to Pain	Respiratory Pattern	Pupil Examination: Light	Size	Vestibulo-Ocular Reflex	Prognosis
Pontine	Decerebration fading	CNH decreases; respiration may appear normal; apneustic breathing	Unreactive	● 4 mm	Absent	Irreversible Coma
Medullary	Flaccid	Brief gasps	Unreactive	● 9 mm	Absent	

NOTE: Each stage of coma is associated with findings caused by dysfunction of progressively lower anatomical structures. During the early diencephalic stages of "coma," the patient is still wakeful, but the process has begun. The uncal syndrome (pp. 170) is not depicted here. Without immediate treatment, the uncal syndrome may lead rapidly to irreversible stages of coma.

expected the discovery of widely disparate findings in metabolic coma, but we would not have recognized them without prior knowledge of the *orderly* nature of structural coma.

Thus, the patient whose respirations are normal, and whose pupils react to bright light, but who has no response to deep painful stimulation is characteristic of surgical stages of anesthesia and of the alcoholic who is "feeling no pain." Clearly, in these two metabolic cases, brainstem postural reflexes have been suppressed much more than the other functions. Various metabolic causes of coma produce somewhat different findings, but the important characteristic is that the patient's findings were not all at a "level of coma" but were dispersed at various levels.

Therefore, the three-minute examination in the emergency room allows the physician to determine whether his patient needs a CT scan for diagnosis, and a neurosurgeon for possible treatment of a mass lesion; or an internist and emergency blood examinations to determine the cause of metabolic coma.

A Note on Therapeutic Urgency

In some cases, the lesion is known, and there is no available treatment from the start. In such cases, the physician may be useful to patient and family by his quiet presence and his suppression of the empty bustle which often surrounds the dying person in the hospital.

But in other cases, the lesion is not known. Patients in the diencephalic stages of coma may recover if the offending supratentorial mass is diagnosed and removed before they descend to midbrain stages of coma or develop uncal herniation (p. 170). The undiagnosed patient who is still in the semiwakeful and stuporous stages of diencephalic coma represents one of the infrequent neurological emergencies.

Some patients in midbrain stages of coma can return to normal life if they are treated promptly, but many are permanently and severely damaged. Patients in pontine and medullary stages of coma due to supratentorial mass lesions have an irreversible process and cannot be salvaged. If the patient first appears in these late stages of coma, or develops these stages despite proper treatment, and if the physician knows with *certainty* that the cause is not metabolic, his job again becomes a passive one for the patient and a preparatory one for the family who must expect a fatal outcome.

Exceptions to the Rule

1) Early Coma

The distinction between metabolic and structural comas may not be made during wakeful or stuporous stages of diencephalic coma as it may once the patient is fully unconscious. The author was fooled twice by an apparent variability of findings in such patients, and made a diagnosis of metabolic precoma. Both had structural, not metabolic disease, and both eventually developed levels of deepening coma, and died.

2) Uncal Syndrome

Occasionally, a patient with a supratentorial mass bypasses the orderly rostro-caudal disintegration and suddenly begins to dilate one pupil. This process may progress rapidly, directly into decerebrate stages of coma, highly asymmetrical paralysis, and death. If a patient, who is suspected of having a supratentorial mass lesion, begins to dilate a pupil, even though he is wide awake and talking with the examiner, his case is a dire emergency, and must receive priority attention, because he may be dead in a few hours if he does not get help. McNealy and Plum called this the "uncal syndrome" because it is caused by the downward herniation of the uncus, which is situated on the medial surface of the temporal lobe, into the posterior fossa where it compresses the third nerve and the midbrain itself. This causes the pupillary dilatation and the sudden progression to decerebrate posturing. McNealy and Plum correlate this syndrome with intraventricular hemorrhage or untimely lumbar puncture, but it may also occur in the normal course of events, related to temporal lobe mass lesions or to subdural hematoma, without outside interference.

3) Posterior Fossa Lesion

Some comatose patients have structural lesions *below* the tentorium. In these cases, the neurological examination in coma discloses evidence of midbrain or pontine disease, and the patient does not deteriorate in an orderly rostro-caudal progression. Acute cerebellar lesions cannot be clearly distinguished from primary brainstem lesions.

Can the reader come to accurate conclusions about the cause of coma in these four cases? The answers are detailed at the end of the four examples.

Example 1: The patient is brought to the emergency room deeply comatose. Response to deep pain is absent. Respirations are shallow, slow and regular. Pupils are widely dilated but respond to bright light. Doll's head eye movements are absent, but vigorous cold caloric stimulation produces conjugate eye movements. Is the coma due to structural or metabolic disease?

Example 2: The patient is brought to the emergency room deeply comatose. Response to pain is decerebrate on the right, absent on the left. Respirations are rapid and noisy. Pupils are 3 mm and do not react to light. Doll's head eye movements are absent, but cold caloric stimulation reveals dysconjugate eye movements with apparent paralysis of medial rectus muscles bilaterally. Is the coma due to structural or metabolic disease?

Example 3: The patient is brought to the emergency room deeply comatose. Response to deep pain is initially absent but eventually produces unformed writhing movements. Respirations are normal. Pupils are in mid-position and respond to light. Cold water caloric stimulation in the left ear produces jerk nystagmus to the right. Is the coma due to structural or metabolic disease?

Example 4: The patient is brought to the emergency room deeply comatose. There is no response to painful stimulation over either orbit. Respirations are rapid, noisy, but irregular. Pupils are pinpoint but react to bright light. Doll's head eye movements are absent. Cold caloric stimulation on the right produces no response. Cold caloric stimulation in the left ear produces abduction of the left eye. Is the coma due to structural or metabolic disease?

 Example 1 is coma of metabolic origin. There is no distinct level of dysfunction. Despite apparently flaccid, unresponsive postural reflexes, pupillary reaction is intact, and respirations are normal.

 Example 2 has a mass lesion in the right hemisphere with a midbrain stage of coma and hemiplegia on the left.

 Example 3 is not comatose at all!

 Example 4. It was unfair to give the reader this example at this point, but it may have been clear that this is a different lesion from the rest, because, despite the fact that the patient was not "at one level" of coma, his examination was asymmetrical, and this should not be the case in metabolic disease. This patient has an acute destructive lesion in the pons and needs a neurological examination to confirm it.

THE NEUROLOGICAL EXAMINATION IN COMA

The neurological examination during coma helps to localize the cause of a structural coma. Sometimes, the neurological examination will verify that there is no evidence of focal structural disease, at all, and will strengthen the conclusions derived from the coma examination that the cause is metabolic or psychiatric.

Many clinicians do not attempt to perform a neurological examination unless the patient is awake and cooperative. By omitting this important part of the physical evaluation, they deny themselves the satisfaction of clinical competence and miss potentially important information. Actually, during all stages of coma except those immediately preceding death, the functions of all major systems may be assessed except cerebellar coordination and the muscles of the mouth and pharynx. Let us briefly consider techniques for these examinations and the reasoning process that allows localizing conclusions to be drawn from the available evidence.

Examination of the Visual Fields

In diencephalic stages of coma, the patient is still wakeful or stuporous. Threatening gestures toward the opened eyes produce a blink response if the threatened visual field is intact. The clinician must be careful to make a movement like a karate chop, not like a slap in the face, because the latter produces a breeze, which may stimulate the trigeminal innervation of the conjunctivae and produce a brainstem "corneal reflex" rather than a response to visual threat.

If there is no blink response to threat, we may assess whether the patient "has vision" by turning on a bright light directly in front of the face and watching for the resultant grimace. Patients do not grimace in response to a flashlight. Use a bright light, and if there is no response to this stimulus in a patient with diencephalic coma, he is blind. In later stages of coma, connections between visual cortex and brainstem structures responsible for the grimace may be interrupted, so lack of a response has no distinct significance.

Response of the pupils to light may be observed at the same time. These too should be tested with a bright light in order to be certain of the response. Many sluggish, but reactive pupils do not appear to constrict to a flashlight beam.

Examination of Eye Movements

The individual extraocular muscles cannot be closely evaluated during coma, but the resting position of the eyes may provide information about weakness of one or another set. Divergent strabismus in the anatomically neutral position does not necessarily mean medial rectus palsy. This is a common finding in metabolic coma (alcohol for instance).

Cold water caloric stimulation is the most potent stimulus to extraocular movements, and clearly demonstrates conjugate or dysconjugate eye movements. Results of caloric stimulation, and analysis of pupillary size and responsiveness, may be used to distinguish an oculomotor paralysis due to midbrain destruction (medial rectus palsy *with* pupillary paralysis, Example 2 above) from a medial longitudinal fasciculus lesion in the pons (medial rectus palsy without pupillary paralysis, Example 4 above).

Examination of Facial Sensation and Muscles of Facial Expression

Examination of facial sensation and facial movement are performed together during the neurological examination in coma. The corneal reflex is easiest to elicit and depends for its reflex arc upon intact trigeminal sensory function, intact facial nerve function, and intact connections between the two in the brainstem. If the corneal reflex is intact bilaterally, the examiner has considerable information about the intact sensory and motor functions in the pons! But touching the cornea with a cotton wisp is a mild stimulus and absence of the corneal reflex carries no definite anatomical significance.

Deep pain is the most adequate stimulus during coma. The examiner's thumbs are pointed toward each other and pressed with increasing force into the substance of the masseter muscle on each side *individually.* If the reader attempts this maneuver on himself, he is likely to grimace, because it produces intense deep pain. Testing facial responsiveness in this manner allows the examiner to assess the symmetry of the facial grimace, and the degree of responsiveness to a given amount of pressure on *each side individually.* This procedure makes unilateral sensory loss or unilateral facial paralysis obvious.

If the lesion is within the brainstem, there may be no response to deep pain from either side, as in Example 4 above.

This is where the clinician must begin to think! Is the lack of facial grimace due to destruction of the facial nucleus with bilateral facial *paralysis* (Figure 8-1a), or to destruction of the trigeminal input with bilateral facial *anesthesia* (Figure 8-1b, c)? Production of deep pain over the sternum with knuckle pressure can help to answer this question. If the lesion is above the facial nucleus, causing trigeminal destruction (Figure 8-1b, c), pain impulses from the sternum can ascend to brainstem levels and be organized into a facial grimace or into decerebrate posturing, even though there had been no response to facial pain. On the other hand, if the lesion is in the lower pons, it has destroyed the facial nuclei and probably all postural reflexes also (Figure 8-1a). In this case, there will be flaccid quadriplegia with no response to deep pain over the masseters or over the sternum.

At this point, it is important to reevaluate the eye findings, because if the lesion is in the upper pons, destroying trigeminal afferrents, it may also have spread destruction to midbrain levels. If so, the pupils are midposition and fixed (Figure 8-1c). But if the lesion is *confined* to the upper pons, the pupils are pinpoint and responsive to light (Figure 8-1b). By analysis of the response to two stimuli *only,* the response to pain and pupillary size and responsiveness to light, the clinician has been able to localize *closely* inside the brainstem!

The reader may imagine a fourth possibility in which the deeply comatose patient *does grimace* and develops decerebrate responses to pain, equal muscle tone or hemiplegia on one side, central neurogenic hyperventilation, dysconjugate doll's head eye movements with intact abduction bilaterally during cold caloric stimulation, and fixed mid-position pupils. This is the classic midbrain stage of coma, but if it appears suddenly, with no orderly rostro-caudal deterioration, it may represent an acute hemorrhage into midbrain

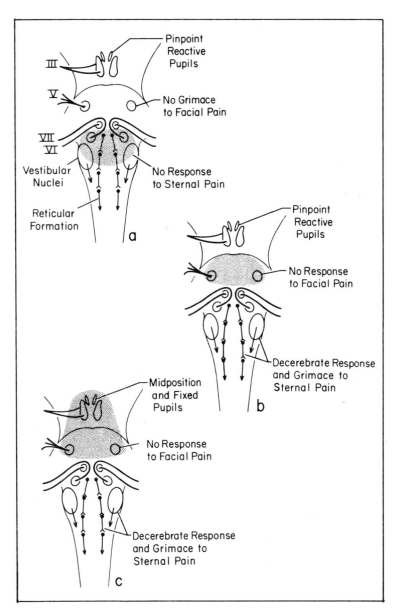

Figure 8-1. *Pupillary size and reactivity and responses to pain in three brainstem lesions. Two functions help to localize closely within brainstem structures.*

structures, not a supratentorial mass. The level of coma *alone* does not establish the cause. The history of its progression remains of vital importance.

Examination for Body Paralysis

The patient's resting bed position tells the examiner a great deal about paralysis. A hemiplegic bed position consists of an upper extremity which is flat on the bedsheet, the lower extremity extended and externally rotated. Head and eyes may be turned to one side, and the response to pain may show definite decorticate or decerebrate posturing on one side; no movement at all on the hemiplegic side. If there is no response in the limbs of either side to painful stimulation over the orbit *or* the sternum, quadriplegia becomes a likely diagnosis.

Examination for muscle tone may be accomplished in the upper extremities by holding the arm vertical and the forearm horizontal over the face. Even patients in midbrain coma still have enough tone in a normally innervated arm to slow the fall of the forearm. The hemiplegic arm falls freely to the face, and the examiner must be careful at this point to catch the hand before it actually hits the face.

Similarly, if the examiner flexes the patient's knees so the heels approach the buttocks, with the patient supine, the paralyzed lower extremity falls to the side farther and more rapidly when the knees are released. Deep tendon reflexes and Trömner's and Babinski's signs may be examined during coma as they are in the normal subject.

Examination for Loss of Body Sensation

Graduated pressure with a pencil or the handle of the reflex hammer over the fingernail or toenail pulp produces graduated degrees of deep pain. If sensory pathways are intact, even patients in midbrain and lower stages of coma respond with facial grimace or with decerebrate or decorticate posturing. The clinician watches for these responses as he gradually increases nail pulp pressure and notes results from stimulation of the two sides of the body.

Family Members and the Examination During Coma

Anxious family members are usually present when the physician makes his rounds on a comatose patient. Once their patient is comatose, they have no means of telling whether he is improving or dying. I usually perform the coma examination and the neurological examination in front of such families and interpret the results directly to them, so they may have a basis for understanding the results in concrete terms, and can participate intelligently in the decisions that must be made about further care.

Examination for the response to deep pain may be performed without alarming the family if the examiner avoids gestures of raw power as he goes about his testing. It is important to avoid maneuvers such as pinching of the skin, because these do not produce as clear a diagnostic response as deep pain, and they leave unsightly bruises on the patient's body. Families understand the need for a diagnostic examination and appreciate interpretation of results, but they are understandably upset by an examination which needlessly disfigures their patient. If the family can help during the examination, such as by holding the head properly for cold caloric stimulation, they are usually grateful for a chance to particpate in the care of their patient. If examinations are done *with* the family in this manner, doctor, patient, and family all benefit, and the author highly recommends that the reader learn to perform his examinations with the family in attendance.

A Special Case: The Locked-In Syndrome

Occasionally an elderly patient is admitted "in coma" or develops a cardiac arrhythmia or cardiorespiratory collapse from which he does not recover, even though cardiac function returns to normal. Examination reveals that he is not comatose but quadriplegic. This is called the "locked-in syndrome" and is caused by infarction of the motor system in the base of the brainstem.

The locked-in syndrome is recognized by the fact that the patient's eyes may be open from time to time and may follow the examiner as he moves about. When the eyes are closed, there may be normal blinking, which is associated with a waking brain. Nurses may report that they feel the patient wakes and sleeps, although they cannot give specific information about how they know it.

As the clinician begins to talk directly to the patient, he may be able to get a "yes-no" conversation going, using blinks or eye movements or residual facial twitches, revealing the presence of a normal thinking brain locked up inside a totally paralyzed body and documenting that auditory stimuli reach an essentially intact consciousness! Examination reveals total flaccid quadriplegia, but there is a change of respiratory rate or a slight grimace visible during deep pain stimulation, indicating that sensory information is also transmitted. This terrible syndrome is almost always fatal, either because of extension of the infarct into critical areas of the brainstem or because of the onset of pneumonia.

SUMMARY

The examination for depth and cause of coma and the neurological examination in coma provide the clinician with a clear window into the structure and function of his patient's brain, through which he can visualize the responsible pathologic process, and from which he can call for the appropriate help to consultants, radiologists, or the laboratory as he needs them.

REFERENCES

1. McNealy, D.E., Plum, F.: Brainstem Dysfunction with Supratentorial Mass Lesions. Arch. Neurol. 7:10–32, 1962.
2. Plum, F., Posner, J.B.: *Diagnosis of Stupor and Coma,* 2nd edition, F.A. Davis Co., Philadelphia, 1972.

CHAPTER 9

Seizure Disorders

INTRODUCTION

Early classifications of the epilepsies were based solely on the external manifestations of seizures, but they proved to be inadequate because they could not distinguish between the various *causes* of the seizure disorders, and did not help to predict the response to treatment. Modern classifications of the epilepsies are based on modern information about the anatomy and physiology of the brain. Clinical symptomatology of seizures remains an important part of seizure classification, but its importance is diminished by the availability of more incisive diagnostic criteria.

New classifications of the epilepsies are modifications of the internationally accepted Classification of Epileptic Seizures and of the Epilepsies, but this listing is more complete than we require for this volume, so the author has chosen the modification of Schmidt and Wilder[7] because it emphasizes the distinction between primary generalized epilepsy, and all other seizure disorders. This distinction is fundamental to an understanding of the epilepsies because it is based on the concept of a central, brain-integrating mechanism, first described by Penfield and Jasper.[6] Malfunction of the central integrating mechanism is the direct cause of primary generalized seizures. A focal seizure, which begins in some specific cortical region, becomes generalized only if it first excites the central integrating mechanism to join in the seizure activity.

This concept arose from analysis of the electrographic characteristics of seizure discharges. Penfield and Jasper found that certain EEGs were punctuated by fairly stereotyped discharges, which burst synchronously and symmetrically from both sides of the brain, and appeared quite similar from patient to patient. Other EEGs displayed greatly variable forms of focal and multifocal discharges. Penfield and Jasper surmised that the generalized sterotyped bursts originated in some deep midline structure, whose function is to integrate brain activity. They named this the "central integrating mechanism," and called this type of seizure "centrencephalic." Although the complexity of the International Classification blurs the outlines somewhat, and uses different terms, it, and all other modern classifications of the epilepsies are based on the distinction between primary generalized (centrencephalic) and partial (focal or multifocal) seizures. The interested reader is invited to compare the simplified version in this volume with the Internation Classification of Epileptic Seizures[3] and the International Classification of the Epilepsies.[4]

New terminology accompanies the new classifications, which avoid words like "petit mal" and "grand mal" because these have become imprecise owing to long and uncritical use. As we proceed, the reader will learn that not all major seizures are "grand mal," and not all minor seizures are "petit mal." Because of the imprecise connotations which have become attached to some older terms, the International Classifications attempted to avoid their use altogether. We shall emphasize the more ponderous modern terminology and use older terms in a more precise manner, indicating them in parentheses.

CLASSIFICATION OF THE EPILEPSIES

Primary Generalized Epilepsy (Centrencephalic Epilepsy)

About 10 percent of seizure patients have primary generalized epilepsy. This is the only seizure disorder which is a specific heritable disease. Other seizure disorders are symptoms of some *other* underlying brain lesion. Primary generalized epilepsy is caused by an autosomal dominant gene with incomplete expressivity.[5] Patients with this disease inherit *only* a tendency to have three specific kinds of seizure. They have no other neurological disability, have normal intelligence, and a completely normal neurological examination. Their seizures consist of: 1) typical absence attacks (*true* petit mal); 2) generalized convulsive seizures (*true* grand mal); and 3) myoclonic and akinetic seizures. These three seizure types represent a *single seizure syndrome*, but because the seizures

TABLE 9-1

Classification of the Epilepsies

I. *Primary Generalized Epilepsy (centrencephalic epilepsy)*

    A. Typical absence attack (*true* petit mal)
    B. Generalized convulsive seizure (*true* grand mal)
    C. Myoclonic seizures and akinetic seizures

II. *Partial Seizures With or Without Generalized Spread (focal or multifocal seizure disorder)*

    A. Partial seizures with simple symptomatology
        Partial motor seizures
        Partial sensory seizures
    B. Partial seizures with complex symptomatology
        Automatisms (psychomotor seizures)
        Psychical (hallucinations and illusions)
        Visceral and autonomic
          Olfactory
          Gustatory
          Visceral sensations
          Affective sensations

III. *Epileptic Syndromes*

    A. Myoclonus syndromes
        Hereditary myoclonus epilepsy
        Myoclonus as an accompaniment of systemic or cerebral disease
    B. Diseases accompanied by seizure activity
    C. Infantile spasms

IV. *Unclassified Seizures*

themselves differ from each other, we shall discuss them individually.

Typical Absence Attacks (*True* Petit Mal)

Typical absence attacks develop between six and ten years of age, and may continue throughout life. Even without treatment typical absence attacks may be infrequent, or they may occur up to several hundred times each day. The electrographic abnormality of

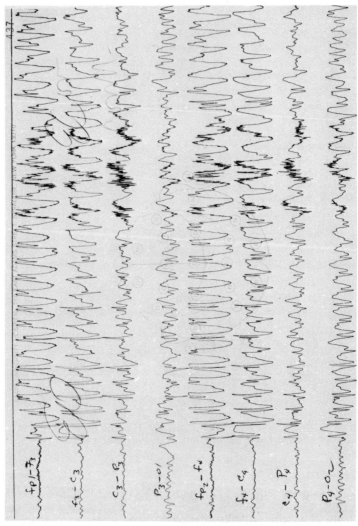

Figure 9-1. *Prolonged burst of 3-Hz spike-wave discharge associated with typical absence attacks.*

typical absence attacks consists of the classic 3-Hz spike-wave discharge, with synchronous and symmetrical bursts from all parts of the calvarium. The voltage is maximal anteriorly. Onset is sudden, and cessation of the discharge is just as sudden. These discharges may be precipitated by repetitive flashes of bright light and especially by forced hyperventilation. In fact, forced hyperventilation is a diagnostic test, because primary generalized epilepsy is the only type of seizure disorder which is precipitated in this manner.

In order to produce a typical absence attack, the child is asked to breathe hard, and the effort is timed. Hyperventilation continues for three minutes unless an attack occurs earlier. A one-minute effort with no seizure is an inadequate test, and so is a three-minute effort unless the child is breathing *hard.* As the child begins to hyperventilate, he is asked to signal each time the examiner snaps his fingers, and this stimulus is given periodically during the test to be sure the child is responsive.

Suddenly, the child stops hyperventilating. He no longer signals to the snapping fingers. He fails to respond to verbal commands. He stares blankly and may blink his eyes rapidly. There are occasional minor twitches of the upper extremities. If he is attached to the machine, the EEG discloses 3-Hz spike-wave discharges during the attack, which cease as he regains consciousness.

The attack usually lasts 3-10 seconds, and unless the examiner is fully alert, he will miss it completely. At the end of the attack, the child resumes hyperventilation as though nothing had occurred. If he is questioned, he is likely to deny that he was unconscious, but he is unable to repeat what was said to him during the attack.

Generalized Convulsive Seizures (*True* Grand Mal)

Usually, generalized convulsive seizures and myoclonic seizures develop in adolescence or in early adult life, as a natural consequence of the genetic inheritance. There is no aura. The seizure itself is symmetrical, and has no sign of a focal onset. The *true* grand mal attack interrupts ongoing activity without warning. The patient is suddenly unconscious and falling. He is rigid for 15-45 seconds in the tonic phase of the seizure, his face is contorted, and he gradually assumes a dusky, then alarmingly purple hue. If his tongue is between his teeth during this phase, it may be badly bitten and flattened because of the prolonged biting during the tonic phase. As the seizure progresses, the tonic phase is replaced by repetitive symmetrical "clonic" jerks of arms and legs. He begins to take short breaths during the end of the clonic phase and gradually loses his cyanosis. Some patients awaken shortly after the seizure ends. During this period they are confused and may be extremely restless. Then they quickly fall asleep again. When they finally recover fully, they do not remember events of this period. When they reawaken 30 minutes to several hours later, mentation is intact, but the patient may be fatigued and sore. Some patients do not display this dramatic seizure sequence during a generalized convulsive seizure. Theirs may be a much more benign-appearing seizure, even though the electrical characteristics are essentially identical.

Myoclonic and Akinetic Seizures

Myoclonic seizures consist of small, symmetrical, rhythmic extensor jerks of the upper extremities. They may cause the person to drop his toothbrush or his coffee cup. They do not cause unconsciousness unless they progress to a generalized convulsive seizure. They frequently occur immediately after awakening from sleep.

Akinetic seizures may be a variant of typical myoclonic attacks. A patient with akinetic seizures drops to the ground suddenly "like a bag of bones," with no loss of consciousness. He is able to rise again immediately. This may occur because of a sudden massive myoclonic jerk of the lower extremities, or because of actual sudden loss of muscle tone.

As the patient with primary generalized epilepsy reaches adolescence and develops the generalized convulsive and myoclonic seizures, his EEG changes to include 4 1/2–5-Hz polyspike-wave discharges, which are still synchronous and nearly symmetrical. By now, they are even more prominent in frontal parasagittal regions of the calvarium and less prominent in temporal and occipital leads. This pattern is still activated by repetitive flashes of bright light and by hyperventilation, but now photic stimulation is more likely to provoke a generalized convulsive seizure, while hyperventilation is likely to produce only seizure discharges on the EEG, unaccompanied by clinical seizure activity.

Partial Seizures With or Without Generalized
Spread(Focal or Multifocal Seizures)

If 10 percent of seizure patients have primary generalized epilepsy, then almost all the rest have partial seizures, which are due, at least in part, to specific brain lesions of many kinds. Most of these lesions are static, related to birth trauma or anoxia; or to infection, trauma, or vascular disease at some other time of life. But in some, there is a progressive etiology, like tumor, degenerative disease, meningitis, or some specific metabolic disease. The manifestations of a focal seizure depend upon the site of the seizure focus, not the pathological process that causes it. Since the age of onset, course of the seizure disorder, and especially the onset and course of permanent neurological disability depend directly on the pathologic process, these clinical features determine what kind of evaluation the physician will recomend, in order to arrive at the ultimate diagnosis.

Whereas primary generalized seizures have no aura at all, partial seizures *may* begin with an aura whose manifestations represent distorted function of the region of the seizure focus. The aura does not warn of an impending seizure; it *is* the seizure itself, beginning locally in the still conscious brain and recorded by still normally functioning portions of that brain. The aura may end with unconsciousness when the central integrating mechanism is activated, spreading seizure activity diffusely and producing a *secondary* generalized convulsive seizure. If the central integrating mechanism is not activated, the aura remains as a localized discharge, and eventually subsides. Like asymmetrical major seizures, and Todd's paralysis, the aura serves to establish that the seizure had a focal origin and to localize the seizure focus. Table 9-2 lists many of the common seizure auras and indicates their usual site of origin.

If it does become generalized, the focal nature of the generalized seizure may continue to be evident as asymmetrical motor activity during the seizure itself, or during the postictal period as transient paralysis on the opposite side of the body from the seizure focus. This is called Todd's paralysis. It usually lasts only a few minutes or a few hours but may remain as long as several days after a seizure. These asymmetrical aspects of secondary generalized seizures (major focal seizures) may be used as localizing information if they occur in a seizure patient who has no aura. They are sure signs that the seizure had a focal onset and serve to alert the clinician to the need for information about the underlying pathological process.

The EEG in focal seizures is quite variable because of the variety of seizure foci and of pathologic etiologies. Some patients with focal seizures have a completely normal waking EEG, and display seizure activity only during sleep. This is especially characteristic of tem-

---

TABLE 9-2

Anatomic Origins of Common Seizure Auras

Prefrontal
  Lesions in prefrontal regions may produce initial unconsciousness with no aura. These seizures may be only slightly asymmetrical. They must be identified by EEG and physical examination.

Frontal
  Head and eye contraversion
  Head and eye ipsiversion (rare)
  Speech arrest

Frontal Parasagittal
  Tonic posturing seizures

Motor Strip
  Elemental muscle twitches in the face, upper or lower extremity, depending on the region of motor strip affected

Sensory Strip
  Rarely produces seizures but may produce localized sensory auras

Occipital
  Rarely produces seizures, but unformed visual hallucinations may occur

Temporal
  Psychic auras
    Emotional (fear, rage)
    Formed visual hallucinations
    Formed auditory hallucinations
    Forced speech (right temporal)
    Speech arrest (left temporal)
    Macropsia, micropsia
    Déjà vu, jamais vu
  Visceral auras
    Unpleasant olfactory and gustatory hallucinations
    Epigastric rising sensations

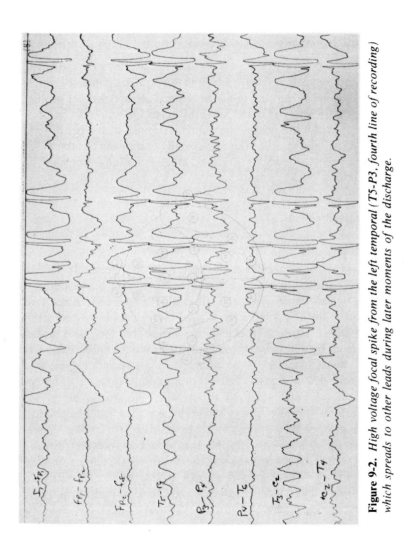

Figure 9-2. *High voltage focal spike from the left temporal (T5-P3, fourth line of recording) which spreads to other leads during later moments of the discharge.*

poral lobe foci. Abnormal wave forms range from occasional sharp waves to frank high-voltage multifocal spikes and slow activity, depending on the ultimate brain pathology.

Epileptic Syndromes

Certain progressive illnesses, like Creutzfeldt-Jakob disease, hereditary myoclonus, epilepsy, and other hereditable metabolic diseases cause major and minor multifocal seizures as part of their symptomatology. These are never mistaken for simple seizure disorders, because the neurological manifestations of the disease are more disabling than the seizures. Usually there is no treatment for the disease, but the seizures may be at least partially controlled by medications.

Semantic Problems

Atypical vs. Typical Absence Attacks

Most clinicians use the term "petit mal" incorrectly. In general medical parlance, it means a "minor seizure," but the reader now knows that we can distinguish various kinds of minor seizures from each other to the patient's advantage. "Atypical absence attacks" are minor seizures with brief unconsciousness, but they are often accompanied by automatic movements of face and limbs. These are usually focal seizures, whose origin is in the temporal lobe, and could properly be termed "minor psychomotor attacks." The patient is usually older than six to ten when the attacks begin, has fewer attacks during the day, and may have a history or a physical examination that suggests focal brain disease. Unlike typical absence attacks, the atypical absence attack may evolve directly into a secondary generalized seizure (major focal seizure). Instead of the diffuse 3-Hz spike and wave of typical absence, the EEG of the patient with atypical absence displays focal or multifocal spikes or focal background slowing.

Lastly, the patient with atypical absence attacks responds best to phenobarbital or phenytoin, and does not respond to ethosuximide or trimethadione, while the child with typical absence attacks responds just oppositely. The importance of distinguishing typical from atypical absence attacks revolves around the different effective treatments and around their distinctly different etiologies. These are important differences, which should be reflected in different terminology.

True Petit Mal vs. Petit Mal *Variant*

Here is more confusing terminology, but this time the confusion originates from the electroencephalographers, not the general medical community. If an EEG report mentions petit mal *variant*, it indicates the electrographic abnormality of 2-Hz spike-wave forms. This electrographic picture has nothing to do with *true* petit mal (typical absence) attacks. It occurs in severely brain-damaged children with major and minor multifocal seizures, mental retardation, and neurological disability. The use of this confusing term is unfortunate for both the clinician and his patient.

LABORATORY EVALUATION OF SEIZURE PATIENTS

We have already emphasized the importance of the EEG in distinguishing primary generalized epilepsy from the partial (focal) seizure disorders. The EEG may disclose the classic forms of primary generalized epilepsy or it may show multifocal seizure discharges, removing anxiety about the presence of a single primary brain tumor. On the other hand, the classic electrographic signs of a mass lesion, a spike focus, accompanied by background slowing, demands diagnostic evaluation. But even the EEG is not an absolutely necessary part of the evaluation of a seizure patient. Decisions about the extent of each patient's workup depend upon the judgment of the physician.

If the clinical evidence suggests that evaluation will reveal progressive treatable disease, the workup must pursue that diagnosis until it is either established or proved wrong. Certainly, all patients with changing neurological symptoms, those whose seizures began after age 25 and those whose seizure disorder is worsening or uncontrollable, need more than a cursory examination. Even so, angiography is not indicated unless there is clinical evidence of structural disease, confirmed by CT or nuclear brain scans.

MEDICINAL MANAGEMENT OF SEIZURE PATIENTS

We may now consider the goal of anticonvulsant therapy, and some problems with management. The goal is clear:

That the patient be seizure-free, and free of toxic side effects from his medications for the rest of his life.

This goal affects the choice of medications, since the patient will take them for many years, and cumulative toxicity is undesirable. It also determines the nature of the relationship between doctor and patient, because the patient needs a comprehensive education in seizure management from the onset of his treatment. The goal cannot always be reached, but it is legitimate to strive toward it, important to recognize failure, and to *act* when failure occurs.

Who should be treated for seizure disorder and for how long? This is a matter of therapeutic philosophy, but I recommend treatment after the first *unprovoked* seizure. An unprovoked seizure is one which arises during the natural course of a person's life, not immediately after an accident or during the natural course of viral encephalitis or some other acute insult. The college student who has been up dancing till dawn and has a seizure, does so in the natural course of his life. Probably even if he lives a more sedate life, he will have more seizures without medication, but in any case, he does not need the danger, embarrassment, and loss of social privileges that result from a seizure, and he may want to dance till dawn again. He can do this without fear if he takes a therapeutic dose of medication.

If the first seizure occurs after puberty, there is a good chance that the person will have seizures later in life if he stops his medication. If absolute seizure control is established with nontoxic, inexpensive medications, there is no need for the physician to experiment further with that life by stopping them. The patient should plan to stay on his pills forever unless taking medications is so onerous to him that he demands to stop. In that case, he may want to stop his pills, at least temporarily, in order to discover whether having seizures or taking medication is worse. When the seizures reappear after he stops, he will be able to decide more clearly.

Once the decision has been made to treat, several essential facts bear directly on the quality of seizure control and plans for treatment.

Blood Anticonvulsant Determinations

Seizure control is directly related to the concentration of anti-convulsant in the blood. This fact is of central importance to the patient who seeks absolute control of his seizures. It has been established for all major convulsants and determines the first steps of treatment. If physician and patient have not resolved that the patient shall always have a blood level in the therapeutic range, they cannot plan to establish permanent control of seizures. If both doctor and patient know the therapeutic range, they can agree together on a desirable blood level and adjust dosage accordingly. This is an important initial part of the patient's education.

"Range of normal" has a different meaning for blood levels than for the value of the blood hemoglobin. It does not mean that any blood level within the range is acceptable for any patient. It means that some patients stop having seizures with as little medication as the lower figure, and most patients are not toxic as long as the levels do not rise above the higher figure. Even so, some patients will develop definite signs of toxicity with levels in the therapeutic range while others, especially patients taking phenobarbital, may need much higher blood levels than the published "therapeutic range" for seizure control, and still not feel toxic.

In nearly all cases, it is best to aim initially for a blood level in the middle of the therapeutic range. This will assure most patients of seizure control and will rapidly identify patients whose seizure disorder will be difficult to control. Figures for the usual therapeutic range of each anticonvulsant are included with discussions of the various available medications.

Biological Half-Life

Most anticonvulsants have a biological half-life of 24 hours or longer. Because of this, the medications accumulate slowly in the body after treatment begins, and finally establish steady-state blood levels when metabolism and excretion equal the daily dose. Blood levels do not drop precipitously if the patient forgets a dose and, by the same token, they do not immediately rise to previous blood levels once he has missed a dose unless he makes it up. Long biological half-life means that dosage schedules for nearly all anticonvulsants may be arranged for the patient's convenience. Nearly all

192 / PRACTICAL CLINICAL NEUROLOGY

may be taken once a day at bedtime or at any other single time of the day. Such a dosage schedule allows the patient better compliance with his prescription. Because seizure control depends on the blood levels and the blood levels rise gradually before they reach a steady state, seizure control cannot be evaluated during the first three weeks after a medication change. On the other hand, *any* seizure which occurs later than that time demands an explanation.

There are several tricks which can help patients toward better compliance with their medication. First is the once-a-day dosage schedule. People forget noon doses but less often forget a once-a-day schedule. Second is to make up missed doses. If an entire day's dose is missed, it may be made up the following day with no danger, and blood levels will be back where they belong. Third is the one-week bottle. Patients buy anticonvulsants once every month, or every three months. These bottles are so large that patients have no accurate knowledge of their daily and weekly compliance, but if they fill a small bottle on each Sunday and see to it that the medication is *gone* by the following Sunday, they have a constant check and know when they have to make up missed doses.

These statements are not valid for patients using valproic acid, which is rapidly and completely absorbed, reaching peak blood levels in about an hour after each dose. Because the biological half-life is only 8-15 hours, valproic acid blood levels fluctuate widely during the day.[8,10] It is not even certain that the blood levels of valproic acid determine seizure control. Perhaps an unknown metabolite acts as the anticonvulsant. The medication may even control seizures by its known effect on critical enzyme systems in the brain. The patient should establish at least a three times-a-day dosage schedule and attempt to keep a steady supply of medication available to his body, making up missed doses from the previous few hours but not from the previous day.

Treatment Plans

If the new seizure patient learns about long biological half-life, and gradually rising anticonvulsant blood levels, he can understand that he may have side effects during the first 2-3 weeks of treatment, but he will know that the eventual blood level, which is taken three weeks hence, will determine the eventual dosage recommendation. This may allow him to comply better with the initial recommendations, at least until the initial blood level has been established. He will understand that a seizure occuring during the three weeks after any medication change will not prompt another change of dose, but he may not understand all this well enough to continue taking his medications indefinitely.

The most common cause for recurrent seizures after a permanent dose is established by these means is that the patient forgot to take his pills. Unless they are on a one-week bottle, people do not believe they have forgotten doses, especially if the next seizure occurs several months later. They need advanced instructions to have blood levels drawn *that day* if they ever have another seizure. When they call with the report of the seizure, immediate blood levels will give the reason. A markedly lower blood level on that day strongly suggests that the patient has forgotten his pills. If the blood level is repeated two weeks later after he *concentrated* on taking his medications and the result is again up to the therapeutic goal, the diagnosis is established. The seizure and resultant blood levels educate a patient rapidly if he is given access to the *entire process* and the *specific results* of his laboratory examinations.

On the other hand, if the blood level after a seizure is again at the initial therapeutic value, this is a clear indication to increase the dose. The strategy for ultimate seizure control involves initial use of a single medication. An initial blood level is established, and the dose is increased each time a seizure occurs until the seizures stop. If the patient becomes toxic before he achieves seizure control on one medication, the dose is lowered slightly and a second medication is added to the first. Initial blood level goals for the second medication are again around the middle range.

Children with primary generalized epilepsy and typical absence attacks are an exception. Ethosuximide stops the typical absence attacks but does not prevent the generalized convulsive seizures which are expected to develop in the future. Ethosuximide and phenobarbital together, each prescribed in therapeutic doses, provide excellent protection against both seizure types.

The patient who continues to have seizures after he has arrived at therapeutic doses of two anticonvulsants has a difficult seizure disorder or perhaps still has unrecognized treatable disease. Neurologists are best equipped to manage such patients.

ANTICONVULSANT MEDICATIONS

In this section, we shall consider some of the available anticonvulsant medications. Some are safe, predictable, and effective. Others are less safe or have more specialized uses. The non-neurological clinician will profit if he learns to use phenobarbital, phenytoin, ethosuximide, and trimethadione effectively. He may decide occasionally to use mephobarbital as a substitute for phenobarbital. If he must go further afield for seizure control in an occasional patient, that patient should be advised to consult a neurologist.

Phenobarbital

How supplied: Tablets: 15 mg, 30 mg, 60 mg, 100 mg
      Elixir: 20 mg/5 ml
      Parenteral: (IM or IV) 130 mg/ml
Biological half-life: 2-6 days
Therapeutic blood levels: 15-30 ng/ml (1.5-3.0 mg/100 cc)

Phenobarbital is an extremely predictable medication, with blood levels and resultant therapeutic effectiveness that rise in direct proportion to the daily dose. Its metabolism is not greatly affected by concomitant use of other medications, so doctor and patient may depend on stable seizure control over long periods of time if the patient takes his medication. It is completely and reliably absorbed via oral, intramuscular, and intravenous routes. While some patients cannot tolerate phenobarbital, because of psychological depressive reaction, allergic reaction, or sedation, even in normal therapeutic doses, most patients have no long-term side effects but do achieve excellent seizure control. Lastly, a patient can get completely effective seizure control for about a dollar a month. This is important for patients who take medications for many years.

Some authors recommend phenytoin as the treatment of choice for most seizure disorders with the exception of typical absence attacks and some of the serious seizure disorders of childhood. But the characteristics of predictability, efficacy, and safety with few side effects and low cost have convinced this author that phenobarbital, not phenytoin, is the drug of choice. If phenobarbital fails, there is time enough to add medications with more side effects and less predictability.

Any medication may affect the fetus during the first trimester of pregnancy. In addition to this, phenobarbital and other anticonvulsants have been implicated as a cause for neonatal hemorrhage. This can be prevented by giving the mother an injection of vitamin K as she goes into labor and giving the baby a similar injection at birth.

Mephobarbital (Mebaral®)

How supplied: Tablets: 32 mg, 50 mg, 100 mg, 200 mg
Biological half-life: 2-6 days (as phenobarbital)
Therapeutic blood levels: 15-30 ng/ml (1.5-3.0 mg/100 cc)
(measured as phenobarbital)

Mephobarbital has limited usefulness, but there are some patients who develop a hyperactivity syndrome on phenobarbital. This is especially prominent among children with "minimal brain damage syndrome," but occasional adults have the same reaction to phenobarbital. Even though mephobarbital is transformed into phenobarbital, some of these patients can derive the anticonvulsant benefits of phenobarbital without the psychological side effects of direct phenobarbital therapy. In those few case, mephobarbital is extremely useful. It is more expensive than phenobarbital, so it is not the barbituate treatment of choice. The dose of mephobarbital is approximately 1 1/2–2 times the dose of phenobarbital in order to produce identical blood phenobarbital levels.

Phenytoin (Dilantin®)

How supplied: Capsules: 30 mg, 100 mg
Chewable tablets: 50 mg
Parenteral (IV only!): 50 mg/ml
Suspension (not recommended): 125 mg/5 ml, 30 mg/5 ml
Combinations with other anticonvulsants (not recommended)
Biological half-life: About 24 hours, may be much longer at higher dose (see below)
Therapeutic blood levels: 15-25 ng/ml (1.5-2.5 mg/100 cc)

At therapeutic blood levels, phenytoin is an excellent anticonvulsant. However, phenytoin metabolism is unpredictable because it is affected by extraneous factors. Concomitant use of many different medications may produce either a toxic rise in phenytoin blood levels, or may drop the level even to the point of seizure! Furthermore, phenytoin blood levels do not increase in direct proportion to the dose; indeed, there is a wide variation of blood levels among patients who begin with standard starting doses. After the dose is increased to a certain point, the liver enzyme system becomes saturated, causing a marked prolongation of the biological half-life and literally staggering increases in blood levels after small changes in dose. All this means that there is no certain correlation between the dose and the seizure control, even if the dose remains unchanged.

Phenytoin should be used orally if at all possible. It is well absorbed by this route. It is poorly absorbed intramuscularly, so parenteral phenytoin is best given intravenously. Intravenous phenytoin is given at 50 mg/minute or less to prevent cardiovascular collapse and to lessen the sclerosing effect of the high pH on the recipient vein.

Gum hypertrophy is a frequent complication of phenytoin therapy. This is occasionally severe enough to interfere with tooth eruption in children and is also disfiguring enough to warrant surgical removal of excess tissues. While medically serious side effects are uncommon, they are manifold. If seizures can be controlled without all the problems associated with the use of phenytoin, there is no good reason for the patient to accept them. An appreciable number of babies born to women who take phenytoin have physical and mental defects that have been attributed directly to the effect of phenytoin on the fetus, so women of childbearing age should avoid its use unless they cannot achieve seizure control without it.

Despite its drawbacks, phenytoin is certainly the medication of second choice. If adequate blood levels are established, the anticonvulsant action is comparable to phenobarbital. Patients need to be educated about the possible effects of other medications on their phenytoin metabolism. If they must take other medications from time to time, they should establish whether they need to change phenytoin dosage when they do. They may need more frequent blood level determinations, and they will have to decide to put up with the common irritations associated with the use of this medication.

Ethosuximide (Zarontin®)

How supplied: Gelatin capsules: 250 mg
            Syrup: 250 mg/5 ml
Biological half-life: Children, 30 hours
            Adults, 60 hours
Therapeutic blood levels: 40-120 ng/ml (4.0-12.0 mg/100 cc)

Ethosuximide is the treatment of choice for typical absence attacks of primary generalized epilepsy. It is generally a safe, effective medication, and blood levels remain stable for long treatment periods if the dose is raised to correct for growth. While ethosuximide has many potentially serious side effects, fortunately they are uncommon. Some children develop gastric distress and cannot tolerate ethosuximide therapy. If the child cannot use ethosuximide, trimethadione is a close second choice.

Children with primary generalized epilepsy who are given ethosuximide or trimethadione for suppression of typical absence attacks, should also receive a therapeutic dose of phenobarbital. It is said that ethosuximide or trimethadione "release" major motor seizures if they are not used in conjunction with phenobarbital. Perhaps those seizures merely appear in the natural course of maturation. In either case, these children all have a high probability of developing generalized convulsive seizures, which are not suppressed by ethosuximide or trimethadione alone. For this reason, they should receive the protection of phenobarbital even though generalized convulsive seizures have not yet occurred.

On the other hand, once the child has become an adult, physicians frequently attempt to remove the ethosuximide or trimethadione, believing it to be unnecessary, because the patient may have "grown out" of the typical absence attacks. When this is done, the typical absence attacks may return. Worse yet, generalized convulsive seizures may become more difficult to control in their absence. If an attempt is made to remove these medications, the clinician must be aware of these possibilities and be prepared to reinstitute treatment immediately.

Trimethadione (Tridione®)

How supplied: Capsules: 300 mg
            Chewable tablets: 150 mg
            Solution: 40 mg/ml

Biological half-life: (as dimethadione, DMO) 6-13 days.
Therapeutic blood levels: (measured as DMO)
above 600 ng/ml (60 mg/100 cc)
(blood levels not easily available)

Trimethadione is also indicated for treatment of typical absence attacks if the patient cannot tolerate ethosuximide. The major drawback to its use is that blood levels are not readily available for DMO (dimethadione), its most active metabolite, so this important aspect of seizure management may not be monitored. The usual dose is 600–1500 mg/day depending on the patient's weight.

The five medications discussed above provide seizure control for most patients. Those who still have seizures despite adequate doses of well-chosen medications have difficult seizure disorders. They and their primary care physician will both benefit by a neurological consultation. There are specific, but infrequent, indications for the use of other anticonvulsants, and the neurologist is more likely to be familar with their indications and side effects.

Mephenytoin (Mesantoin®)

How supplied: Tablets: 100 mg
Therapeutic blood levels: 10-16 ng/ml (1.0-1.6 mg/100 cc)

Mephenytoin is closely related to phenytoin. If a hydantoin medication is indicated, but allergic response or gum hypertrophy prohibits the use of phenytoin, this is an excellent substitute. Potentially serious side effects are more common with mephenytoin, which prevents its use as the hydantoin of choice.

Primidone (Mysoline®)

How supplied: Tablets: 50 mg, 250 mg
Suspension (not recommended): 250 mg/5 ml
Biological half-life: primidone 3-24 hours
phenylethymalonamide (PEMA) 24-48 hours
phenobarbital 2-6 days
Therapeutic blood levels: (measured as phenobarbital)
15-30 ng/ml (1.5-3.0 mg/100 cc)

Primidone has anticonvulsant effects of its own, but the principal anticonvulsant effect derives from its biotransformation to phenylethymalonamide (PEMA) and phenobarbital. It is extraordinarily expensive and is more irritating to the stomach than phenobarbital. For these reasons, it should not be used as a phenobarbital substitute unless there is a specific neurological indication. If primidone is prescribed, phenobarbital is discontinued.

Carbamazepine (Tegretol®)

How supplied: Tablets: 200 mg
Biological half-life:15-72 hours
Therapeutic blood levels: 6-10 ng/ml (0.6-1.0 mg/100 cc)

Carbamazepine has had only about 15 years of general use abroad and much less in this country, so long-term side effects are not yet known. Short-term side effects of carbamazepine include leukopenia and more serious indications of bone marrow depression. Carbamazepine is recommended for treatment of tic douloureux and of seizures that cannot be controlled by other measures.

Clonazepam (Clonopin®)

How supplied: Tablets: 0.5 mg, 1.0 mg, 2.0 mg
Biological half-life: 20-40 hours (adult)
Therapeutic blood levels: 10-50 ng/ml. (1.0-5.0 mg/100 cc)
                         (blood levels not easily available)

Clonazepam is useful in the treatment of myoclonus seizures, and some of the severe minor seizures associated with diffuse brain damage in childhood. It may have some application in treatment of typical absence attacks if routine medications fail. It is a new medication, therefore long-term side effects are not known.

Valproic Acid (Depakene®)

How supplied: Capsules: 250 mg
              Syrup: 250 mg/5 cc
Biological half-life: 8-15 hours

Valproic acid was introduced in 1967 for general use in France. It is newly released in this country. The short biological half-life and rapid absorption cause marked fluctuations in blood levels even if it is taken on a three-times-per-day schedule. Investigators have not found good correlation between blood levels of valproic acid and seizure control.[8,10] Frequently, there is a lapse of a week from onset of treatment to beginning of seizure control, which suggests that either an undetected metabolite or the known inhibition of certain enzyme systems may be acting indirectly to produce the anticonvulsant effect. Valproic acid appears best suited to the treatment of typical absence attacks and treatment of some other minor seizures. Until this medication is better understood, and the cumulative side effects of long use are known, it is best withheld unless other medications have failed.*

STATUS EPILEPTICUS*

Status epilepticus describes continuous seizure activity or seizures that recur so frequently that the patient fails to recover between attacks. It is usually a sign of serious intracranial disease or a sign that the seizure patient has neglected his pills. It is of prime importance to discover the cause for status epilepticus when it occurs, as well as to treat the seizures.

Intravenous diazepam (Valium®) is the treatment of choice for status epilepticus. As little as 2 mg may stop the seizures permanently. Other patients continue to have seizures after many doses, each up to 20 or 30 mg. Phenobarbital or some other long-acting anticonvulsant should be started at the same time diazepam is given to provide long-term control of seizures.*

Occasionally, patients with aggressive brain disease, such as drug or alcohol withdrawal seizures, meningoencephalitis, or other toxic-metabolic encephalopathies, continue to have frequent major seizures despite the use of large doses of diazepam and other anticonvulsants. Because of the constant major seizure activity, body temperature rises, further aggravating the situation. Untreated, this syndrome may be rapidly fatal.

In such cases, controlled hypothermia may be lifesaving and usually stops the seizures completely. Such patients are already admitted to the intensive care unit, with respirator and cardiac

*See addendum on page 204.

monitors connected. A constant rectal temperature monitor is inserted, and an initial temperature goal of 90-93°F (32-33°C) is usually sufficient to stop the seizures. If the process is reversible, seizures may be controlled with limited hypothermia; but when this procedure is instituted as a measure of desperation in patients with progressive disease, hypothermia merely delays death.

Cooling blankets may *maintain* lowered temperatures, but they are usually inadequate to lower the temperature initially; ice is usually necessary for initial cooling. Rub the skin over the entire body first, so it glows with increased perfusion. Then apply moistened bath towels, cover these with generous quantities of ice, and continue rubbing to hasten body cooling. Be certain that the skin remains red and that ice gets to all areas effectively. Usually, the fever may be reduced by 10°F in about 30 minutes. Icing should stop three or four degrees before the goal is reached, because the temperature will continue to drift downward after the ice is removed.

Controlled hypothermia may be maintained for 24 hours or longer, depending upon the clinical situation. Body temperature may be lowered further; but at some point, the clinician must decide between the danger of death by cardiac arrhythmia, and the discomfort of watching his patient develop continuous seizures that lead to death. Usually, in such cases, the disease process is known, so family and physician know that the prognosis is hopeless in any case.

During hypothermia, medication doses may be reduced if seizures stop, and blood levels should be monitored carefully so that dosage may be reduced to compensate for slowed drug metabolism. As temperature is raised, it is important to be certain that blood levels remain in the high therapeutic range. If seizures remain under control, the blood levels may be reduced later.

Patients with status epilepticus, especially those who need controlled hypothermia, are comatose and cannot take medications by mouth. Rather than give repeated doses of highly irritating phenytoin by vein, it is better to insert a nasogastric tube and give all anticonvulsants by this route. This allows the clinician to monitor stomach contents for stress hemorrhage, and provides the best route of administration for all anticonvulsants except diazepam, which must be given intravenously.

The seizure patient who has forgotten his medications may be known to the physician. In this case, the patient whose normal medications are phenobarbital or phenytoin may receive these medications intravenously to restore therapeutic blood levels rapidly, and stop the seizures. Thereafter, the situation needs a serious discussion with patient and family in an attempt to avoid a repetition. In a previously healthy patient, status epilepticus is a serious symptom which demands prompt and complete evaluation to discover the cause.

ALCOHOL WITHDRAWAL SEIZURES

"Rum fits" generally occur during the 24-48 hours after the chronic alcoholic has sharply decreased his dose of spirits. Treatment with intravenous diazepam or phenobarbital, followed by oral or intramuscular phenobarbital during the next 72 hours is generally adequate to prevent more seizures.

Alcohol withdrawal seizures may be a prelude to delerium tremens, so it is valuable to observe the patient during the next several days in order to treat DT's promptly if they do appear.

It is generally of little value to prescribe chronic use of anticonvulsants to the alcoholic, because he will have more trouble staying on steady doses of medication than a normal person and will not have therapeutic blood levels when he needs them.

Alcohol withdrawal seizures are primary generalized seizures with no aura and no focal sign. The alcoholic who has focal seizures has a focal brain lesion and needs a diagnosis.

SEIZURES VS. SYNCOPE

It is usually easy to distinguish seizure from syncope. The usual syncopal attack occurs while the patient is standing or sitting. He usually is warned by a dizzy spell or lightheadedness and has had that symptom before without becoming unconscious. He knows that sitting or lying down usually stops the symptoms, and realizes that this time he did not get down fast enough. Frequently, syncope patients report visual blackout before the loss of consciousness, which does not occur with seizure. Syncope due to heart disease is generally accompanied by a history of cardiac disease or arrhythmia on examination. The Holter monitor has been of great service in the documentation of occasional arrhythmias when it is used over a period of time at home and interpreted after a monitored attack has occurred.

On the other hand, most seizure patients have a clear and diagnostic history. There is a standard aura, or a convulsive component to the attack, or, despite lack of history, the tongue has deep ridges on the edges and flattening where the teeth bit down on it during the seizure. This appearance is diagnostic of a major motor seizure, since it is not duplicated by the tongue laceration, which occurs if the patient falls, striking his jaw and biting the tongue in that manner.

What of the person whose attack occurred without witness, who reports no postictal confusion, no aura, and a brief or untimed period of unconsciousness? The EEG may be of help if the history points toward a diagnosis of seizure, but if the clinician leans toward a diagnosis of syncope, even an abnormal EEG should not change his mind without more evidence. The poorly described syncopal attack should not consign a patient to life-long use of phenobarbital. It is worthwhile to *establish* the diagnosis. The patient can usually live carefully for a time, and be aware that descriptive information will be of great value. Usually only one or two more attacks are sufficient to establish the diagnosis and then appropriate treatment can begin.

SUMMARY

The interested reader will find a rich literature concerning the clinical, social, and electrophysiologic aspects of seizure disorders. The author would suggest that further reading begin with one of the monographs listed in the references at the end of this chapter.[1,2,7,9] Fortunately, most patients with seizure disorder can be treated successfully if they and their physician cooperate in the management of their disease.

REFERENCES

1. Aird, R.B., Woodbury, D.M.: *The Management of Epilepsy.* Charles C Thomas, Springfield, Ill.,1974.
2. Eadie, M.J., Tyrer, J.H.: *Anticonvulsant Therapy.* Churchill, Livingstone, Edinburgh, London, 1974.
3. Gastaut, H.: Clinical and Electroencephalographical Classification of Epileptic Seizures. Epilepsia 11:102–113, 1970.
4. Merlis, J.K.: Proposal for an International Classification of the Epilepsies. Epilepsia 11:114–119, 1970.

5. Metrakos, J.D.: Heredity as an Etiological Factor. In: *Disorders of the Developing Nervous System.* Fields, W.S. and Desmond, M.M. (Eds): Charles C Thomas, Springfield, Ill.,1961.
6. Penfield, W., Jasper, H.: *Epilepsy and the Functional Anatomy of the Human Brain.* Little, Brown and Co., Boston, 1954.
7. Schmidt, R.P., and Wilder, B.J.: *Epilepsy.* F.A. Davis Co., Philadelphia, 1968.
8. Simon, D., Penry, J.K.: Sodium Di-N-Propylacetate (DPA) in the Treatment of Epilepsy: A Review. Epilepsia, 16:549–573, 1975.
9. Woodbury, D.M., Penry, J.K., Schmidt, R.P.: *Antiepileptic Drugs.* Raven Press, New York, 1972.
10. Wulff, K., Flachs, H., Wúrtz-Jorgensen, A., Gram, L.: Clinical Pharmacological Aspects of Valproate Sodium. Epilepsia, 18:149–157, 1977.

ADDENDUM

While the volume has been in production, valproic acid has proved itself to be an excellent anticovulsant, despite several deaths that have occurred in children.

Valproic acid blood levels are now available. It appears that an effective therapeutic range is 50–100 ng/ml.

Patients in status epilepticus may come under complete seizure control through the use of retention enemas composed of valproic acid syrup diluted in small quantities of water, or given through a nasogastric tube in doses of 250–500 mg every six hours. Valproic acid delivered in this manner may effectively stop status epilepticus even when massive doses of intravenous diazepam and other anticonvulsants have failed. In such cases, valproic acid may be unaccompanied by the severe respiratory depression that is so troublesome after large doses of intravenous diazepam.[1,2]

Valproic acid still should not be used as a first choice in epilepsy, because long-term side efefcts are unknown. Phenobarbital is effective, cheap, and safe; and it should not be abandoned. Nonetheless, valproic acid is highly effective in the control of both minor and major seizures, and it should be prescribed by the neurological consultant if other anticonvulsants have failed to provide complete seizure control.

REFERENCES

1. Barnes, S.E., Bland, D., Cole, A.P., Evans, A.R.: The Use of Sodium Valproate in a Case of Status Epilepticus. Dev. Med. Child Neurol. 18:236–238, 1976.
2. Thorpy, M.: Rectal Valproate Syrup and Status Epilepticus. In preparation.

CHAPTER 10

Adult Dementias

INTRODUCTION

Dementia is a symptom of diffuse cerebral dysfunction. It is common among adults, especially among the aged, but during the past few decades, advances in the scientific aspects of medical practice have provided diagnosis and even treatment for some dementing diseases. Because we now know that Creutzfeldt-Jakob disease, progressive multifocal leukoencephalopathy, and subacute sclerosing panencephalitis are caused by infection, not "degeneration," these diseases are no longer included in the discussion of dementia. Instead, they comprise major topics in the chapter on the Slow Viral Infections (pp. 251ff). Normal pressure hydrocephalus is a relatively newly recognized entity, whose pathogenesis and treatment are at least partially understood. It, too, is discussed elsewhere (pp. 28-31). Systemic diseases, which occasionally cause dementia, are usually recognized and treated before the dementia appears.

This means that we are left with a limited number of common, but untreatable dementing diseases, whose etiology is unknown; and with a large number of potentially treatable diseases which only rarely produce dementia as an initial symptom.

We shall also distinguish between dementia, which is a symptom of diffuse brain disease, and the amnestic syndrome, which is distinct and caused by focal pathology.

THE AMNESTIC SYNDROME

In the section on mental status examination (pp. 13ff), we discussed the differences between hysterical concern about dementia, dementia itself, and the amnestic syndrome. The amnestic syndrome was defined as an *isolated inability to make new permanent memories.* The amnestic syndrome is also accompanied by some loss of previously made permanent memories; however, this feature does not distinguish the amnestic syndrome from the other dementias. Differential diagnosis for the amnestic syndrome is limited anatomically to bilateral, focal cerebral lesions which destroy structures of the medial temporal lobe, the fornix, and mamillary bodies. Victor et al[10] have shown that Korsakoff's psychosis, the amnestic syndrome of alcoholics, is caused by bilateral damage to medial thalamic structures. In addition to alcoholism, the amnestic syndrome may infrequently result from bilateral metastases, midline tumors, cysts of the third ventricle, stroke syndrome from the posterior circulation to both temporal lobes, and bilateral surgical intervention.

There is an amnestic syndrome which lasts only hours or days, and it is called transient global amnesia. The precise etiology of this syndrome is unclear, but it probably represents a form of transient ischemic attack. Surprisingly, transient global amnesia does not carry a serious prognosis for frequent recurrence, nor for permanent memory loss due to ischemic stroke.

ADULT DEMENTIAS

Progressive dementia is a devastating syndrome. Nursing homes, state hospitals, acute care hospitals, and family homes contain large numbers of patients who are receiving terminal care for their dementia or treatment for its complications. The majority suffer from Alzheimer's disease–senile dementia, which is not treatable.

Some dementias actually are treatable, so we shall use the criterion of treatability in our discussion. Since the untreatable dementias are the most common, we shall begin with them. If the clinician can be certain that he has made an accurate diagnosis of one of these diseases, he can spare his patient the expensive laboratory workup aimed in other directions.

The Untreatable Dementias

Alzheimer's Disease—Senile Dementia

Alzheimer's disease is the most common dementing illness of adult life. Formerly, this diagnosis was arbitrarily limited to patients whose dementia began before age 65. Dementia that began after age 65 was labeled senile dementia. This artificial barrier is falling. With the rare but distinct exception of familial Alzheimer's disease, the clinical and pathological pictures of Alzheimer's disease and senile dementia are identical, so ' it appears now that Alzheimer's disease is simply the same illness with earlier onset.

Intellectual failure is hardly noticeable at first. The initial warning may be that the patient missed a promotion at work because he lacked precision and dependability. Later, he is fired. After a time at home, his friends and family recognize that the diversity of his interests has shrunk progressively to the immediate present and to a limited number of stories from the past, repeated over and over. Eventually, these too are forgotten, and he even forgets habits of careful dressing and eating and becomes generally confused. Even now, he may remain alert to his immediate environment and may be able to converse. At this stage, he may wander away from home and be injured or killed accidently. When he finally becomes inconti-

---

TABLE 10-1

"The Untreatable Dementias"

"Degenerative" Diseases
  Alzheimer's disease-Senile Dementia
  Pick's lobar atrophy
  Parkinson-dementia complex
  ALS-dementia complex
  Progressive supranuclear bulbar palsy

Heritable Diseases
  Huntington's chorea
  Neuronal storage diseases and leukodystrophies
  Hereditary myoclonus epilepsy
  Down's syndrome

Infectious Diseases
  Creutzfeldt-Jakob
  Progressive multifocal leukoencephalopathy
  Subacute sclerosing panencephalopathy

Trauma
  Single acute trauma
  Dementia pugilistica

nent, frequently the family can no longer care for him and places him in a chronic care facility. At this stage, the disease may be quite asymmetrical; hemiparesis, focal seizures, and aphasia become prominent.

The entire disease lasts five to ten years from noticeable onset to death due to pneumonia or septicemia. Generally, the family brings their patient for diagnosis after two to four years of symptomatic dementia, and by that time the dementia is far advanced. After he dies, the family is left with memories of his progressive dissolution rather than with memories of the previous 50 vigorous years; a terribly distorted immortality!

If the history consists of gradually progressive dementia without signs of systemic illness, the diagnosis may be established by CT scan or pneumoencephalogram, which discloses diffuse cerebral atrophy with ventricular enlargement commensurate with the degree of cortical atrophy. Once this is accomplished, no further workup is necessary.

There is a constellation of pathologic abnormalities that is most prominent in the brains of Alzheimer's disease but is also present to a lesser extent in normal aging brain and is found in abnormal amounts or in distinctive distributions in several others: Parkinson-dementia and ALS-dementia complex of Guam, Down's syndrome, postencephalitic Parkinsonism, progressive supranuclear bulbar palsy, Pick's disease and dementia pugilistica.

The pathologic findings include senile plaques, neurofibrillary tangles, granulovacuolar degeneration of nerve cells, and eosinophilic rods (Hirano bodies). Interestingly, the popular conception that neuronal loss is a major cause of dementia is not confirmed by painstaking cell counts[3,4,9] and histochemical analysis of demented brains. There may be as much as a five percent per year increase in cell loss in dementia, but the dramatic changes consist of shrinkage of neurons and loss of dendritic spines.[6,7] Neurons of demented people, like the people themselves, show shrunken spheres of interest and respond to more and more limited sources of stimulation.

Parkinson-Dementia and ALS-Dementia Complex of Guam

The indiginous population of the Mariana Islands has a greatly increased risk of dying from neurologic deterioration. Clinically, these appear to be two different diseases: either a classic Parkinsonian syndrome with progressing dementia or a classic amyo-

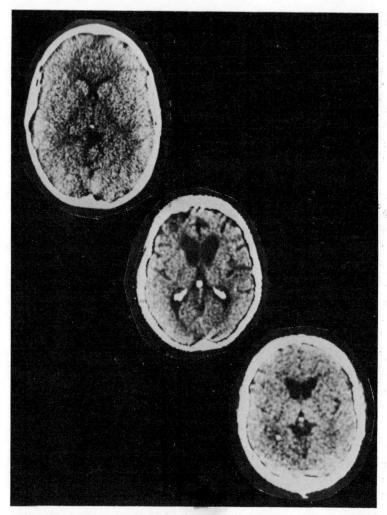

Figure 10-1. *Top: Normal CT scan. Middle: CT scan in Alzheimer's disease. Note ventricular enlargement with marked atrophy of brain substance and enlargement of sulci on the surface. The pineal and glomera of the choroid plexus are visible. Bottom: CT scan in Huntington's chorea. Note that the ventricles are not actually enlarged nor is there marked cerebral atrophy. The ventricles appear enlarged because of atrophy in the head of the caudate nuclei. Compare these scans to Figure 2-1 (page 30) in a patient with normal pressure hydrocephalus, marked enlargement of the ventricles, and no cerebral atrophy.*

trophic lateral sclerosis syndrome with progressing dementia. The etiology is not known, but the pathology of these two syndromes is quite similar, and there is no certainty that they actually represent two distinct diseases.

Parkinsonism in this country is not considered to be one of the major dementing diseases, but the physician who examines numerous Parkinsonian patients recognizes that, as a group, they are considerably more demented than normal people of their age or other sick people with similar degrees of neurologic disability.

Progressive Supranuclear Bulbar Palsy

This disease is usually recognized by the clinican who finds atypical abnormalities in a patient he has diagnosed as Parkinsonian. The patient develops slowed stiff movements and altered voice but little tremor. Early in the course of the disease, the patient complains of having trouble seeing. Examination discloses limited eye movements, especially in the vertical direction. With the passage of time, the eyes become fixed in a dysconjugate stare. Gay et al[5] state that the initial ocular abnormality consists of loss of vertical, especially downward, saccades. This is most easily demonstrated by testing for optokinetic nystagmus, but the clinican who does not have an optokinetic tape can easily test this function by placing his two hands above and below the line of vision and asking the patient to look rapidly back and forth between them. Normal saccades occur rapidly and accurately. Vertical eye movements in progressive supranuclear bulbar palsy are slow, like following movements, or absent, and are more affected than horizontal saccades even in early stages of the illness.

In addition to their Parkinsonian features and abnormal eye movements, patients with progressive supranuclear bulbar palsy develop snappy reflexes, Babinski's signs, dysphagia, dystonic posturing, and progressive but not overwhelming dementia. The course is usually less than ten years to death. Treatment with levodopa preparations may relieve the rigidity to some extent but does not produce dramatic relief of disability. The best description of this disease is still be be found in the original paper by Steele, et al[8] who described the clinical syndrome in nine patients and gave detailed pathological findings in four of seven fatal cases.

Huntington's Disease

The hallmark of Huntington's chorea in the adult is a combination of progressing dementia and chorea-athetosis. Occasionally, the movement disorder is difficult to detect even though the dementia is severe. On other occasions dementia appears only after severe chorea-athetosis is established. Huntington's disease is only one cause of chorea-athetosis. The other conditions are not accompanied by dementia and are discussed with the movement disorders (pp. 155).

Chorea consists of brief, nonrepetitive jerks of fingers, extremities, face, and trunk. Its presence is frequently missed unless the patient is directed to sit still, because, in the normal course of conversation, choreiform movements may look like exaggerations of normal gestures. During the screening examination, they become obvious when the patient is asked to sit, arms outstretched, eyes closed. Normal children under the age of 10-12 all have minor choreiform twitches in this posture. These should not be confused with pathological chorea.

Athetosis refers to recurring postural attitudes, primarily in the upper extremities. Athetotic postures are best observed in people with dystonic cerebral palsy, but the same postures recur repeatedly in Huntington's disease. The best recognized of these consists of sharp flexion at the wrist, extension of the fingers, and flexion and apposition of the thumb. If the reader imitates this attitude with his own hand in an imitation of dystonic cerebral palsy, he will recognize the posture again when it appears momentarily in the hands of his patient with advanced Huntington's disease.

Huntington's disease is inherited as an autosomal dominant gene with complete penetrance if the person lives long enough. Symptoms frequently do not appear until age 30 and may not first appear until after age 50. The heritable characteristic means that each of the children of an affected person has a 50 percent chance of developing the disease and transmitting it to half of his or her children. The affected person may not know that he has the disease until after he has passed middle life. Unfortunately, many children of Huntington's disease patients raise families of their own despite this risk, so the disease is perpetuated.

Huntington's Disease and the Family History. If all the information is available, there is always a family history of Huntinton's disease because the mutation rate for this gene is extremely low, but frequently the history is not available. There may be vague references to a parent who died with psychosis in the state hospital, or there may be no history at all. Why is the history not available in so many cases? Some affected people die before they develop symptoms of the disease. If this occurs in two successive generations, the family might not know about it. Some families are ashamed and do not tell the children, or the affected spouse may not have told the marriage partner before the illness began and is now too demented to remember. Lastly, we do not all know our biological fathers; but illigitimacy should not account for the frequent absence of the family history!

At any rate, the clinician who is faced with an absolutely typical case of Huntinton's disease need not be dissuaded from his diagnosis for lack of a family history. The major structural change in the brain consists of an isolated atrophy of the head of the caudate nucleus. This produces the characteristic picture of essentially normal-sized ventricles with localized dilatation of the anterior horn where the caudate nucleus used to be. The CT scan displays this change with a minimum of discomfort. If the CT scan is not available and radiographic confirmation is required, the brow-up view in the pneumoencephalogram clearly shows the abnormality.

Medicinal Treatment of Huntington's Disease. Haloperidol (Haldol®) in gradually increasing doses up to 7-10 mg per day is frequently an effective treatment of chorea. Haloperiodol has a long biological half-life, so a given dose may produce sedation during the first several weeks of treatment. Some patients refuse to take it for that reason. If the chorea is less bothersome than the side effects, haloperidol may be stopped until the patient or the family change their mind. No medicinal treatment stops the progression of the dementia and the general decline.

Creutzfeldt-Jakob Disease (pp. 254-258)
Progressive Multifocal Leukoencephalopathy (pp. 258-259)
Subacute Sclerosing Panencephalitis (pp. 261-264)
  Although there is still no treatment for these important diseases,

the question of their etiology is partially solved. They are discussed in the chapter on Slow Viral Infections.

Treatable Causes of Dementia

The treatable causes of dementia are usually diagnosed before dementia ever appears, because they cause other symptoms first. In such cases, when dementia develops, the cause is not in doubt, or dementia is completely prevented by adequate treatment. The unusual patient who does present with progressive dementia usually has a history that distinguishes his case from that of the patient with Alzheimer's disease and the other specific untreatable dementing diseases. Patients with the following uncharacteristic symptoms need more complete evaluation:
1) The clinical picture does not fit nicely into the description of any of the specific untreatable dementias described above.
2) Rapidly progressing dementia without signs of Creutzfeldt-Jakob disease.
3) Marked fluctuations in the degree of dementia, with periods of completely normal mental status.
4) Psychosis was a prominent early symptom.
5) Focal neurologic signs preceded the dementia.
6) Systemic disease already diagnosed (i.e., systemic lupus, liver, kidney, thyroid, cancer, tuberculosis, syphilis.)
7) Acute delirious state, somnolence, or coma preceded dementia.
8) History of toxic exposure.
9) History of severe dietary deprivation.

This list emphasizes that cerebral syndromes associated with treatable illnesses are not the usual picture of dementia. The patient may feel sick and spend much time in bed early in the course of the disease. Drug addiction produces wide fluctuations between somnolence, apparent dementia, and normal. This is usual in alcoholism, but we tend to forget that glutethimide, oxycodone, barbiturates, bromides, and many other prescription drugs produce the same symptoms, occasionally even accompanied by withdrawal seizures. If the clinician is alert to this possibility, a blood sample drawn during an "attack" can frequently document the presence of specific drugs.

Fever may not be recognized at home but is rapidly documented in the hospital as a specific sign of chronic infection. A careful neurologic examination may first uncover focal neurologic signs. A history of exposure to industrial toxins or heavy metals suggests that

---

TABLE 10-2

Causes of Treatable Dementia

Toxic and Metabolic Diseases:
Organ failure
  Thyroid (myxedema)
  Liver (pre-coma)
  Kidney
  Lungs (CO_2 narcosis and anoxia)
  Parathyroid
  Hypoglycemia
  Hyponatremia-Addison's disease
Toxins
  Heavy metals
  Drug abuse (even prescribed medications)
  Industrial toxins
Vitamin deficiencies
  B_1 (beriberi and Wernicke-Korsakoff)
  Niacin (pellagra)
  B_{12} (pernicious anemia)
Heritable diseases
  Wilson's disease
  Porphyria

Infections
  Syphilis
  Tuberculous meningitis
  Fungal meningitis

Tumor
  Primary frontal lobe glioma
  Metastatic tumors
  3rd ventricular tumor with hydrocephalus
  Subdural hematoma

Vascular
  Carotid artery occlusion
  Systemic lupus erythematosus
  Arteriovenous malformation

Unclassified
  Normal pressure hydrocephalus (pp. 28-31)

an aliquot of the 24-hour urine from the Schilling test should go to the laboratory for heavy metals and abnormal porphyrin excretion to help diagnose lead poisoning. The characteristic basophilic stippling of red blood cells may already have been reported on the CBC, awaiting incisive thought.

The clinician earns his keep by recognizing when things are not "right" and discovering why. If the demented patient does not fit nicely into a preconceived diagnosis, it is likely that he will fall easily into some other category. If such a patient is evaluated for treatable disease, the family, patient, and physician must be satisfied at the end that treatable causes have been sought and not found, or that a specific diagnosis has been established. The diagnostic process takes the patient through most of the laboratories in the hospital.

Clinical Pathology

Routine blood and urine examinations can immediately rule on a host of possible diagnoses:

CBC
Urinalysis (and 24-hour urine for heavy metal poisoning)
Electrolytes
BUN, creatinine
Liver battery
Ca, PO_4, alkaline phosphatase
T_4 (thyroid scan and uptake in nuclear medicine)
VDRL, FTA-ABS
Lumbar puncture results.

Ceruloplasmin for Wilson's disease is not routine and should be ordered only if dementia is accompanied by movement disorder or concomitant liver disease.

Porphyrin studies for acute intermittent porphyria are not routine, but this illness appears in such varigate form that it must be kept in mind. This cause of fluctuating cerebral syndromes and even fatal peripheral nerve disease will go undiagnosed unless it is considered and sought.

Lumbar Puncture

If meningitis is a reasonable part of the differential diagnosis, it becomes an absolute indication for immediate lumbar puncture. When the presenting complaint is dementia, the acute meningitides are not in question, but tuberculous and fungal meningitis and tertiary syphilis are all indolent infections which can be diagnosed and effectively treated. If there is serious question about fungal meningitis, repeated lumbar punctures, large volumes of fluid and examination of centrifuged specimens may be necessary before the organism can be visualized and cultured.

Radiology

The radiology department is especially useful in the workup of demented patients because of the frequency of Alzheimer's disease-senile dementia. If the CT scan or pneumoencephalogram discloses diffuse cortical atrophy and ventricular enlargement commensurate with the amount of cortical disease, and if the patient's history suggests that diagnosis, the workup is complete. On the other hand, radiological examinations establish other diagnoses with certainty. Brain tumors and subdural hematomas are obvious in appropriate examinations. The widely dilated ventricles *without* cortical atrophy, characteristic of normal pressure hydrocephalus, are easy to visualize. The chest x-ray and other studies in the rest of the body may give evidence of more generalized disease.

Nuclear Medicine

In addition to the brain scan, which is discussed in some detail in Chapter 2, the nuclear medicine department offers a wide variety of specific organ function evaluations. Liver-spleen scan, thyroid scan and uptake, kidney scan, bone scan, lung scan, and gamma cisternogram are all available in the workup of certain patients. They are. not all required in the evaluation of each demented patient but must be chosen with forethought.

Vitamin B_{12} blood levels may not be used to rule out the diagnosis of pernicious anemia because of the widespread misuse of B_{12} shots for all manner of irrelevant conditions. The only diagnostic examination for pernicious anemia is the Schilling test. Occasionally, neurological and mental symptoms may precede the characteristic changes in white cells and the anemia, so the Schilling test has become a standard procedure in the dementia workup even though it is almost never abnormal.

ARTERIOSCLEROSIS VS. DEMENTIA

Arteriosclerosis and dementia both occur in older people but they are not the same. The degree of intellectual deterioration does not correlate well with the severity of atherosclerosis. Patients with stroke develop aphasia, paralysis, and many mental symptoms related to multifocal brain infarction, but these are not the same as dementia. Patients with carotid artery occlusion and rapidly progressing dementia have been reported, but this syndrome, developing without focal abnormalities, must be very rare indeed. Dementia and senility must not be equated with vascular disease even as an easy way to talk to families!

REFERENCES

1. Bowen, D.M., Smith, C.B., White, P., Goodhardt, M.J., Spillane, J.A., Flack, R.H.A., Davison, A.N.: Chemical Pathology of the Organic Dementias. I. Brain. 100:397–426, 1977.
2. Bowen, D.M., Smith, C.B., White, P., Flack, R.H.A., Carrasco, L.H., Gedye, J.L., Davison, A.N.: Chemical Pathology of the Organic Dementias. II. Brain. 100:427–453, 1977.
3. Brody, H.: Organization of the Cerebral Cortex. III. A Study of Aging in Human Cerebral Cortex. J. Compr. Neurol., 102:511–556, 1955.
4. Brody, H., Aging in the Vertebrate Brain. In: *Development and Aging in the Nervous System*. Rockstein, M., (Ed.) Academic Press, New York, 1973, pp. 121–133.
5. Gay, A.J., Newman, N.M., Keltner, J.L., Stroud, M.H.: *Eye Movement Disorders,* C.V. Mosby, St. Louis, 1974, pp. 129–130.
6. Mehraein, P., Yamada, T., Tarnowska-Dziduszko, E.: Quantitative Study on Dendrites and Dendritic Spines in Alzheimer's Disease and Senile Dementia. Adv. Neurol., 12:453–458, 1975.
7. Scheibel, M.E., Scheibel, A.B.: Structural Changes in the Aging Brain. In: *Aging*, Vol. I. Brody, H., Harman, D., Ordy, J.M., (Eds.) Raven Press, New York 1975, pp. 11–37.
8. Steele, J.C., Richardson, J.C., Olszewski, J.: Progressive Supranuclear Palsy. Arch. Neurol. 10:333–359, 1964.
9. Terry, R.D.: Personal communication of unpublished results.
10. Victor, M., Adams, R.D., Collins, G.H.: *The Wernicke-Korsakoff Syndrome.* F.A. Davis Company, Philadelphia, 1971.

CHAPTER 11

Ischemic and Hemorrhagic Cerebrovascular Disease

Death by stroke ranks third in the United States, after heart disease and cancer. Proper treatment of ischemic cerebrovascular disease remains the most controversial topic in clinical neurology because, while we now understand the pathogenesis of stroke better than we did 30 years ago, our track record in the treatment of symptomatic patients has changed very little. We shall focus primarily on ischemic cerebrovascular disease, because this most common cause of stroke requires attention.

ISCHEMIC CEREBROVASCULAR DISEASE

Introduction

Symptoms of atherosclerosis usually do not appear until the disease is far advanced, so if we are to provide significant prolongation of life, effective treatment must begin long before symptoms appear. There is a voluminous and strident literature concerning the evaluation and treatment of the various symptoms of brain ischemia. This literature is unsatisfying because it fails to provide clear information about the effective prevention of ischemic stroke in the symptomatic patient.

There is also a growing literature concerning the treatment of risk factors for atherosclerosis. Hypertension, obesity, smoking, marked elevations of serum cholesterol in patients under 65, and diabetes mellitus are well-defined precursors of atherosclerosis. Reduction of systolic and diastolic blood pressure reduces the risk of stroke at all levels of blood pressure, at all ages, and at all stages of the disease. Non-smoking and weight reduction also correlate with decreased stroke incidence. There is still no proof that reduction of elevated serum cholesterol prevents stroke, but treatment of elevated blood lipids should be offered until definitive information becomes available.

Individual doctors and the health professionals as a whole could be of tremendous service to their patients and to the general population by stressing these facts, and by instituting indicated treatment of risk factors early in life, rather than waiting for the disease to progress to its symptomatic stages before becoming concerned.

In this section of the chapter, we shall examine first the evidence concerning risk factors in cerebral atherosclerosis. Then we shall discuss the immediate pathophysiology of an acute stroke and consider the treatment of stroke patients and prospective stroke patients with anticoagulants, antiplatelet drugs, and vascular surgery. Last, we shall outline the management of acute ischemic stroke in terms of diagnosis, and the multitude of available treatment possibilities for the hospitalized patient.

Risk Factors for Ischemic Stroke

For 30 years, citizens of Framingham, Massachusetts, have participated in a long-term prospective study designed to identify causative factors in atherosclerosis. We shall discuss only the information pertinent to cerebrovascular disease in Framingham, since it differs in some respects from the information about heart disease. The Framingham study has demonstrated that the two greatest factors in the development of ischemic stroke are advancing age, and hypertension.[24,25]

After 16 years of follow-up, only 15 percent of ischemic stroke patients had normal blood pressure before their initial stroke![35] At all ages, men and women are equally prone to the adverse effects of rising blood pressure, and at all blood pressures and all ages, rising systolic and diastolic blood pressure are accompanied by a rising risk of stroke. This negates two pieces of medical lore: first, that women tolerate hypertension better than men; and second, that the diastolic pressure is a stronger determinant of atherogenesis than the systolic. The various components of blood pressure are all about equally effective predictors of stroke incidence; thus, systolic blood pressure, diastolic blood pressure, pulse pressure, or mean arterial pressure may be used interchangeably in the establishment of risk. For patient screening, it is easiest to use a casual systolic blood pressure if it is taken during a less stressful part of the interview. At *all* levels of blood pressure, the risk of ischemic stroke increases by about 30 percent with each 10 mm Hg rise in the systolic blood pressure. Using the arbitrary figure of 160/95 as a criterion for hypertension, about 20 percent of the population is hypertensive. This 20 percent accounts for 50-60 percent of all ischemic strokes, even if no other risk factors are considered.[25]

Cardiac complications of hypertension greatly increase the risk of stroke. At the 16-year stage of the Framingham study, it is clear that electrocardiographic evidence of left ventricular hypertrophy (ECG-LVH), or symptomatic coronary heart disease (CHD), produces a threefold increased risk of stroke, independent of the blood pressure measurement. Definite enlargement of the heart as seen on chest x-ray doubles the risk of stroke regardless of the blood pressure. Of course, these complications correlate highly with increased blood pressure, so the risks for any patient are actually additive. As a group, those with ECG-LVH carried a ninefold increased risk of stroke, and those with CHD carried a fivefold increase because of their associated higher blood pressures.[35]

Treatment of Hypertension Reduces Risk

It is no longer "true" that reduction of blood pressure is dangerous in the hypertensive patient. Precipitous lowering of very high blood pressure may cause a stroke, but the gradual reduction of blood pressure to normal levels, and the continued rigid maintenance of normal blood pressure for the *rest of the patient's life* reduces the incidence of hypertensive complications regardless of the presence or absence of previous stroke.

The Veteran's Administration Cooperative Study Group on Antihypertensive Agents showed that treatment of even mildly hypertensive patients, whose diastolic blood pressures were between 90-114 mm Hg before randomization, reduced the death rate from hypertensive complications by half. Hypertension-related incidents like heart attack, sudden death, and ischemic stroke were reduced in the treatment group. Direct effects of hypertension like cerebral hemorrhage, dissecting aneurysm, congestive heart failure, hypertensive encephalopathy, and hypertensive retinal disease were completely abolished in the treatment group. During the five years of this study, the risk of a morbid event related to hypertension was reduced from 55 percent in the controls to 18 percent in the treatment group.[32] Studies of more seriously hypertensive patients have shown similar dramatic effects of treatment.

Treatment of hypertension after the first stroke effectively prevents further strokes and postpones death. Merrett and Adams[28] found otherwise, but theirs was a retrospective analysis of the charts of stroke patients followed "from time to time" after their stroke. Their study is based on "casual" blood pressures without proper protocol or controls. Other investigators have provided strong confirmation for the statement that antihypertensive therapy prevents stroke recurrence.[5,9,22,26] Carter studied severe hypertensives whose systolic and diastolic blood pressures remained above 160/110 before randomization. In this study, "good control" consisted of lowering systolic and diastolic blood pressures only to 160/90-100. Even with this relatively meager treatment, Carter discontinued his study after four years, because, he concluded, "It would be wrong to deny hypertensive patients the benefits of hypotensive therapy after a stroke." During that four years, 46 percent of controls and 26 percent of treated patients had died. Non-fatal recurrences were 23 percent in the controls, 14 percent in treated patients.

The Framingham study has documented four other risk factors for ischemic stroke, but their individual influence is not as great as the impact of hypertension. Heavy smoking,[24] elevated serum cholesterol in persons under the age of 65[23] and obesity, especially in women, are decreasingly important in that order. Glucose intolerance almost doubles the risk of ischemic stroke over the entire range of risk. In the person with no other risk factors, this is a small increment; but in the high-risk group, with hypertension, elevated serum cholesterol, and ECG-LVH, the added problem of glucose intolerance adds significantly to the risk of stroke.

The American Heart Association, in cooperation with the Framingham group, has compiled two booklets that allow computation of the risk of heart attack or stroke for various ages and various combinations of risk factors.[1] Using age, systolic blood pressure, serum cholesterol, evidence for glucose intolerance, electrocardiogram, and the smoking history, the physician may immediately identify the risk of these complications in men and women and determine which of his patients are in high-risk categories. Twenty percent of the population in these high-risk groups develop 80 percent of ischemic strokes or heart attacks. These are the patients who have the most to lose and may gain the most from education, treatment of hypertension, reduction of obesity, and cessation of smoking.

Symptomatic Atherosclerotic Cerebrovascular Disease

Introduction and Terminology

We shall now turn to ischemic symptomatology in far-advanced and end-stage atherosclerosis to understand the available treatments for prevention of ischemic stroke at this stage of the disease. This topic has a special vocabulary, so let us begin with a glossary.

"Ischemic stroke" describes an area of brain necrosis in the distribution of one artery of any size. Necrosis may have resulted from thrombosis in the end artery just proximal to the stroke, or from atheroma in a brachiocephalic vessel that caused diminution of blood flow or generated a platelet or cholesterol embolus. Emboli from the heart may also cause ischemic stroke. In each case, tissue necrosis is caused by ischemia; clinical assessment and even sophisticated laboratory examinations cannot always distinguish between the various specific etiologies. Between 60-80 percent of stroke patients have ischemic stroke.[24,27]

"Cerebral hemorrhage" encompasses several other stroke syndromes. Some intracranial hemorrhage originates in the subarachnoid space and may be caused by structural vascular abnormalities like berry aneurysm or arteriovenous malformation. Intracerebral hemorrhage may also originate from structural vascular disease in small arteries. About 15 percent of stroke syndromes are caused by hemorrhage, one half to two thirds of these by completely preventable hypertensive hemorrhage.

"Cerebral emboli" are diagnosed if there is a definite source of emboli such as rheumatic heart disease or bacterial endocarditis, and if several lesions appear simultaneously in the brain and elsewhere in the body. Although some ischemic strokes are undoubtedly caused by cardiac emboli, the diagnosis is uncommon since the advent of effective cardiac surgery. Treatment of embolic stroke is directed to the original cardiac pathology and therefore will not be discussed further in this chapter.

"Cerebrovascular accident" (CVA) is a bad word, and should be dropped. The Framingham study clearly demonstrates that stroke syndromes are no accident, and the variety of pathology among the stroke syndromes precludes the use of a single blanket term. Treatment varies for the various kinds of stroke syndrome, and specific terminology for each kind of stroke helps to keep etiology, pathology, and treatment clearly in mind.

"Transient Ischemic Attack," "stroke in evolution," ("progressing stroke"), and "completed stroke" are the three major stages of ischemic cerebral symptoms. *TIA* consists of neurological deficit from the distribution of one artery of any size caused by ischemia, which clears completely in 24 hours or less. Specific symptoms of TIA, and the significance of TIA as a warning of impending stroke vary depending upon the affected artery. TIA implies that no permanent damage has occurred, but the techniques of physical examination are relatively insensitive, so this is not always the case.

"Stroke in evolution" or "progressing stroke" describes stepwise increments of neurological deficit over a period of hours or a few days. This is an uncommon stroke syndrome. It is frequently caused by tight stenosis or thrombosis of an internal carotid artery in the neck, rather than by small vessel disease in the brain. Stroke in evolution frequently begins with a flurry of TIAs and incomplete recovery from one of these. Over the next few hours or days, there may be dramatic fluctuation of neurological deficit, but each worsening is followed by more incomplete recovery, until finally the deficit is stable. At this point, the patient has a completed stroke.

"Completed stroke" refers simply to fixed ischemic neurologic deficit. It does not refer to the *degree* of impairment. A very severe fixed deficit or a very mild fixed deficit are both completed strokes.

"Stenosis" and "occlusion" of arteries are important subjects of discussion that help to dramatize the unpredictability of the symptoms of cerebral vascular disease. A stenotic artery usually does not decrease blood flow unless there is more than 70 percent narrowing of the normal lumen, but an artery with any degree of stenosis may pass platelet or cholesterol emboli to the brain and cause TIA or completed stroke. Some patients whose TIAs are caused by a stenosing atheroma in the internal carotid artery stop having TIAs when the artery becomes completely occluded and they do not develop a stroke. Indeed, occlusion of the internal carotid artery may occur in middle life and remain completely asymptomatic until stenosis in collateral vessels produces symptomatic brain ischemia. On other occasions, patients of any age may develop fulminating cerebral edema and die within hours after acute occlusion of the same vessel.

"Brachiocephalic vessels", or *the great vessels*, consist of the two common carotid arteries, both vertebral arteries, the right innominate artery, and the proximal left subclavian artery. Some of the brachiocephalic vessels are available to surgical procedures for interarterial shunts or the removal of atherosclerotic plaques.

"Amaurosis fugax" is one form of transient visual loss. It is caused by ischemia to one retina due to carotid artery disease on that side, and consists of blindness in one eye, usually lasting several minutes. Vision eventually returns to normal. Examination of the retina after an attack of amaurosis fugax occasionally discloses shiny cholesterol emboli at branch points of retinal vessels. These are called Hollenhorst plaques after their discoverer.[21]

With this glossary, the reader should be able to navigate the rest of this chapter without going aground. Let us first consider the pathogenesis of ischemic stroke.

Pathogenesis of Ischemic Stroke

The immediate cause of ischemic symptoms may be related to a number of different events: an ulcerated atheroma, thrombosis of brachiocephalic, or small intracranial arteries, diminished cerebral perfusion to part of the brain or to the entire brain, or to individual processess associated with systemic disease

The Ulcerated Atheroma. As atherosclerotic material forms in the arterial wall, the endothelial surface may slough off baring collagen, cholesterol crystals, and other components of the atheroma to the passing blood. When atheromatous material breaks off, it floats into terminal vessels where it may cause TIA, amaurosis fugax, or ischemic stroke. Thus, Hollenhorst plaques are an important diagnostic discovery, because they signal internal carotid artery disease even in the absence of a bruit. When platelets make contact with the ulcerated atheroma, they adhere to it and begin the process of thrombosis.[2,29] Eventually, the entire surface of the ulcer may become covered by a platelet and fibrin thrombus. The entire vessel may be occluded by thrombosis or parts of the thrombus may break off and cause TIA. Cholesterol and platelet emboli are thought to be the two most common causes of TIA. Prevention of thrombosis is the theoretical basis for the use of anticoagulant and antiplatelet agents.

Intravascular Thrombosis. Before 1950, ischemic stroke was properly called "cerebral thrombosis" because stroke was thought to originate from thrombus formation in the middle cerebral or other intracerebral arteries. In 1951, Fisher challenged this concept because, he said, after examining the brains of 200 people who died with cerebral vascular disease, he found not one instance of a thrombus in the middle cerebral artery, even though the diagnosis had often been made clinically.[18] That article is still worth reading because of the careful clinical description of the syndrome of internal carotid artery occlusion, and because it is the first article that stresses the importance of great vessel disease in cerebral vascular symptomatology.

The frequency of great vessel disease was recognized about the same time that surgeons learned to operate on those vessels, and it seemed highly probable that removal of stenosing and occluding lesions in the brachiocephalic vessels, or the prevention of thrombosis with anticoagulants, would provide the much needed breakthrough in the treatment of this disease. Large cerebrovascular disease studies were launched, which required complete angiography of the brachiocephalic as well as the intracerebral vessels. These confirmed Fisher's contention that atherosclerosis in the internal carotid artery is an important cause of ischemic stroke.

The Joint Study of Extracranial Arterial Occlusion collected fairly complete angiographic evidence about the brachiocephalic and intracranial circulation in 3,788 patients who had symptoms of cerebrovascular disease and normal spinal fluid.[13,20] Three quarters of them had stenotic or occlusive lesions in the brachiocephalic vessels. Nearly 70 percent of stenotic lesions and 17 percent of occlusions in the brachiocephalic vessels occurred at the bifurcation of the common carotid artery in the neck

However, small vessel occlusions must not be forgotten simply because great vessel lesions are frequent. Modern radiographic equipment provides much greater resolution of small arteries than was available in the 1960s, but even in their 1968 report, Fields et al found that 40 percent of their patients had lesions in small, surgically inaccessible arteries.[13] Terminal branches of the intracerebral circulation were barely visible then. Currently, there is increasing interest in the terminal branches. Better radiographic equipment allows detailed visualization of smaller and smaller structures, and branch occlusions are frequently identified, coinciding with the position of ischemic stroke at brain scan, CT scan, or autopsy. Fisher's failure to find occlusive lesions results from the fact that he examined only larger intracerebral vessels. Recently, painstaking postmortem dissection of small arteries known to have been occluded at angiography has disclosed the lesions in smaller vessels, demonstrating their importance to the symptomatology and pathology of ischemic stroke.[33] The lesions are presumed to be *in situ* thromboses in some cases, and emboli from great vessel disease in many others.

Decreased Blood Flow. Stenosis and occlusion of great or small vessels causes decreased cerebral blood flow. This may be thought of, at least partially, as a problem in faulty brain plumbing, a problem familiar to residents of older houses. Angiography demonstrates frequent stenosing and occlusive lesions in vessels of all sizes. A lesion that produces 70 percent or greater reduction of the lumen causes significant reduction of blood flow. If the internal carotid artery is occluded or markedly stenosed, circulation from the external carotid artery, or from the other side, or via the circle of Willis, may compensate for the lost blood flow. However, when collaterals also become diseased, symptoms may develop solely on the basis of ischemia.

Increased blood viscosity due to polycythemia, macroglobulinemia, or dehydration can aggravate ischemic symptoms. More commonly, brain ischemia is precipitated by a sudden drop in perfusion pressure during orthostatic hypotension, cardiac arrhythmia, congestive heart failure, or surgery. Interest in great vessel surgery is based on considerations of cerebral blood flow as well as on the prevention of thrombosis by removal of offending lesions.

As we have noted, the pathogenesis of an ischemic stroke is highly complex, because it relates to many combinations of structural disease on both sides of the neck, and within cerebral vessels. Thrombotic and embolic events, and moment-to-moment variations of cardiac output, or changes in the physical characteristics of the blood all impinge upon the aging vascular system to produce a given stroke at some particular time.

Prevention of Ischemic Stroke in Symptomatic Patients

Occasionally patients develop devastating ischemic stroke with little or no evidence of atherosclerosis, but they are the exceptions. The presence of far advanced and disseminated atherosclerosis in most patients with early symptoms of cerebrovascular insufficiency, is a tribute to the excellent construction of the cerebral vasculature. It is remarkable that so many people can function with so few symptoms, despite stenosis or occlusion of one or more of the brachiocephalic vessels. On the other hand, it is not surprising that patients who already have symptomatic cerebral atherosclerosis carry a dismal prognosis for longevity and for recurrent vascular insults.

The vast bulk of research time, money, and controversy has been spent on the evaluation of various treatments for symptomatic patients with far advanced disease, rather than on the prevention of atherosclerosis by public and professional education and by life-long treatment of known risk factors. Since the available treatments attempt only to correct one or another kind of complication of established disease but do not address the basic biochemistry of atherosclerosis, it is to be expected that they might, at best, have only marginal effects on the eventual outcome of the disease. Most of the studies have been directed toward anticoagulation and carotid endarterectomy. Recently, antiplatelet drugs and microvascular surgery have become available for evaluation.

Anticoagulant Therapy

Evaluation by individual investigators, by groups, and by large cooperative studies among groups has produced sharply divergent conclusions about the value of anticoagulants in the prevention of ischemic symptomatology. As a result, the profession still has neither clear evidence that anticoagulants affect the prognosis of cerebrovascular disease nor clear indications for using or withholding anticoagulants. Even Dr. Toole, who is known for his work on cerebral atherosclerosis, had to admit that he "selects for each patient the medical or surgical treatment that seems best suited for his or her problem, taking into account systemic disease, [his] guess as to the likelihood of finding an operable lesion, and the patient's desires."[31] Each case must still be handled individually.

Most of the information we *think* we have about the use of anticoagulants in the treatment of ischemic cerebrovascular disease comes from large studies, the results of which were published in the 1960s. These anticoagulant studies have suffered from some insurmountable diagnostic problems and from others of a purely statistical nature. If we examine the problems themselves, it becomes obvious why the conclusions that were drawn are still controversial.

Diagnostic Problems. Every clinician can appreciate the diagnostic difficulties presented by patients with cerebral symptoms if he has been fooled by a patient who seemed to have an ischemic stroke, but later developed clear signs of brain tumor or some other disease. The anticoagulant studies used the best tools available in the 1960s, but at that time neuroradiologists were mainly interested in larger vessels, because radiographic equipment could not provide the detailed resolution available today. Nuclear brain scanning was in its infancy. Lumbar puncture helped to rule out cerebral hemorrhage. These were the best examinations available. Since the advent of the CT scan, we have learned how inadequate those tools really are, even now, in the detection of small, intracerebral hemorrhages whose symptoms mimic those of a branch occlusion. They do not produce bloody spinal fluid, displace arteries and veins on the angiogram, or change the nuclear brain scan. Such hemorrhages are uncommon, but by no means rare. The case of the unfortunate patient with such a hemorrhage who worsened and died during anticoagulant treatment, would be very likely to color the conclusions reached by the investigator who treated him for ischemic stroke with anticoagulants and later found massive hemorrhage at the autopsy! One firm conclusion from all the major anticoagulant studies is that anticoagulants are contraindicated in hypertension and in completed stroke, because they occasionally "cause" fatal cerebral hemorrhage. In all probability, at least some of the cerebral hemorrhages diagnosed at autopsy resulted from continued bleeding in a small primary cerebral hemorrhage perhaps aggravated by the anticoagulant. Lack of accurate diagnosis on admission to the hospital may have driven the investigators to the wrong conclusion after the patient died.

Other diagnostic problems arose from differences in the definition of terms. When is an event termed a TIA? What are the criteria for the diagnosis of a completed stroke? Who should be excluded from the study? How much warfarin (Coumadin®) is adequate treatment, and how closely should treated patients be followed to insure that they actually take their medication? Above all, who evaluates the results? Different studies differed in their answers to these questions, so comparison of results among them is difficult.

Statistical Problems. Some of the published studies were retrospective chart reviews, or lacked proper controls. Some seem to have been written to prove a point. None of them was initiated and controlled by a trained statistician; on the contrary, the statistical analysis was simply done on the available evidence. By this criterion, all were retrospective.

Although each study has been criticized by its own authors or by other investigators immediately after oral presentations or in print, they have all become part of the quotable literature regardless of their scientific value. Thus, a proponent of either side of almost any question can find published conclusions to confirm his opinion. Fortunately, continuous dissatisfaction with the statistical inadequacies of the anticoagulant studies has forced modern researchers to conform more closely to the known needs of statistical analysis even if it has not stilled the controversy about the conclusions reached in the 1960s.

Complexity of the Disease and Unpredictability of Individual Clinical Course. Research errors are not the only cause of divergent conclusions. We have already considered a number of important factors that have determined either the development of atherosclerosis, or the occurrence of an individual symptom, once the disease is established. The variablity of clinical course among individual patients is so dramatic, that the literature is not even unanimous about the natural history of some symptoms of TIA. If treatment actually provided only a small margin of benefit, under certain limited circumstances, enormous numbers of patients would be required to provide the needed number of clinical categories for treatment and control groups, and this number of patients is not available for controlled study.

But if a treatment truly provides a breakthrough, its effects should be visible despite bad studies. There is no argument about the effect of hypertension on atherogenesis. There is no question about the effectiveness of penicillin in the treatment of pneumococcal pneumonia, even though millions of dollars have not been spent on its evaluation. There never has been a controlled study of the effect of phenobarbital on epilepsy, but we do not need one. If we wished to state whether phenobarbital is more or less effective than phenytoin, we would need such a study, but that is a totally different problem from the one we face in the anticoagulant treatment of cerebrovascular disease.

Is there evidence that supports the use of anticoagulants in the treatment of symptomatic cerebrovascular disease under any circumstances? The answer is of necessity a biased one. I believe the best evidence supports the use of anticoagulants in the treatment of TIA to prevent further TIA, but I do not believe the evidence supsupports the contention that anticoagulant therapy prevents stroke.

The complications of long-term anticoagulation are appreciable: cerebral hemorrhage, subdural hematoma, epidural spinal hematoma, joint, urinary tract, and gastrointestinal hemorrhages, and a host of other kinds of bleeding. For this reason, I would limit the use of anticoagulants to those patients with incapacitating TIA who have not responded to aspirin, and who, for whatever reason, are not candidates for surgery.

There is a new class of articles about anticoagulation in cerebrovascular disease. The reader who is interested in reading further about the problem would profit by beginning his studies there [7,10] because they contain references to all the primary research. These articles have analyzed the primary studies from the standpoint of their statistical validity and their individual answers to a number of related questions. Each concludes that there is no proof that anticoagulants are of any value in the treatment of TIA or in the treatment of cerebrovascular disease in general. They do not even support this author's contention that an occasional patient with incapacitating TIA might benefit from anticoagulation. But this is not a burning problem, since such patients are vanishingly rare anyway.

Aspirin, Sulfinpyrazone, and Platelets

If platelet aggregation initiates the process of intra-arterial thrombosis, prevention of platelet aggregation might prevent TIA or ischemic stroke. Various agents limit platelet aggregation and serotonin release *in vitro*.[37] Scanning electron microscope examination of platelets discloses dramatic morphologic changes in response to thrombin, epinephrine, and aspirin.[3] An early short-term, double-blind, crossover study of the effects of sulfinpyrazone (Anturane®) or placebo on the prevention of amaurosis fugax disclosed a definitely decreased frequency during sulfinpyrazone treatment.[11,12]

Two prospective controlled studies on the effect of antiplatelet drugs in symptomatic cerebrovascular disease developed from these and other considerations. One controlled trial of aspirin in cerebral ischemia reported a significant decrease in the frequency of carotid artery TIA, but a less significant decrease in stroke, retinal infarction, and death in the treatment group after only six month's follow-up.[16]

The Canadian Cooperative Study has examined the effect of aspirin and sulfinpyrazone, individually and in combination, against placebo.[8,19] The descripton of this study reflects the care that must be taken if results are to become valid. Specific clinical criteria for patient eligilibty were established before the study began. Protocols of patients who were considered for the study but then were excluded were also examined to determine that the study population was not contaminated by selection bias from individual study centers. Strictly double-blind medication regimens were established, and patient compliance was monitored at each visit. Because of the ubiquitous nature of aspirin, patients were cautioned to avoid all other aspirin-containing preparations and were withdrawn from the study if they did not comply. We may only hope that careful statistical analysis of such controlled data has provided accurate conclusions that may be used in future clinical situations.

The Canadian Cooperative Study demonstrated a clear reduction in stroke and death among men who took aspirin, 325 mg four times each day. This was especially true of men who had no previous history of myocardial infarction. Women did not benefit from aspirin therapy. Sulfinpyrazone had no effect on morbidity or mortality, and did not appear to interact with aspirin either favorably or unfavorably. The results of this study provide a clear indication for treatment with aspirin for men who have transient ischemic attacks or minor stroke, providing they can tolerate the medication.

Carotid Endarterectomy

Patients who survive carotid endarterectomy have fewer strokes and TIA during follow-up than medically treated controls, and if carefully defined preoperative criteria are used, those who survive surgery live longer than their medically treated counterparts.[4,17]

But cerebrovascular surgery is quite different from other surgical procedures: devascularization of a small part of the stomach or omentum usually has transient and insignificant consequences, but the devascularization of small parts of the brain may produce devastating stroke or kill the patient. Thus, cerebrovascular surgery may be performed with relative safety only if the surgeon is especially trained and experienced in the operative techniques of these special procedures. Otherwise, the mortality and operative morbidity figures preclude a recommendation for surgery under any circumstances. This problem is aptly illustrated by the results of treatment of TIA in the Joint Study of Extracranial Arterial Occlusion.[14] Patients who survived the surgery fared better than those who were treated medically, but the surgical mortality and morbidity was so high that the total result in the randomized surgical group was worse than the results of medical treatment. This occurred partly because the patient sample was collected before 1968, when operative techniques were not as well developed as they are now, partly because of highly variable mortality figures representing variations in surgical competence among the cooperating institutions,[6] and partly because endarterectomy was performed on patients with many degrees of advanced atherosclerosis.

The indications for carotid endarterectomy cannot be listed like the indications for appendectomy because of the variable mortality and morbidity associated with the technical problems and variations of surgical expertise. But if the patient can travel to a center where cerebrovascular surgery is performed frequently and competently, there are considerations that make it more likely that he will survive surgery with a favorable result.

The best candidate is relatively young and otherwise healthy. He has an ulcerated or stenosing atheroma in one carotid artery in the neck which is causing TIA, but he has made complete recovery after each attack. He has no other evidence of cerebrovascular disease in the great or small vessels and has no underlying illness. Such patients are rare.

Variations on this theme do occur. Patients with bilateral carotid artery stenosis, whose TIA come from one side, have a better prognosis if endarterectomy is done on that side than medically treated patients, or than patients whose surgery is done on the opposite side, regardless which side has the tighter stenosis.[17] If one carotid artery is occluded, the risks of carotid endarterectomy on the other side are proportionately higher because blood flow is even more compromised while the surgeon is removing the lesion. This situation seems especially well suited to the use of new procedures that connect branches of the external carotid artery directly to branches of the middle cerebral artery. Such a shunt would provide increased blood flow to an ischemic hemisphere without compromising blood flow during the procedure. If TIA originate in the vertebrobasilar system owing to diminished blood flow, and there is tight stenosis of an internal carotid artery, surgery may relieve the symptoms. As operative techniques and competence improve, other indications for cerebral vascular surgery may appear.

There are major contraindications to endarterectomy; these may become less important if new techniques prevent intraoperative stroke and operative mortality. Disseminated great and small vessel disease produces greater risk in proportion to the severity of the disease. At present, carotid artery surgery is contraindicated in patients with severe disseminated disease. By the same reasoning, plans for multiple-stage procedures, each with its own risks, should be approached advisedly. Patients with tight stenosis of the carotid artery above the operative site do not develop increased blood flow after surgery. Severe neurological disability and clouding of consciousness are definite contraindications to carotid endarterectomy. If the patient has has an ischemic stroke within six weeks of surgery, carotid endarterectomy proximal to the stroke site is likely to produce fatal cerebral hemorrhage. Mortality due to cerebral hemorrhage contributed to the dismal results of endarterectomy for carotid artery occlusion as reported by the Joint Study,[4,15] but need not represent mortality figures for the same procedures performed by a highly skilled surgical team who waited the requisite six weeks or more after a stroke and used different criteria as an indication for surgery. Chronic occlusion of the internal carotid artery is an absolute contraindication for endarterectomy on that side because the thrombus usually cannot be removed, or, if it is removed, the artery thromboses again.

Atherosclerosis is a disseminated disease. The Joint Study showed that most categories of atherosclerotic patients continued to die of heart attack and stroke, whether they were in the medical or surgical groups, because of the dissemination of their lesions. The quality of life was improved in successful surgical survivors because they had fewer TIA and strokes from the operated arteries, but patients with other progressive diseases like cancer, heart disease, and dementia have more operative complications and additional operative and postoperative mortality from their second disease. These are further contraindications to carotid endarterectomy.

Surgeons disagree about these indications and contraindications. For instance, Sundt et al. recognized the high risk of brain hemorrhage following the repair of an acutely thrombosed internal carotid artery, but they recorded gratifying reversal of hemiplegia in a few patients when the thrombosis was removed within hours of the onset of symptoms.[30] Is the tremendously increased risk of surgery acceptable in light of the occasional tremendous increased quality of postoperative life? The patient should have the prerogative to make that decision after mature reflection, but at that point he and his family face sudden frightening disability and a continuous series of emergency procedures from the instant of arrival in the emergency room. Under such circumstances, there is no such thing as informed consent, let alone mature reflection!

There are other points of contention among surgeons, but the non-surgical clinician cannot make his decision about surgical management by perusal of the literature. His decision depends upon the availability of expert surgical care. Under most circumstances, when he makes the diagnosis of an acutely occluded internal carotid artery, he and his patient must simply ride out the consequences of this lesion with his best medical management. If the situation is not an emergency, he may evaluate the availability of skilled care locally, and recommend appropriate consulation, or suggest that his patient travel for the necessary evaluation and treatment.

Microvascular Surgery: The Extracranial-Intracranial Shunt

The surgical microscope has made microvascular surgery available to some patients with vascular disease. Yasargil first introduced the technique of anastomosing a branch of the external carotid artery to a branch of the middle cerebral artery in order to improve blood flow to an ischemic hemisphere.[36] This technique is currently undergoing careful evaluation through a cooperative study.[34] Clinicians must await the results of this study and the developing expertise of their own surgical teams in order to decide how to use this promising procedure.

Summary. Carotid endarterectomy, and the less frequently performed great vessel shunt procedures, have provided confirmation of the importance of great vessel disease in the production of ischemic stroke. They offer a partial answer to a minority of patients with atherosclerotic cerebrovascular disease, but most patients first seek medical care after their first completed stroke. Some appear after TIA, but already have disseminated disease or associated illnesses, or they complete their stroke before the surgery is accomplished. For the present, we must continue with attempts to correct individual lesions in a small proportion of affected patients and to treat the rest with the best medical management, but the real breakthrough that would attack the disease over the entire body is not in sight. The best service physicians can render their patients now, is to take blood pressures on everyone, at every age, and to provide education and life-long treatment of known hypertension and of other known risk factors.

Hospital Management of the Acute Stroke Patient

Before management begins, the clinical diagnosis must be confirmed by CT or nuclear brain scan. Occasionally, lumbar puncture is valuable to document the presence or absence of blood in the spinal fluid. Angiography is indicated only if the diagnosis is still in doubt, because there is no adequate surgical treatment for acute ischemic stroke. Unless there is evidence for a cardiac source of emboli, consideration of treatment with anticoagulants is probably irrelevant. The electrocardiogram, chest x-ray, and various blood and urine studies help to focus diagnostic and therapeutic concern on associated pathology that may have contributed to this stroke, or which may complicate and prolong the hospital stay. Initial blood studies help to determine the doctor's future orders for the maintenance of metabolic balance.

Once the diagnosis is firmly established, health professionals working for the patient and family develop simultaneously a number of treatment goals. As the ultimate prognosis becomes clearer, these may change somewhat, but they usually can be stated with some accuracy on admission. If the patient is lucky, he and his family confront a team of professionals who talk with each other, at least occasionally, about their various goals and problems, so that the patient receives coordinated services. The physician has prime responsibility for this coordination. He must manage prescriptions, diagnose and treat complications, and see to it that the patient remains in metabolic balance, but above all, the physician's job is to lead patient and family through the available hospital and community resources by introducing them to professionals in a number of different fields, and helping them to implement recommendations from all sources.

Numerous goals reflect the multiplicity of services available to neurological patients. The goals determine the treatment.

a) Prevention of Cerebral Edema

Patients with large ischemic stroke die because of massive cerebral edema. Cerebral edema increases permanent brain damage in patients with smaller strokes. Edema may be suppressed to some extent during the first week after a stroke with dexamethasone (Decadron®), 16-20 mg per day, orally or parenterally, in divided doses. After the first week, the dose may be tapered rapidly to zero.

b) Maintenance of Normal Metabolic Balance and Nutrition

Cerebral edema increases progressively during the first 3-5 days after a stroke, then subsides slowly. During this acute period, the patient should be kept on the "dry" side with moderate fluid restriction. Unless there are unusual circumstances, intravenous therapy is unnecessary during the first 24-36 hours. When intravenous therapy is begun, free water and sodium loads should be limited. Repeated serum electrolyte determinations and BUN or creatinine values can guide the clinician toward accurate intravenous therapy prescriptions. Salt and water restriction must not be so stringent that it causes abnormalities in laboratory results.

A decision needs to be made between intravenous and oral intake as soon as possible. If the patient has severe dysphagia, or prolonged unconsciousness, nasogastric tube feedings may be appropriate. Gastrostomy is a measure of desperation and should be recommended exceedingly sparingly.

c) Prevention of Decubitus Ulcers

Proper bed position, regular and frequent turning from *one* side *all the way to the other side*, careful attention to reddened areas of skin, and clean, dry, unwrinkled sheets are the best defense against bedsores. If the patient is incontinent, he should be offered a urinal or bedpan every two hours. If he cannot remain continent with this regimen, he should be catheterized. External drainage may be adequate for some men. The complications of catheter care are not nearly as serious as the chronic decubitus ulcer that results from chronic wetness. Alternating pressure mattresses are an adjunct to, not a replacement for, excellent nursing care.

d) Prevention of Pneumonia

Most stroke patients die of pneumonia, not of the stroke, during the acute hospitalization. Regular turning helps to prevent pneumonia, but it is even more important to have the patient get out of bed as soon as possible. Once the electrocardiogram and blood studies have ruled out the possibility of myocardial infarction and the patient is awake, he should spend time, at least twice a day, in a high-backed chair with full arms to support him. His chair time will be brief at first, but it may be increased as rapidly as he can tolerate it. When indicated, the respiratory therapist may be requested for chest percussion or for more aggressive pulmonary toilet.

e) Prevention of Pulmonary Emboli

Turning in bed, time in a chair, and thigh-high support stockings are all of value. All bedridden patients benefit from support stockings, and these must be replaced after each treatment or examination, not left at the bedside!

f) Prevention of Contractures, Development of Mobility, and Learning to Eat and Dress

Passive joint motion by physical therapists helps to prevent contractures and may be instituted at least once each day from the time of admission. Active range of motion may begin as soon as some voluntary muscle power returns. Once the patient is able to cooperate with active physical therapy, he may travel to the PT suite for gait training and exercises to increase muscle power and coordination of spastic limbs. While he is confined to bed, a foot board to prevent foot drop and finger extension splints to maintain useful hand position may be valuable. When he is up in a chair, the patient should have a sling to support the paralyzed upper extremity. This will help to prevent shoulder subluxation.

Occupational therapists assist in helping the patient to adjust to his disability and to adapt his life activities so that he can attain his highest functioning level. Many self-help devices are available to the patient, and these help to increase his independence. During OT sessions, the therapist works with the patient on using such devices as a rocker knife, plate guard, buttonhook. In addition, the therapist teaches the patient new ways of performing daily tasks that can no longer be done normally with his new disability.

Some patients need braces to immobilize weak joints. These are obtained from the orthotics department. Braces should not be used while muscle strength is returning, but only to correct permanent disabling weakness

Physical therapists, occupational therapists, and orthotists are professionals who can offer special expertise to doctor and patient. The physician should ask for consultation, not order services from these specialists unless he has advanced training in their field, because they usually know better than he how to apply the entire range of their services to individual problems.

g) *Recovery of Language*

If aphasia is severe, the speech therapist may be of value in teaching techniques for the recovery of communication. Speech therapy is of especial value for patients with some kinds of dysarthria and dysphonia as well as aphasia.

h) *Education of Family Members*

Families are frequently absent during the day so they may not witness treatments or recognize problems when they arise. If the patient is planning to return home, the family needs to be educated in the management of new disability. Families need to know how much improvement they can expect and how they best can help. If the prognosis points toward a nursing home or to an extended care facility, the family should participate in the development of these plans.

i) *Discharge Planning*

Although discharge planning is last on this list, the process is best begun during the early stages of hospitalization, even before the physician knows the precise prognosis. Specific plans depend upon family adjustments and financial resources. Hospital social services make contact with a variety of community agencies as they plan for post-hospital care in nursing homes, extended care facilities or in the patient's home. This takes time, and the plans cannot be developed suddenly in the last days of a hospital stay. If the social service department is involved from the beginning, they and the community resources can make much more effective plans with patient and family. A planned home visit by members of the physical and occupational therapy departments may be very helpful to both patient and family, because adaptive equipment such as commode chairs, shower tub seats, and safety bars can be purchased and plans may be suggested for improving the access to kitchen facilities or constructing a wheelchair ramp if this is needed.

The Fatal Stroke

The plans discussed above are not appropriate for all stroke patients. In some cases the stroke is so massive that death is inevitable despite all available help. The principal attention in these cases is directed toward the family who must understand their situation and prepare for the patient's death.

In other cases, patients develop potentially fatal stroke with a hopeless prognosis for returning home. Many patients and families abhor the idea of nursing home existence and want no part of it. The patient would rather die. Others want heroic intervention to maintain life, despite the disability. Families of each kind should have the opportunity to talk with their physicians and make their wishes known. They must be allowed to make the ultimate decisions if they wish, based upon the physician's best estimate of the prognosis. if the patient is able to participate in these discussions, he usually appreciates being included in the consultation, and his wishes must be respected above everyone else's.

Each clinician decides for himself how to manage ethical problems in his own practice. I have found it valuable to provide patients and families with an open, direct discussion of all possible treatment options from only keeping the patient comfortable, if that is appropriate, to heroic measures. I give family and patient my own opinion about the best course of action. If family members disagree among themselves about these recommendations, I send them away to settle their differences, and we meet again to come to a more nearly unanimous decision. If even only one close family member votes strongly for treatment, even if the case is hopeless, I recommend aggressive treatment.

Nurses are the backbone of the total treatment plan. They spend 24 hours a day with the patient, while doctors and other health professionals are mere transients. They implement orders and treatments. They care for physical needs. They get the patient up in a chair and see to it that he gets back to bed again when he is tired. They are the first to note complications when they develop and if they communicate this knowledge immediately, everyone's job is smoother and easier. They are the sole determinants of skin care and bowel and bladder training. They perform physical therapy when the therapist is elsewhere, and they teach patient and family how to use newly acquired techniques from occupational and physical therapy. They listen when things are bad. They talk to families in the evening.

A neurological service stands or falls on the excellence of its nursing care, and the physician who institutes training sessions or provides bedside teaching for nurses can help them to improve their care even more as their knowledge of neurology increases. Additionally, the physician who listens carefully to his nurses during daily rounds receives important information about his patient's changing situation.

HEMORRHAGIC CEREBROVASCULAR DISEASE

Hemorrhagic cerebrovascular disease is divided into four types: 1) primary intracerebral hemorrhage, 2) subarachnoid hemorrhage, 3) subdural hemorrhage, and 4) epidural hemorrhage. It is important for the clinician to recognize these conditions and to establish his diagnosis, because in some cases, direct neurosurgical intervention is mandatory to preserve life or to prevent complications. In other cases, other therapies may prevent further bleeding or eradicate an intracerebral arteriovenous malformation. In patients who are fatally injured by their hemorrhage, neurological or neurosurgical consultation may still be appropriate so that the patient's family may have confirmation that there is nothing more to do.

Intracerebral Hemorrhage

The frequency of intracerebral hemorrhage is largely related to the adequacy of antihypertensive therapy. Although other causes exist, such as previously unrecognized brain tumor, arteriovenous malformation, cranial arteritis, blood dyscrasia, and excessive anticoagulant therapy, the incidence of all these entities is small compared to the incidence of hypertensive cerebral hemorrhage, and this complication simply does not occur in persons who maintain excellent control of their blood pressure.

Uncontrolled hypertension causes hyaloid degeneration in the walls of arterioles, which predisposes cerebral vessels to the development of microscopic aneurysms, visible only in specially prepared specimens. Their occurrence is directly related to the degree and the duration of hypertension, and their rupture is the probable cause of hypertensive intracerebral hemorrhage.

The most frequent sites of hypertensive hemorrhage are the basal ganglia, the thalamus, and deep within the frontal lobe. Hemorrhages in these sites are usually inaccessible to surgery. Commonly, they are large and rapidly fatal. They begin with a momentary complaint of severe headache, but the patient quickly falls hemiplegic. Within minutes, he is comatose. When he arrives in the emergency room, such a patient is frequently at a midbrain stage of coma (p. 167) and may die within hours or a few days.

The CT scan is the best tool for diagnosis of intracerebral hemorrhage. Lacking the CT scan, the nuclear brain scan may show apparently decreased blood flow on the side of the hemorrhage, and the spinal fluid may be bloody. Lumbar puncture is hazardous because of the danger of brain herniation, but if the CT scan is not available to make the diagnosis, lumbar puncture is justified. Cerebral angiography discloses a large cerebral mass in patients with massive intracerebral hemorrhage. Unfortunately, the CT scan may provide the *only* evidence of small intracerebral hemorrhage, and without this tool, the diagnosis may easily be missed.

It is frequently impossible to distinguish, on clinical grounds alone, a large cerebral hemorrhage from total occlusion of the middle cerebral artery. Both produce destruction of an entire hemisphere, rapidly developing hemiplegia, coma, and death. Total occlusion of the middle cerebral artery is more lethal in younger patients than in elderly ones, because in old age, there has been enough cerebral atrophy that the resultant massive cerebral edema does not cause an abrupt rise in intracranial pressure or herniation and brainstem compression. For this reason, the older person may survive total occlusion of the middle cerebral artery, while the person of 40 or 50 years of age almost invariably dies within a day or two because of uncontrollable cerebral edema.

There is no treatment for a massive intracerebral hemorrhage. Small intracerebral hemorrhages do not need treatment and may be managed like ischemic stroke once the diagnosis is established. Medium-sized intracerebral hemorrhage may occur with little clouding of consciousness and mild or moderate neurological deficit. If the site of hemorrhage is superficial and located in frontal, temporal, or parietal lobes, the clot may be removed surgically. If it appears that the mass effect is contributing to continued neurological disability, or if the patient's condition worsens during the recovery period, he should be transferred to neurosurgical care for consideration of a craniotomy to remove the clot.

Congenital arteriovenous malformation is another cause of primary intracerebral hemorrhage. These may be so small that they are obliterated by their own hemorrhage, or so large that they replace large portions of the cerebral hemisphere. Bleeding from these lesions need not be massive. They may bleed repeatedly with few symptoms, or they may remain completely silent until they suddenly burst with fatal consequences.

Patients who recover from a ruptured arteriovenous malformation, and some patients with unruptured malformations, may become candidates for complete eradication of their lesions. Arteriovenous malformations may be excised completely at craniotomy, or by a recently developed neuroradiological technique, which involves embolization of the malformation with plastic spheres through an angiographic catheter. The spheres are of graded size so they progressively obstruct blood flow to the lesion as they are injected into feeder vessels. By this technique, the malformation may be completely obliterated without causing further neurological deficit. This procedure is not universally available, but its potential benefit is so great that patients who have recovered after a hemorrhage, and patients whose arteriovenous malformations have not yet bled, should be referred for neurosurgical consultation to consider ablation of the lesions. These patients should be warned in advance that they may not be candidates for treatment, but the non-neurosurgical clinician should request consultation rather than attempt to make that determination alone.

Arteriovenous malformations produce premonitory symptoms more commonly than berry aneurysms. Focal seizures may begin in childhood or during the teens. Some malformations are large enough that they interfere with brain function. The person may grow up with hemiatrophy on the opposite side of the body or "cerebral palsy" with hemiparesis. Further examination discloses a smaller hand or foot and smaller fingernails on the hemiatrophied side. The patient may be aware that he must buy shoes for the larger foot, or gloves for the larger hand if they are to fit. Careful auscultation of the head, the eyes, and the neck may reveal a bruit caused by increased blood flow to the malformation. The diagnosis may be established by nuclear brain scan, CT scan, arteriography, or sometimes even by plain skull x-rays.

Headache is a troublesome symptom, because it is so common, and usually so innocuous. But headache may be a premonitory symptom of either an arteriovenous malformation or a berry aneurysm. Sometimes it exactly mimics all the other headaches which have passed through the physician's office, and the diagnosis is not made until the cerebral hemorrhage occurs. If doctor and patient are fortunate, the headache may become the first clue which eventually leads to a successful diagnosis and treatment. Headache is more likely to represent serious intracranial disease if it is always unilateral, never switches to the opposite side, and if it is unaccompanied by specific symptoms that proclaim it to be migrainous. If such a headache is accompanied even by minute neurological abnormalities appropriate to the site of the headache, it should be followed up first with CT or nuclear brain scan, and eventually with cerebral angiography.

Sometimes the clinician is unable to find neurological abnormalities in a patient with atypical headaches. Berry aneurysm and arteriovenous malformation are unusual causes of chronic headache even among patients whose symptoms do not fall easily into the description of a routine headache variety. Once the CT scan and other noninvasive studies have been performed for such a patient, angiography is the only remaining precise diagnostic study; but angiography carries risk, so it is not indicated in every atypical case, even though its omission may cause us to miss potentially treatable disease. At this juncture, either decision, for or against angiography, becomes painful; and a wrong decision sometimes results in disability or death for the patient. But it is the doctor's job to make the best recommendations possible on the basis of the available facts and to give his decision all the care and cogitation he can. If the result is disaster, he must go on and do his best job again, even though he has been shaken.

Subarachnoid Hemorrhage

Congenital berry aneurysms and acquired arteriosclerotic or mycotic aneurysms may cause subarachnoid hemorrhage. Mycotic aneurysms are caused by infected emboli, usually from subacute bacterial endocarditis. Most patients with ruptured berry aneurysms have not consulted a doctor for premonitory symptoms. Suddenly, they develop a headache that may radiate down the back. If the hemorrhage is massive, if the jet of blood is directed toward the brain, where it penetrates like a knife, or if there is severe arterial spasm in cerebral vessels, the patient lapses quickly into hemiplegia and coma, quite resembling the patient with severe intracerebral hemorrhage. Such subarachnoid hemorrhage is rapidly fatal.

Fortunately, aneurysms may rupture so that the jet of blood is directed away from the brain. Some patients do not develop hemiplegia or even clouding of consciousness, but they do complain of severe headache which began suddenly, and they may already have a stiff neck when they arrive in the emergency room, even if there are no other neurological abnormalities. These patients provide an absolute indication for CT scan, if available, and lumbar puncture. If the fluid is bloody, they represent another of the infrequent neurological emergencies. In this case, the emergency involves immediate admission to the neurosurgical service, because such a patient can survive workup and surgery with a minimum of morbidity and mortality, but he is at risk of a second potentially fatal hemorrhage in the next two weeks.

Other subarachnoid hemorrhage patients are less fortunate. They have definite focal abnormalities on examination or are confused or somnolent. Some are comatose and hemiplegic. Each increment of neurological damage adds a large component to the mortality and morbidity of surgery. Such patients quickly cease to be surgical candidates, but if they respond to treatment and improve, they may again benefit from an operation, so they, too, should be admitted immediately to the neurosurgical service, where their progress may be monitored and decisions may be made about further treatment.

Presurgical treatment of berry aneurysms has changed since the advent of antifibrinolytic agents. Use of these agents is based on the theory that re-bleeding during the acute illness is caused by dissolution of the clot which stopped the bleeding during the original hemorrhage. Antifibrinolytic agents help to prevent this dissolution, decrease the incidence of re-bleeding, and allow more complete healing to occur. The effectiveness of these agents is still under investigation, but preliminary results are encouraging.

Constant monitoring of the subarachnoid hemorrhagic patient's mental and physical status may allow the detection of normal pressure hydrocephalus (pp. 28-31) before it produces permanent brain damage. Angiography may disclose the aneurysm and allow the surgeon to plan definitive surgical treatment.

Aneurysms of the carotid siphon within the cavernous sinus do not cause subarachnoid hemorrhage. If they rupture, they cause a carotid-cavernous sinus fistula which is difficult to obliterate. These aneurysms may reach enormous size with few symptoms, or they may cause ophthalmoplegia and facial pain because they press on oculomotor nerves or branches of the trigeminal nerve within the cavernous sinus. Patients with these symptoms may have other lesions in the cavernous sinus or in the middle fossa, but in any case, they need accurate diagnosis and should be referred to a neurologist or neurosurgeon for definitive evaluation.

Subdural Hematoma

Chronic subdural hematoma may occur after a seemingly inconsequential history of trauma. Cough headache may be the only symptom. This is a sudden lancinating head pain which occurs only during a cough, sneeze, or while straining at stool. Cough headache occurs in a variety of intracranial disease states and should always be followed up with further evaluation. Mental dullness may alternate with somnolence or coma. Progressive hemiparesis, coma, and death may occur if the hematoma continues to enlarge and is not diagnosed. Alcoholics are particularly prone to chronic subdural hematoma because of their frequent falls and brawls.

Two useful neurological adages concern subdural hematoma, the most important of which is that the diagnosis must first be considered, so appropriate studies can be done or the hematoma will be missed entirely. Even the CT scan is fallible in subdural hematoma. Usually, it shows diagnostic changes, but if it does not, the nuclear brain scan may be abnormal. The only definitive examination in this situation is cerebral angiography. If the clinician is convinced that subdural hematoma is a likely diagnosis, he must order angiography.

Secondly, chronic subdural hematoma affects consciousness more severely than movement, sensation, and vision. This is because symptoms usually result from general pressure on the brain, rather than from focal brain destruction. This adage is especially useful for the patient who arrives without much history, who might otherwise be labeled "stroke." If there is marked clouding of consciousness or coma without severe hemiparesis or hemianopsia, the cause is unlikely to be ischemic stroke. Subdural hematoma is more likely to be the right diagnosis.

There is legitimate controversy about the proper treatment of chronic subdural hematoma. In the past, surgical removal has been proper; but it appears that cerebral edema, not an enlarging hematoma, may be responsible for increasing disability in many cases, so hospitalization, vigorous treatment with dexamethasone and careful observation may be appropriate in these cases. Such treatment provides time for the subdural hematoma itself to be resorbed or to reach equilibrium with the rest of the intracranial contents. If the patient continues to worsen despite medicinal treatment, burr holes or formal craniotomy is indicated.

Acute subdural hematoma accompanies severe head injuries. Because of the associated direct brain injuries, and the rapid development of a large hematoma, this complication is frequently fatal. Treatment consists of rapid surgical intervention if the patient arrives in time for help.

Chronic subdural hematoma may occur as a terminal event during the course of otherwise fatal diseases like leukemia, Hodgkin's disease, and renal failure. While the subdural clot itself may be evacuated, the patient may not be salvagable. The clinician faced with such a patient should think twice before recommending surgery, because the patient may not recover from the triple insult of his original disease, the subdural hematoma, and the surgery. There can be no firm rule at this point, only a serious consideration of the risk factors balanced against the possible benefits.

Epidural Hematoma

The middle meningeal artery and its branches travel in a groove on the inner table of the skull. If the skull is fractured across this

248 / PRACTICAL CLINICAL NEUROLOGY

groove, the artery may tear, releasing blood under arterial pressure
into the epidural space. Because of the high pressure, a large mass
may develop rapidly and kill the patient if he does not reach a surgeon in time.

The typical story is that of a head unjury with initial unconsciousness. The patient wakes, apparently unhurt, but within 10-30
minutes again becomes confused, lapses into unconsciousness,
dilates one pupil, and may eventually die. Treatment consists of instant neurosurgical consultation and drainage of the hematoma. If
done in time, this can completely reverse the symptoms and save a
life.

REFERENCES

1. American Heart Association. *Coronary Risk Handbook and Stroke
   Risk Handbook* Available free from: American Heart Association,
   44 E. 24th Street, New York, New York 10010.
2. Barnett, H.J.M.: Platelets, Drugs, and Cerebral Ischemia. In:
   Platelets, Drugs, and Thrombosis, Hirsh, J., et al., (Eds.) S. Karger,
   Basel, 1975, pp. 233-252.
3. Barnhart, M.I., Walsh, R.T., Gilroy, J.: Formal Discussion. In: *Cerebral Vascular Diseases,* 8th Conference. McDowell, F.H., Brennan,
   R.W., (Eds.) Grune & Stratton, New York, 1973, pp. 300-306.
4. Bauer, R.B., Meyer, J.S., Fields, W.S., Remington, R., Macdonald,
   M.C., Callen, P.: Joint Study of Extracranial Arterial Occlusion. III.
   Progress Report of Controlled Study of Long-Term Survival in Patients With and Without Operation. J.A.M.A. 208:509-518, 1969.
5. Beevers, D.G., Fairman, M.J., Hamilton, M., Harpur, J.E.: Antihypertensive Treatment and the Course of Established Cerebral
   Vascular Disease. Lancet I:1407-1409, 1973.
6. Blaisdell, W.: Extracranial Arterial Surgery in the Treatment of
   Stroke. In: *Cerebral Vascular Dieeases,* 8th Conference. McDowell,
   F.H., Brennan, R.W., (Eds.) Grune & Stratton, New York, 1973, pp.
   3-15.
7. Brust, J.C.M.: Transient Ischemic Attacks: Natural History and
   Anticoagulation. Neurology 27:701-707, 1977.
8. Canadian Cooperative Study Group: A Randomized Trial of Aspirin
   and Sulfinpyrazone in Threatened Stroke. N. Eng. J.Med. 299:53-59,
   1978.
9. Carter, A.B.: Hypotensive Therapy in Stroke Survivors. Lancet
   I:485-489, 1970.
10. Cervantes, F.D., Schneiderman, L.J.: Anticoagulants in Cerebro-

vascular Disease. A Critical Review of Studies. Arch. Intern. Med. 135:875–877, 1975.

11. Evans, G.: Effect of Platelet-Suppressive Agents on the Incidence of Amaurosis Fugax and Transient Cerebral Ischemia. In: *Cerebral Vascular Diseases,* 8th Conference. McDowell, F.H., Brennan, R.W., eds. Grune & Stratton, New York, 1973, pp. 297–299.

12. Evans, G., Gent, M.: Effect of Platelet Suppressive Drugs on Arterial and Venous Thromboembolism. In: *Platelets, Drugs, and Thrombosis.* Hirsh, J. et al., (Eds.) S. Karger, Basel, 1975, pp. 258–262.

13. Fields, W.S., North, R.R., Hass, W.K., Galbraith, J.G., Wylie, E.J., Ratinov, G., Burns, M.H., Macdonald, M.C., Meyer, J.S.: Joint Study of Extracranial Arterial Occlusion as a Cause of Stroke. I. Organization of Study and Survey of Patient Population. J.A.M.A. 203:955–960, 1968.

14. Fields, W.S., Maslenikov, V., Meyer, J.S., Hass, W.K., Remington, R.D., Macdonald, M.: Joint Study of Extracranial Arterial Occlusion. V. Progress Report of Prognosis Following Surgery or Nonsurgical Treatment for Transient Cerebral Ischemic Attacks and Cervical Carotid Artery Lesions. J.A.M.A. 211:1993–2003, 1970.

15. Fields, W.S., Lemak, N.A.: Joint Study of Extracranial Arterial Occlusion. X. Internal Carotid Artery Occlusion. J.A.M.A. 235:2734–2738, 1976.

16. Fields, W.S., Lemak, N.A., Frankowski, R.F., Hardy, R.J.: Controlled Trial of Aspirin in Cerebral Ischemia. Stroke 8:301–315, 1977.

17. Fields, W.S.: Formal Discussion. In: *Cerebral Vascular Diseases,* 8th Conference. McDowell, F.H., Brennan, R.W., (Eds.) Grune & Stratton, New York, 1973, pp. 15–19.

18. Fisher, M.: Occlusion of the internal Carotid Artery. Arch. Neurol. & Psychiatr. 65:346–377, 1951.

19. Gent, M.: Canadian Cooperative Study of Recent Recurrent Presumed Cerebral Emboli (RRTCE). Design and Organization of the Study. In: *Platelets, Drugs, and Thrombosis.* Hirsh, J. et al., (Eds.) S. Karger, Basel 1975, pp. 253–257.

20. Hass, W.K., Fields, W.S., North, R.R., Kricheff, I.I., Chase, N.E., Bauer, R.B.: Joint Study of Extracranial Arterial Occlusion. II. Arteriography, Techniques, Sites, and Complications. J.A.M.A. 203:961–968, 1968.

21. Hollenhorst, R.W.: Neuro-ophthalmologic Aspects. In: *Cerebral Vascular Diseases,* 3rd Conference. Siekert, R.G., Whisnant, J.P., (Eds.) Grune & Stratton, New York, 1961, pp. 8–12.

22. Hypertension-Stroke Cooperative Study, University of Michigan: Stroke Recurrence after Antihypertensive Therapy. Circulation (Suppl. IV) 1973, p. 84.

23. Kannel, W.B., Gordon, T., Dawber, T.R.: Role of Lipids in the

Development of Brain Infarction: The Framingham Study. Stroke 5:679–685, 1974.

24. Kannel, W.B., Wolf, P.A., Dawber, T.R.: An Evaluation of the Epidemiology of Atherothombotic Brain Infarction. Milbank Mem. Fund Quart. 53:405–448, 1975.

25. Kannel, W.B., Dawber, T.R., Sorlie, P., Wolf, P.A.: Components of Blood Pressure and Risk of Atherothrombotic Brain Infarction: The Framingham Study. Stroke 7:327–331, 1976.

26. Marshall, J., Kaeser, A.C.: Survival After Non-Haemorrhagic Cerebrovascular Accidents. A Prospective Study. Br. Med. J. 2:73–77, 1961.

27. Matsumoto, N., Whisnant, J.P., Kurland, L.T., Okazaki, H.: Natural History of Stroke in Rochester, Minnesota, 1955 through 1969: An Extension of a Previous Study, 1945 through 1954. Stroke 4:20–29, 1973.

28. Merrett, J.D., Adams, G.F.: Comparison of Mortality Rates in Elderly Hypertensive and Normotensive Hemiplegic Patients. Br. Med. J. 2:802–805, 1966.

29. Nachman, R.L.: The Platelet as an Inflammetory Cell. In: *Cerebral Vascular Diseases*, 8th Conference. McDowell, F.H., Brennan, R.W., (Eds.) Grune & Stratton, New York, 1973, pp. 281–285.

30. Sundt, T.M., Jr., Houser, O.W., Sharbrough, F.W., Messick, J.M., Jr.: Carotid Endarterectomy: Results, Complications, and Monitoring Techniques. In: *Advances in Neurology* Vol. 16. Thompson, R.A., Green, J.R., (Eds.) Raven Press, New York, 1977, pp. 97–119.

31. Toole, J.F.: Management of T.I.A.s and Acute Cerebral Infarction. In: *Advances in Neurology* Vol. 16. Thompson, R.A., Green, J.R., (Eds.) Raven Press, New York, 1977. pp. 71–80.

32. Veterans Administration Cooperative Study Group on Antihypertensive Agents: Effects of Treatment on Morbidity in Hypertension II. Results in Patients with Diastolic Blood Pressure Averaging 90 through 114 mm Hg. J.A.M.A. 213:1143–1152, 1970.

33. Waddington, M.M.: *Atlas of Cerebral Angiography with Anatomic Correlation*. Little, Brown and Co., Boston, 1974.

34. Whisnant, J.P.: Extracranial-Intracranial Arterial Bypass. Neurology 28:209–210, 1978.

35. Wolf, P.A., Kannel, W.B., McNamara, P.M., Tordon, T.: The Role of Impaired Cardiac Function in Atherothrombotic Brain Infarction: The Framingham Study. Am.J.Public Health 63:52–58, 1973.

36. Yasargil, M.G., Krayenbuhl, H.A., Jacobson, J.H., II.: Microneurosurgical Arterial Reconstruction. Surgery 67:221–233, 1970.

37. Zucker, M.B.: Pharmacology of Agents Which Affect Platelet Adhesiveness and Aggregation. In: *Cerebral Vascular Diseases* 8th Conference. McDowell, F.H., Brennan, R.W., (Eds.) Grune & Stratton, New York, 1973. pp. 287–295.

CHAPTER 12

Slow Viral Infections

INTRODUCTION

In previous chapters, we have outlined some aspects of the evolution of neurological diagnosis and treatment. In this chapter, we shall discuss information that has revolutionized our knowledge of the pathogenesis of a number of diseases. Despite advances in pathology, microbiology, and biochemistry, there remains a core of diseases, especially in the brain, that are not associated with structural abnormalities or with obvious infectious processes. Some of these are abortive biochemical experiments of nature, but the causes of others have eluded us, such as Parkinson's disease, amyotrophic lateral sclerosis, Alzheimer's disease, multiple sclerosis, many of the sporadic adult dementias, and some hereditary dementias, like Huntington's disease. They show "degeneration" of tissue elements under the microscope.

What is "degeneration"? Gowers' early 20th century concept of "abiotrophy" was useful in the past. Abiotrophy meant that degeneration occurs when some cell systems in the body simply have not been constructed to last as long as others. The cells degenerate, and the result is perceived as disease. Abiotrophy explained many diseases, especially the hereditary ones.

But during the last 30 years, degeneration and abiotrophy have failed us because, one by one, diseases which have been classified as degenerative dementias, hereditary abiotrophies, or metabolic remote effects of cancer have been revealed as infectious, due to transmissible agents that may be isolated and characterized.

The story begins in 1954, when Bjorn Sigurdsson[61] published lectures on three diseases of Icelandic sheep. Two of these had arrived with 20 healthy sheep from Germany in 1933, apparently the first purchase of foreign sheep for Iceland in many years.

251

Five years later, *paratuberculosis* was discovered in Icelandic sheep exposed to five of the immigrant sheep. It is caused by an acid-fast bacillus, and Sigurdsson had already shown that a vaccine helped to prevent the disease.

Six years after importation of the new sheep, *maedi* appeared in flocks exposed to five other members of the 20 immigrants. Maedi is a progressive inflammatory pneumonitis. Neither of these diseases occured in sheep from German flocks, but in susceptible Icelandic sheep, they killed up to 10 percent of the population per year! The cause of maedi has since been identified as an RNA-containing virus that also causes a meningoencephalitis, *visna*. Sigurdsson did not know they were the same disease.

Rida is a chronic encephalitis whose incubation period is about 8-18 months. Sigurdsson commented that rida is similar to scrapie. We now know that it is the same disease.

Sigurdsson documented that all three diseases are transmissible. He commented that these three diseases are different from other infectious processes because of three characteristics:
1) A very long period of latency, lasting several months to several years;
2) A regular protracted course, once clinical signs have appeared, leading to serious illness or death;
3) Limitation of the infection to a single host species, and anatomical lesions only in a single organ or tissue system.

These were not characteristic of other known infectious diseases, and he proposed to call them "slow infections."

Three years later, Gajdusek and Zigas published the first description of an apparently unrelated degenerative disease kuru which they thought most probably reflected a toxic or dietary factor.[23] They discounted a possible infectious etiology because there was no evidence of fever, leukocytosis, or histologic inflammatory response, only widespread neuronal degeneration. There was no apparent seasonal incidence, and no preceding epidemic or acute individual illness. The disease was confined to an isolated inbred tribe in New Guinea, the Fore, and only affected members of neighboring tribes who intermarried with the Fore people. It was apparently a disease of recent onset, perhaps 25-30 years, but had not been described elsewhere in the world. It could not have been introduced by white explorers, because the Fore had only trifling exposure to the white man. Only 1-5 percent of the population was affected by the disease, and lastly, attempts to isolate a virus from refrigerated samples of brain, blood, and spinal fluid had failed.

Medical and veterinary physicians rarely read each other's literature, so it was not until 1959 that Hadlow[26] wrote a letter to the editor of "Lancet," detailing the similarities between scrapie in sheep, and kuru in New Guinea Fore tribesman. Both diseases are endemic in a limited population, and the incidence in the population is small. In sheep and people the symptoms may appear months after they are removed from sick contacts. Scrapie may first appear in a healthy flock after an apparently healthy member of an affected flock joins them; and kuru occurs in members of unaffected tribes only if they marry into the Fore. Neuropathological changes are remarkably similar in the two diseases, showing neuronal degeneration, marked astrocytic gliosis, multiloculated "soap bubble" vacuoles in the cytoplasm of nerve cells, and a complete absence of conventional inflammatory response. These changes had long been regarded as characteristic only of scrapie.

Hadlow did not describe the focal lesions of scrapie, which closely resemble the senile plaques of aging brains, Alzheimer's disease, Down's syndrome, and a number of other human diseases. The presence of these plaques has provoked discussion about the possible infectious nature of these diseases, although they lack the other characteristic vacuolar changes in scrapie brain that gave scrapie and related diseases the name "spongiform encephalopathies."

Hadlow pointed out that the cause of both scrapie and kuru was obscure. Scrapie had been transmitted to healthy sheep and to goats by intracerebral or subcutaneous inoculation of brain suspensions from scrapie-affected animals, but clinical disease did not appear before three months after inoculation, and sometimes appeared only after 30 months. Both scrapie and kuru are rapidly fatal once symptoms have begun.

Partially as a result of Hadlow's stimulus, Gajdusek and his coworkers, especially Dr. C. J. Gibbs, determined to launch a long-term project involving the inoculation of many different primates with extracts of kuru brain, and the observation of those animals until either they died of old age or developed a disease. Gibbs inoculated the first chimpanzee at the National Institutes of Health in August, 1963, and a major workshop and symposium on *Slow, Latent and Temperate Virus Infections* was scheduled for early December, 1964, 15 months later.[20] Gibbs' disappointment is palpable, as we read his description of the concepts involved, and the process of investigations, and learn that there were no positive results from small animal inoculations since 1957, Rhesus monkey inoculations nearly two years before, numerous tissue culture lines that did not even display a cytopathogenic effect, or from chimpanzee inoculations 16 months previously.[24] The monograph makes excellent reading, because, in addition to the sense of disappointment, there is excitement and expectancy in these papers. Although they had not yet been confirmed, the authors were discussing new, vigorous ideas about the pathogenesis of disease, and only one of these was kuru. During the ensuing years, some of the excitement has waned as the old facts are reiterated and new facts have simply provided an evolving understanding of concepts that were revolutionary in the early 1960s.

While the symposium proceedings were being prepared for publication, the first chimpanzee inoculated with kuru developed apathy, lassitude, and progressive ataxia. This event was included as an addendum to the conference publication[25], and was fully reported a year later[21]. Neurological nosology has changed as a direct result of that addendum. This chapter attempts to outline the changes in an understandable manner

THE SPONGIFORM ENCEPHALOPATHIES

Since the spring of 1965, when the first chimpanzee became apathetic with kuru, we have learned that there are four diseases caused by similar agents, two diseases in man, and two in lower animals:

1) *Kuru* develops as a progressive ataxia, producing cerebellar, Parkinsonian, and spastic symptoms.
2) *Creutzfeldt-Jakob* disease usually presents as a rapidly progressive dementia with associated findings of spasticity, fasciculations, tremor, ataxia, and myoclonus seizures.
3) *Scrapie* produces ataxia and rubbing activities in sheep which gives the disease its name because the pelt may be scraped off, exposing raw skin before the animal dies.
4) *Transmissible mink encephalopathy* occurs only on mink ranches and causes locomotor incoordination, somnolence, and prolonged biting of inanimate objects.

Once symptoms begin, all four diseases are relentlessly progressive and rapidly fatal. All display widespread neuropath-ological changes within the central nervous system, but there are no abnormalities in other organs of the body. All are caused by a trans-missible agent which is completely unlike conventional virus parti-cles because this agent is associated with cell *membranes*, not with the cytoplasm or the nucleus. It contains little or no nucleic acid.[32] The agents of Creutzfeldt-Jakob disease and kuru are larger than the scrapie agents and transmissible mink encephalopathy agents, but all are much smaller than even the smallest of the previously known viruses. The agent is more resistant to heat than con-ventional viruses and is unaffected by formaldehyde. Proteolytic en-zymes, deoxyribonuclease (DNA-ase) and ribonuclease (RNA-ase) destroy the structure of conventional viruses but do not damage this agent. The agent is susceptible to chemicals that do not normally destroy virus particles, such as detergents, ether, acetone, chloro-form, potassium permanganate, and several others.

The agent grows and multiplies in tissue cultures. Explants from affected brain show abnormal astrocytic growth, but there are none of the usual cytopathogenic effects caused by conventional viruses. These agents do not produce any known inflammatory or immune response in their hosts, and can be identified only if they are inocu-lated into an animal who later dies with characteristic neuropatho-logical changes or provides inoculum that kills a second animal.

When this agent is inoculated intracerebrally, intraperitoneally, intramuscularly, subcutaneously, or even into the anterior chamber of the eye of a susceptible host, it multiplies, apparently in thymic-origin lymphocytes of spleen, lymph nodes, and other organs before it eventually becomes numerous enough to damage the central ner-vous system. Newborn mice have no thymic-origin lymphocytes. If these neonates are inoculated with scrapie agent, the organism apparently lives as a latent virus in other tissues of the body and does not begin to multiply until much later in the life of the animal. Newborn mice inoculated with mouse scrapie virus never develop scrapie before they die of old age, but at some time during middle age, the scrapie agent begins to multiply in their bodies and may be transmitted to other mice by the inoculation of cerebral tissue.[30] The agent apparently never reaches high concentrations in blood because it is not transmitted by blood transfusions from affected animals, but large quantities of the agent are present in spleen, lymph nodes, liver, kidney, and brain. It has even been transmitted from scrap-ings of corneal epithelium.[46]

Of the four, Creutzfeldt-Jakob disease is of special interest to medical doctors. Its frequency in the population is reported to be about one per million, but this undoubtedly is too low, because the disease is being recognized and diagnosed more frequently since it has become scientifically important. It is a dangerous disease, because it may be transmitted accidentally from a patient to his neurosurgeon during a brain biopsy procedure, or from patient to patient if surgical instruments are not heat sterilized, or from cadaver donor to transplant recipient.

The first human-to-human transmission of Creutzfeldt-Jakob disease was reported in a patient of mine who was the recipient of a corneal transplant for keratoconus. Eighteen months after her operation, she developed intense vertigo, ataxia, and dysphagia, resembling a rapidly progressive cerebellar lesion; but she quickly also lost language and became demented. Within a matter of a month, she was so sick that she would have died then but for artificial means of support. After the autopsy, her daughter asked me whether I thought the transplant could have caused this terrible result, and I suddenly remembered the work of Gajdusek and Gibbs, phoned the hospital where she had had her transplant, and found that the donor had died of Creutzfeldt-Jakob disease! Since then, tissue from my patient has transmitted Creutzfeldt-Jakob disease to a chimpanzee, even though it had been preserved in 10 percent formol-saline at room temperature for seven months before inoculations.[22]

The infectious agents of the spongiform encephalopathies are also of special interest because they have been successfully transmitted from the brains of kuru, Creutzfeldt-Jakob, scrapie, and transmissible mink encephalopathy infected hosts to a large number of primate and subprimate species, where they change during serial passage in each new species by developing a shorter incubation time with each passage, being therefore more malignant for the new host species.

Scrapie is an old disease. It was recognized over 200 years ago in Europe and has continued to decimate sheep flocks since then. Its natural mode of transmission is still not completely understood, although it is possible that the dam transmits the disease to her lamb either during gestation, or during birth. Gajdusek has postulated that scrapie agent is the direct forebear of all spongiform encephalopathy agents. Creutzfeldt-Jakob disease in man may result from infection during butchering or from inadequate cooking of sheep products. If a Fore tribesman "spontaneously" developed Creutzfeldt-Jakob disease and died, his tribe's custom of smearing brain and internal organs on themselves, and eating parts of the deceased as a mark of respect, could have infected them in turn through open sores on the skin or directly through the alimentary tract. The mink that contracted mink encephalopathy had eaten carcasses of scrapie sheep and certainly suffered from mink-scrapie.

If it is true that butchering accidents cause Creutzfeldt-Jakob disease, why is it so rare? In fact, infection with human scrapie agent may *not* be rare. We identify subclinical infection by conventional viruses with rising antibody titers, tissue culture, or transmission experiments, but the host does not make antibodies to the agent of the spongiform encephalopathies. The agent does not produce cytopathogenic changes in tissue culture, and widespread inoculation of chimpanzees is impracticable. Perhaps the usual route of inoculation provides only a minute dose of scrapie agent in man, so the incubation period may be many years rather than the 15-20 months required when one is accidentally exposed to more agent during funeral rites, neurosurgery, or transplantation. Perhaps, instead, we are all infected with scrapie agent, which takes the form of senile plaques in aging brains, of Alzheimer's disease in some of us, of Creutzfeldt-Jakob disease in others, and of no disease at all in genetically insusceptible hosts. Recent work has demonstrated that, like maedi and paratuberculosis in German sheep, virtually dozens of infectious agents have adapted themselves to living with human and subhuman species, where they cause no disease in the host except under exceptional circumstances.

Gajdusek led us through the intricacies of these questions and with Gibbs and other co-workers elucidated the basic facts of the spongiform encephalopathies. Because of his work, the Fore now bury their dead without the ritual self-infection they once practiced, and kuru has vanished. Physicians are careful about the care of their patients so they do not transmit Creutzfeldt-Jakob disease to themselves or to other patients. The facts surrounding the spongiform encephalopathies have raised far-reaching questions about the pathogenesis of other diseases and about normal aging. Because of his pioneering thinking and his persistent work over many years, Gajdusek was awarded the Nobel Prize in Medicine for 1976.[66] The literature on spongiform encephalopathies is too enormous to detail in this volume, but the reader will find Gajdusek's Nobel Laureate address

good reading, and it will lead him deeper into this fascinating literature.[19]

PROGRESSIVE MULTIFOCAL LEUKOENCEPHALOPATHY

In 1958, Åström et al[7] described three patients, two with chronic
lymphatic leukemia, and one with Hodgkin's disease. Each of these
patients developed rapidly and relentlessly progressive central nervous system symptomatology that eventually displayed multifocal
distribution as the disease progressed. Although subsequently
patients have lived longer, the three patients in this first communication died within four months of the onset of their neurological illness. There was no fever, no leukocytosis, and the spinal fluid was
always normal. The authors considered this to be a newly recognized disease, but they found descriptions of five similar cases in the
literature and emphasized that two of these previous cases also occurred coincidentally with Hodgkin's disease, one with miliary
tuberculosis, and one with sarcoidosis. One of the previous patients
may have been otherwise healthy.

Microscopic examination of the brains of these first three carefully described cases revealed a primarily destructive, demyelinating
lesion without a conventional inflammatory response. In the early
demyelinating lesions, the investigators found abnormal
oligodendroglia with eosinophillic intranuclear inclusion bodies in
them. When they examined obviously more advanced lesions, they
found strikingly gigantic, malignant-looking astrocytes with giant
nuclei, multiple nuclei, and mitotic figures. Despite the presence of
intranuclear inclusion bodies, the authors avoided consideration of
an infectious etiology, but postulated the response was somehow
related to the associated chronic diseases.

This disease, too, remained an enigma for many years until
ZuRhein and Chou[69] focused interest upon it once more in 1965.
They published electron micrographs of virus particles resembling
papovavirus in the formalin-fixed brain of a patient who had died
two years previously of the disease. Perhaps because multifocal
leukoencephalopathy is very rare, no virus cultures were reported
until 1971 when Padgett et al[51] inoculated trypsinized brain biopsy
material from their patient, J.C., into tissue cultures. They successfully isolated a hitherto unknown papovavirus, which they named
after their patient. Eight months later, Weiner et al described the

isolation of a virus closely resembling SV40 virus from two patients with progressive multifocal leukoencephalopathy.[68]

Although J.C. virus has been identified much more frequently than SV40 from brains of subsequent patients with this disease, both viruses are recognized causes for the illness. This is important because neither virus is normally pathogenic in any known host. The many simian viruses, of which SV40 is only one, were discovered unexpectedly in normal monkey kidney cell cultures when large quantities of polio vaccine were first prepared in this medium.[31] Neither of Weiner's cases had been exposed to polio vaccine, so the source of their SV40 virus is unknown. Papovaviruses in general are not pathogenic to man with the single exception of human wart virus, and this agent never produces systemic disease. One might think that J.C. virus is an unusual infection that produces fatal illness only in selected patients, but this is not the case, because further investigations by Padgett and Walker[50] have shown that nearly 70 percent of adults in their Wisconsin sample had neutralizing antibodies to J.C. virus!

It appears that the viruses that cause progressive multifocal leukoencephalopathy belong to the enormous number of viruses of many kinds that are well adapted to peaceful coexistence within many different kinds of host. Under abnormal circumstances, such as leukemia or Hodgkin's disease, miliary tuberculosis or sarcoid, where the immune response is deficient, or under circumstances of induced immunosuppression for treatment of lupus erythematosus, or suppression of transplant rejection, the normal balance between virus and host is upset and the virus escapes to kill both the host and itself. The conditions that allow such an escape do not appear to be specific for the J.C. and SV40 viruses, so there is reason to expect that future cases of progressive multifocal leukoencephalopathy may be caused by others of the papovaviruses, or even by completely different viruses.

MEASLES VIRUS INFECTIONS

We shall discuss the conventional and the "slow" manifestations of measles virus in continuity because measles may be only one of many viruses that can produce acute illness as well as long-delayed slow infections. Measles has long been a dread disease of childhood because it produces permanent, even fatal, cerebral complications associated with the acute rubeola infection. As our understanding of this virus has matured, we recognize the disease as even more dreaded, because it is also the cause of subacute sclerosing panencephalitis, and quite possibly of multiple sclerosis as well.

Measles Encephalitis

Adams emphasized that subclinical measles encephalitis may be extraordinarily common during acute rubeola.[2] Clinical measles encephalitis is unpredictable. It may be mild. It may kill a child even before the rash is fully developed. If the child lives, he may recover completely from a serious bout of encephalitis, or he may be left permanently blind, paretic, demented, epileptic. When measles encephalitis develops concomitantly with the rash, it is directly caused by measles virus invading the brain.

Postinfectious Encephalomyelitis

Postinfectious encephalomyelitis develops several weeks after the acute infection by measles virus and as a sequel to many other acute viral infections. Seemingly spontaneous acute disseminated encephalomyelitis also occurs, although this may well represent a response to previous unrecognized viral infection. The onset is frequently abrupt, with clouding of consciousness or coma, fever, stiff neck. There is a lymphocytic pleocytosis of several hundred cells in the spinal fluid. The spinal fluid sugar is normal. The spinal fluid protein may be normal or mildly elevated. Such a patient completely mimics one with acute viral encephalitis. In such cases, the diagnosis of postinfectious encephalomyelitis may be made only if there are definite multifocal neurological abnormalities. Some patients develop paraplegia due to transverse myelitis, or dysconjugate eye movements due to brainstem involvement, or blindness in one or both eyes due to optic neuritis. These are uncommon accompaniments of acute viral encephalitis but occur frequently in acute disseminated encephalomyelitis because it is a rapidly developing demyelinating encephalitis, and the symptoms reflect the location of some of the individual demyelinating lesions.

If the patient has a recent history of viral infection or of immunization, this helps to confirm the diagnosis. On the other hand, if the patient develops dramatic neurological abnormalities and few signs of encephalitis, it is impossible to determine initially whether he has acute disseminated encephalomyelitis or a first bout of acute multiple sclerosis.

Acute disseminated encephalomyelitis usually lasts 4-12 weeks with the same uncertain prognosis as acute measles encephalitis. It may result in crippling residua, or the patient may recover completely, even though he appeared desperately ill during the acute stages of his disease.

Acute disseminated encephalomyelitis resembles its counterpart in the peripheral nervous system, Guillain-Barré syndrome, in its postinfectious character, its course and its pathogenesis. It appears that both diseases represent a perversion of the immune response to the previous infection. Myelin protein from the brain or from peripheral nerves is somehow liberated into the body during the acute illness, where it is recognized as "foreign" by the immune system, which then becomes sensitized, tries to destroy the protein where it finds it, and precipitates the clinical disease.

Subacute Sclerosing Panencephalitis (S.S.P.E.)

In 1933, J.R. Dawson [14] described the case of a 16-year-old boy who developed a form of "encephalitis lethargica" that was different from the usual case. The disease began about two weeks before the patient was admitted to the hospital and killed him in about two months. First, his personality changed. He became verbally abusive to his father, changed his sleep pattern, became restless, and refused to sit down. Next, he developed convulsive twitching and double vision. When he was admitted to the hospital, his reflexes were hyperactive, his movements were slowed, and his posture was abnormal. He developed fine tremor of the fingers and eventually lapsed into coma and died. Dawson found intranuclear and cytoplasmic inclusion bodies in the brain and postulated that the disease was infectious. This early description matches the usual clinical development of the disease in most patient as described in detail by Freeman.[18]

The clinical diagnosis of S.S.P.E. is usually not difficult because this disorder resembles no other illness of childhood and adolescence. A previously normal child develops a personality change which is usually first recognized at school. He is forgetful, apathetic, or psychotic. Teachers become concerned about emotional problems. By the time the physician first sees the child the history of personality change is available and, in addition, the child usually has developed second-stage signs such as myoclonus seizures, definite spasticity, rigidity, and frank dementia. The disease develops to this stage in a matter of weeks, or a few months, much more rapidly than the hereditary leukodystrophies and other "degenerative" diseases of childhood.

That history – rapid deterioration, beginning in the intellectual sphere and progressing to seizures and definite neurological abnormalities – should suggest the diagnosis of S.S.P.E. Then the diagnosis may be established by lumbar puncture and serum examinations. The spinal fluid gamma globulin is markedly elevated, and when measles antibody titers return, they too are markedly elevated in spinal fluid and blood. When spinal fluid and blood are reexamined a week or 10 days later, rapidly rising measles antibody titers establish the diagnosis.

There is no treatment for the child or adolescent with S.S.P.E. By the time the diagnosis is established, the patient is usually too demented or somnolent to care, so treatment is directed primarily to the parents who need to know they are dealing with a fatal disease. The course may last weeks or may be prolonged for many months, but death is the only outcome. Death may be further delayed by nasogastric tubes and other extraordinary means, and some parents want such treatment, even in the face of a hopeless prognosis. Others need time to think, because they have never considered the question before. Still others want no extraordinary means used if the prognosis is hopeless. Parents must have as much time as possible to come to their decision about terminal care. They may want consultation with a neurologist, but usually it is not necessary to transfer care from the family doctor, because no one else has anything better to offer the child, and the family physician may be best able to care for the family.

Pathogenesis of S.S.P.E.

We know, now, that S.S.P.E. is a slow viral infection caused by measles virus. Dawson noted that the CSF globulin in his case, was "positive," and soon it was known that this globulin was measles antibody. Vigorous attempts were made to identify measles virus, but these failed until 1969, when, almost simultaneously, a number of different investigators reported the growth, isolation, and identification of measles virus in tissue culture, which could be transmitted to weanling ferrets or to Rhesus monkeys. Free transmissible measles virus could be found only after serial transmission through green monkey kidney and HeLa cell cultures.[12,29,53]

In 1968, Katz et al[35] had transmitted to ferrets a slow virus infection by inoculation of brain biopsy tissue from a case of S.S.P.E., but they were not definitely able to identify the agent as measles virus. A number of other experimental animals developed acute measles encephalitis after inoculation with S.S.P.E. brain, but the clinical picture of S.S.P.E. was not reproduced in primates until 1977.[4] This is important, because only man and primates are susceptible to measles infection under normal circumstances, and without an equivalent experimental model, it was more difficult to study S.S.P.E.

The Rhesus monkeys that finally did develop clinical S.S.P.E. were preimmunized against measles, or had been exposed to measles and had recovered from the acute infection. Then these especially prepared monkeys were inoculated with measles virus that had gone through numerous subcultures in green monkey kidney and VERO cell tissue culture before finally passing once or twice through suckling hamsters! If unimmunized monkeys were exposed to this same modified virus, they promptly developed acute measles encephalitis and died in a matter of weeks, but preimmunized monkeys developed a slow viral infection!

How does this relate to the pathogenesis of S.S.P.E.? Why is it that only the monkey who has successfully repulsed measles can develop S.S.P.E. when he is challenged with the virus? Why is it that S.S.P.E. develops 5-7 years after a child successfully repulses acute measles and develops neutralizing antibodies? We know that the virus is unchanged. We know that the child's measles antibodies are intact, effective antibodies. One suggestion was that the T-cells, lymphocytes responsible for killing virus-infected cells of the body, are defective in cases of S.S.P.E. If this were true, defective T-cells might not identify infected cells or might not be able to kill them.

Kreth and co-workers recently addressed this problem with fascinating results.[37,38] They had previously shown that T-cells may not be responsible for identification and lysis of infected cells in S.S.P.E. There are actually three different kinds of killer cells in the cellular immune system: 1) the T-cells, which originate from thymic lymphocytes and produce rapid destruction of infected body cells, 2) "armed" macrophages, which can also identify and lyse infected cells, and 3) a newly described subpopulation of B-lymphocytes, tentatively called K-cells, which are sensitive to one portion of the gamma globulin molecule.[11]

K-cells identify infected body cells by the gamma globulin attached to abnormal surface membrane antigens specifically related to the viral infection. The K-cells may be the primary cytotoxic agents in measles infection, but because of the tremendous antibody response in the already sensitized host, Kreth and terMeulen postulate that they may be "blinded" and unable to identify and kill affected cells because of the profusion of gamma globulin in the tissues. As a result, the infection is allowed to smolder. Viruses may be able to escape from one cell to another through the tightly packed neuropil of the brain, and escape from the lethal effects of antibody present in the extracellular spaces of other tissues. This hypothesis opens obvious doors to the experimental treatment of S.S.P.E. through antibody suppression or plasmapheresis. Information about such experiments may soon be available.

Pathogenesis of Multiple Sclerosis (MS)

The pathogenesis of multiple sclerosis (MS) is more complex. Multiple sclerosis, too, is probably caused, at least in part, by chronic infection with measles virus. There is evidence that the virus resides in the jejunum, and perhaps elsewhere in the body. But there is also evidence of a strong genetic factor that permits a person to "catch" MS only if he has the "MS gene." Then there is an element of bad luck: the age of first exposure to measles infection partially seems to determine whether a susceptible person will eventually develop multiple sclerosis.

There have been many dead-end issues in MS research. In its turn, each has provided apparently hopeful advances in knowledge, only to be contradicted by later investigation. This volume is not large enough for an encyclopedic discussion of all previous avenues of investigation, so your author has chosen to lead you on the most direct path to the answer which seems best at this time. The answers are not all in, and the reader will want to follow the developments as the current answers evolve to a more complete understanding of the disease.

Epidemiology

Examination of epidemiologic features of MS began in 1947 when the National Multiple Sclerosis Society, the National Public Health Service, and eventually the Canadian Ministry of Health and Welfare launched a project together to determine the prevalence of MS, and to study the influence of climate and race on its distribution.[41] They examined the populations of Winnipeg and New Orleans and found that MS was about six times more prevalent in the northern city than the southern. There were similar, but less dramatic contrasts between the prevalence in New Orleans and Denver, Boston, and San Francisco. An attempt to discover racial or genetic influences on the disease led to the incorrect conclusion that these must be insignificant factors.

This study led to examinations of other populations in the world with the same result: in the Northern and Southern hemispheres, the incidence and prevalence of MS increases in direct proportion to the distance from the equator.[40] Many studies attempted to explain this geographical variation by implicating the number of days of cloudiness, the amount of ultraviolet in sunlight, and even the gluten content of local wheat. One suggestion was that upper respiratory infections occur more frequently in temperate climates, and this might represent a reason for the apparent effect of latitude upon the incidence of MS.

Does this mean that a person with MS who lives in Winnipeg should move to New Orleans? The authors thought not, because numerous MS patients who had moved south in the past had continued to deteriorate.

But could a person move from a northern city to a southern one and prevent the *onset* of multiple sclerosis? Israel was the ideal country to search for an answer to this question. It had an immigrant population from all over the world whose chances of developing MS in their native lands were known. Additionally, every resident of Israel had access to excellent medical facilities, and up-to-date, demographic data were available for the whole population.[6]

The study showed, as expected, that immigrants from Europe had 6-10 times greater prevalence rates for multiple sclerosis than those who immigrated from Afro-Asian countries. Next, the authors analyzed the age of immigration to Israel. They found that

European immigrants who moved to Israel after they were 15 years old maintained a markedly increased risk of developing MS, but European immigrants who were younger than 15 when they moved to Israel had only a 1.7 times greater incidence than their Afro-Asian counterparts. This meant that adult Europeans had "caught" their disease in Europe before they reached age 15. If they moved to Israel in childhood, their chances of "catching" the disease approached the incidence of their new home. This study was repeated in the United States and in Hawaii with similar results.

The reader must not leave this discussion of migration studies thinking that he has the key to an understanding of the incidence of MS through changes in latitude, because the situation is a great deal more complex than that. Even though latitudes of origin remain a factor in the incidence of MS, higher latitudes are also associated with more temperate climate, usually more adequate sanitation facilities, different rates and ages of first infection with various viruses, and markedly different population genetics. In fact, latitude itself is probably not the primary cause for the differences in the incidence of MS at all. For instance, Japan, whose latitudes approximate those of southern Europe, has a surprisingly low incidence of MS by comparison, if latitude were the sole factor. Other known factors still remain to be discussed.

Questions of heredity and infection remained important even in the early investigations. Cendrowski[10] found that the incidence of MS in relatives of MS patients is about seven times higher than the incidence in the rest of the population. Dizygotic twins and siblings of patients had about 10 times more MS than other relatives. He did not examine monozygotic twins, and he concluded that the figures indicated a shared infectious process. Other investigators suggested a genetic factor from similar data.

Abnormal Immune Responses

At about the same time the epidemiological studies became available, immunological research disclosed characteristic abnormalities in MS patients. In 1962, Adams and Imagawa,[3] reported that measles antibody titers in the serum of MS patients were likely to be higher than in controls. Furthermore, 75 percent of MS patients had measurable measles antibodies in the spinal fluid, while none was ever found in the controls. Adams and Imagawa argued that both MS and measles are associated with optic neuritis, both produce similar symptoms from the central nervous system, and they referred to previous studies suggesting that children who develop optic neuritis during an acute attack of measles might later develop multiple sclerosis. Adams and Imagawa already knew that MS patients have increased gamma globulin in the spinal fluid. They suggested that this probably represented the increased measles antibody titer of spinal fluid. They speculated that gamma globulin may have been made in the central nervous system.

This proved to be a controversial paper because various laboratories attempting to duplicate the work, either confirmed or denied the findings of Adams and Imagawa to such a degree that Adams published a partial retraction in 1967,[1] reviewing reports subsequent to his first article and considering whether his original patient population may have been biased. His retraction was unnecessary because, since 1967, the discoveries of Adams and Imagawa have been amply confirmed. However, their conclusion that the antibody elevations are a direct reflection of measles infection remains unsettled.

Tourtellotte[64,65] soon showed that the excess gamma globulin in spinal fluid actually does originate in the brain, and further, that it is probably manufactured in the MS plaques, because gamma globulin concentrations are about eight times higher in plaque tissue than in adjacent normal brain. Further analysis of spinal fluid gamma globulin (IgG) disclosed that it is oligoclonal IgG with two or more distinct bands present in about 90 percent of MS patients.[45] Oligoclonal IgG is characteristic of the antibody response to infection, as opposed to the monoclonal gamopathies of multiple myeloma and related cancers.

The oligoclonal IgG proved more enigmatic than expected. It does not disappear when it is absorbed with high-titer measles antigen, although a small amount of spinal fluid globulin does precipitate, indicating the presence of small quanities of specific measles antibody.[49] Similar oligoclonal IgG is also found in the spinal fluid of S.S.P.E. patients and it, too, fails to absorb easily to measles antigen, even though we *know* that S.S.P.E. is caused by measles infection. The data suggested that there is continuing antigenic stimulation within the central nervous system of MS patients and that measles virus probably plays a role in the process. The authors were unable to state whether the virus might be incomplete or present as virus-antibody complexes. Even now, the problem of measles antibody in MS is not completely solved. Haire[27] has written an excellent review.

The genetic problems arose again during analysis of antibody results. It is true that MS patients have higher measles antibody titers than controls, and they have higher measles antibody titer than their life-long friends, but siblings, born within three years of the MS patient, have measles antibodies that are equivalent to the patient's, suggesting a familial characteristic which cannot simply be explained by prolonged, close physical contact.[28]

Heredity: The Histocompatability Determinants

Multiple sclerosis research has benefited from a totally different series of immunological problems related primarily to human kidney transplantation and the problems of transplant rejection by the host. Both circulating antibodies and delayed cellular hypersensitivity, the two major divisions of the immune system, are involved in transplant rejection. Furthermore, there are at least four genetic loci, located on one chromosome, that largely determine whether a tissue graft will be accepted by both components of the immune system.

Circulating antibodies are easiest to study. These were examined first, and given the designation of HL, for *histocompatibility locus* antigens. There are two gene loci on the chromosome for the HL determinants, and many, many alleles, so each person may have up to four different HL determinants on the two loci of both of his two matching chromosomes.

Delayed cellular hypersensitivity to a tissue graft or to any other antigenic challenge, is also determined by alleles on two loci of the same chromosome. The alleles that *determined lymphocyte* response to the antigen were originally named LD. An individual may have four of many LD determinants as well. Because they are close together on the chromosome, certain of the HL and LD determinants are frequently found together.

It was easy and natural to test populations of patients other than transplant donors and recipients. A striking relationship between HL-A27 and ankylosing spondylitis was discovered. Indeed, a person can hardly develop that disease unless he has HL-A27![9] Other close associations between various histocompatability determinants and specific disease appeared, and in 1972, Bertrams and

Kuwert[8] reported that a comparison of 200 MS patients and 225 controls disclosed a significantly higher frequency of HL-A3, HL-A10, and W5 antigens among the MS patients.

This was the first direct evidence of a genetic factor in multiple sclerosis. The genetic factor is associated with the individual's immune response capabilities for all immunological events of the organism, and MS already had strong associations with an abnormal immune response to measles virus. The results of Bertrams and Kuwert have not been completely substantiated. Since their first paper, it has become clear that MS patients and their families have a higher frequency of HL-A3, HL-A7, and LD-7A (since renamed HLA-DW2) than the general population. This is especially true of the DW2 allele.[33,42] S.S.P.E. has been less well studied, but a preliminary report indicated that S.S.P.E. patients have a preponderance of W29 instead of the HLA determinants commonly found in MS patients.[39]

Multiple sclerosis patients are genetically different from other people, and the difference relates to the immune response genes. Other evidence points to chronic, unrepulsed infection, probably with measles. Are the HL and LD genes themselves the cause of multiple sclerosis? Clearly not, because even though the frequencies of these alleles among MS patients are significantly higher than among controls, the differences are not nearly as dramatic as they are in ankylosing spondylitis. It appears that the HL and LD alleles, which we can identify by their antigenic characteristics, are closely linked to a gene that specifies the appearance of MS under still undetermined circumstances.

The tremendous power of genetic analysis is evident in papers which address the problem of locating the MS gene. We have already seen that this gene is situated on a chromosome which frequently also carries HL-A3 and HL-A7, and DW2 alleles.[15,16,62,63] How can that be? It *can be* if at sometime in the distant past a single gene on that chromosome in a single person, generations ago, developed a mutation at that locus that allowed the development of MS, and on the other loci that person *chanced* to carry the HL-A3, HL-A7, and DW2 alleles.[62]

What a stupendous conclusion! Patients with multiple sclerosis are related to each other through some ancient ancestor whose DNA has come down to them unchanged by time and chemistry, through the replications of the generations and population migrations all over the world. This conclusion relates to Watson and

Crick's discovery of the structure of the DNA molecule and to studies of classic genetics, but the significance of the information is brought home to us only when we consider the enormity of its implications to human populations over the centuries! The *rest* of the progenitor's chromosome descended to MS patients more or less intact because there has been limited crossing over between portions of the chromosome during meiosis. Genes distantly separated from each other along the chromosome, like the HL-A3 and the MS gene, are less likely to stay together than adjacent genes like DW2 and the MS gene.

Taking the problem one step further, Terasaki and Mickey argue that the progenitor must have been a Northern European, because MS is most frequent in Northern European peoples, and the particular chromosome configuration of HL-A3, HL-A7, and DW2 with MS is most common in Northern Europeans. The infrequency of MS in Japan probably relates to the relatively insignificant contacts between Japanese and Europeans until recent times, and it may even be that Japanese MS represents a second independent mutation.[62]

Furthermore, African Negroes do not develop MS, but American Negroes do. American Negroes with MS fail to show the HL-A3 and HL-A7 alleles, but 30 percent of them carry DW2. None of these alleles is present in the normal population of American or African Negroes. Remember that DW2 is the allele closest to the MS gene. It must have descended among American Negroes from an ancestor whose chromosome had traded his progenitor's HL-A3 and HL-A7 portions for other histocompatibility alleles through crossing-over, but had not traded away the progenitor's trademark series of DW2-MS! The other 70 percent of American Negroes with MS may have lost their DW2 through crossing over, or they may be descendents of yet another ancestor.

If we are to understand the pathogenesis of MS, we must discover how the MS gene malfunctions, and we do not yet know. There is a growing literature that indicates that lymphocytes from MS patients may be selectively deficient in their response to myxovirus antigens (measles, parainfluenza), and to some other virus antigens.[13,67] Unfortunately, there is also a distinct literature that indicates that *normal* people with HL-A3, HL-A7, and DW2 genotypes show decreased lymphocyte responses to immunological challenge.[34,43,56] This information demands that experiments involving lymphocyte responsiveness in MS be repeated using MS patients mismatched for their immune response alleles and controls matched to each series.

Most distressing are the findings in the literature which indicate that normal people with HL-A3, HL-A7, and W-18 have an increase in various circulating antibody titers. Multiple sclerosis patients with these genotypes have elevated antibody titers to measles; MS patients without them do not.[52] Remember that family members of MS patients tend to have higher-than-normal measles antibodies, and that the controversy over elevated measles antibodies got us into this discussion in the first place. This new information indicates that in all probability, those increased antibodies were an effect of unrelated genetic markers on the MS chromosome, not directly related to the pathogenesis of the disease itself!

Nonetheless the original epidemiological studies are valid, irrespective of immune response genes. People do "catch" multiple sclerosis. Tourtellotte's work on the origins of spinal fluid gamma globulin in MS plaques must still be significant. The information about lymphocyte unresponsiveness and serum antibodies may still be important to a modern understanding of the pathogenesis of MS, but this work must be clarified by studies of the relatives of MS patients and controls matched for HL-A genotypes before its significance can be determined.

Meanwhile, treatment with measles transfer factor is based on the *increased* responsiveness of MS lymphocytes *in vitro* when transfer factor is added; while treatment with immuno*suppressive* agents is based in part on the excessive production of antibodies in patients with multiple sclerosis. Such treatments may prove to be effective, but future research may reveal that the data which prompted them were the result of irrelevant alterations in lymphocyte activity caused by immune response genes related to MS only by their chance position on a chromosome hundreds of years ago. If measles virus is eventually established as the infectious factor in the pathogenesis of MS, it would not be the first time in history that right conclusions were reached for completely wrong reasons!

Direct Evidence of Chronic Measles Infection in Multiple Sclerosis

The search for measles may have begun for the wrong reasons;

but even so, there may be definite confirmation of chronic measles infection in MS patients. In 1972, Prineas[59] published electron micrographs of paramyxoma-like particles in nuclei of MS brain cells. The finding was confirmed by Raine et al, two years later.[60] Paramyxovirus has been recovered from two MS brains, but the significiance of this discovery to the pathogenesis of MS is doubtful, because this virus is not universally recovered from MS brains.

In the fall of 1976, Pertschuk et al[54] first recorded that all 24 MS patients whose jejunal biopsies were examined had measles antigen present in the lamina propria, while none of the 20 controls did. Additionally, they found components of complement and various immune globulins in jejunal biopsies from some of their MS patients that were not present in control jejunal biopsies. In a second article,[55] they demonstrated measles antigen in all of 20 further cases of MS, and in one case of ALS. Surprisingly, three others of their seven ALS patients had poliovirus antigen, herpesvirus in one, and no viral antigen in a last case. More recently, they have reported the recovery of a paramyxovirus from the tissue culture of six consecutive cases of MS, which presumably is measles virus by its antigenic characteristics.[58]

Two laboratories in Europe have attempted to duplicate the findings of Pertschuk's group but have failed to do so even though one of these laboratories used test reagents sent directly from Pertschuk's laboratory.[17,36] Is the dramatic sequence of papers from this group merely another dead-end mistake in a long list of mistaken conclusions which have accompanied MS research over the years? Possibly, but these results may be confirmed by new evidence that may even be available before the reader finds this chapter. If the work of Pertschuk's group is confirmed, how can we account for the central nervous system disease? Is the jejunum only an easy place to discover and culture the virus? Does it also grow in brain, or does it cause MS through distant effects of a toxic nature or by circulating antigen-antibody complexes?*

Age-Dependent Host Responses to Measles Virus Infection

Children who develop acute measles before the age of two are much more likely to develop S.S.P.E. than children whose measles occurs in later childhood.[48] Measles encephalitis occurs more frequently during acute measles in adolescents. Multiple sclerosis may

*See Addendum, Page 279

also represent one host response to primary measles infection in later childhood.

Poskanzer et al[57] emphasized the striking epidemiologic similarities between poliomyelitis and multiple sclerosis. Both paralytic polio and MS are more common in temperate regions; both are more common in upper socioeconomic groups; and both are more common within a family than in the general population. Paralytic poliomyelitis was rare in tropical countries because of inadequate sanitation so that infants acquired immunity to poliovirus early in life, whereas in developed temperate regions, infection with poliomyelitis virus was delayed until later childhood when the host was, for some reason, more susceptible to the paralytic complications of the infection.

Leibowitz et al[44] re-interviewed the Israeli population that had been studied in the early epidemiologic studies of MS, to determine whether similar factors of sanitation could be implicated in the pathogenesis of this disease. They found that during childhood their MS patients had had statistically better water supplies, toilet facilities, and less family crowding than the controls.

Alter's 1976 discussion is a most complete exposition of the age-dependent host response.[5] He emphasizes the known relationship between early measles infection and S.S.P.E. and late childhood measles infection with acute measles encephalitis, and suggests that MS is a second central nervous system complication of *late* childhood measles infection. A retrospective study had suggested that acute measles had occurred later in MS patients than in controls. Population studies in areas of high or low MS prevalence disclosed that measles immunity is acquired earlier in areas of low MS prevalence, than in areas of high MS prevalence.

Measles inoculation has been widespread in this country since 1965, and Alter predicts a beginning decline in the frequency of MS in about 1980, because that generation of children will have acquired their measles immunity as infants, rather than later in childhood.

But if S.S.P.E. is an aftereffect of *early* measles infection, such inoculation might be expected to increase the incidence of S.S.P.E. This does not seen to be the case. S.S.P.E. became a medically interesting disease in the mid-1960s, and its reported incidence increased steadily until 1970, but has dropped since then. This may indicate that inoculation with modified measles virus early in life actually helps to prevent S.S.P.E.[47,48]

SUMMARY

Multiple sclerosis is, in part, an infectious disease, and now it appears that the agent is measles virus. Other factors are critical to the development of MS, because a person can develop MS only if he is a direct genetic descendant of some early progenitor whose mutation produced a gene allowing its development. It appears also that a maturational factor determines the appearance of MS, because the age of first measles infection bears on the later development of multiple sclerosis.

We do not yet know the significance of the apparent discovery of measles antigen, and the apparent isolation of measles virus from the jejunum of MS patients, but the report is provocative. We do not know whether the immunologic abnormalities in circulating antibodies and delayed cellular hypersensitivity bear directly on the pathogenesis of MS or only reflect a shared genetic background in MS patients. We can expect rapid enlightenment on these issues in future years.

Research into the slow virus infections has provided tremendous insight into the process of immunity, genetics, biochemistry, and microbiology. An understanding of their mechanisms may open doors to treatment of such diverse conditions as premature senility and cancer. This is the newest field of medical endeavor and as a result, it has been the most exciting one during the past 15 years.

REFERENCES

1. Adams, J.M.: Measles Antibodies in Patients with Multiple Sclerosis. Neurology 17:707–710, 1967.
2. Adams, J.M.: Clinical Pathology of Measles Encephalitis and Sequelae. Neurology 18:52–56, 1968.
3. Adams, J.M., Imagawa, D.T.: Measles Antibody in Multiple Sclerosis. Proc. Soc. Exp. Biol. Med. 111:562–566, 1962.
4. Albrecht, P., Burnstein, T., Klutch, M.J., Hicks, J.T., Ennis, F.A.: Subacute Sclerosing Panencephalitis: Experimental Infection in Primates. Science 195:64–66, 1977.
5. Alter, M.: Is Multiple Sclerosis an Age-Dependent Host Response to Measles? Lancet I:456–457, 1976.
6. Alter, M., Leibowitz, U., Speer, J.: Risk of Multiple Sclerosis Related to Age at Immigration to Israel. Arch. Neurol. 15:234–237, 1966.
7. Åström, K.-E., Mancall, E.L., Richardson, E.P., Jr.: Progressive

Multifocal Leuko-Encephalopathy: A Hitherto Unrecognized Complication of Chronic Lymphatic Leukemia and Hodgkin's Disease. Brain 81:93-111, 1958.

8. Bertrams, J., Kuwert, E.: HL-A Antigen Frequencies in Multiple Sclerosis. Europ. Neurol. 7:74-78, 1972.

9. Brewerton, D.A., Caffrey, M., Hart, F.D., James, D.C.O., Nicholls, A., Sturrock, R.D.: Ankylosing Spondylitis and HL-A 27. Lancet I:504-907, 1973.

10. Cendrowski, W.S.: Multiple Sclerosis in Twins and Other Relatives. Acta Neurol. Scand. 49:552-556, 1973.

11. Cerottini, J.-C., Brunner, K.T.: Cell-Mediated Cytotoxicity, Allograft Rejection and Tumor Immunity. Adv. Immunol. 18:67-132, 1974.

12. Chen, T.T., Watanabe, I., Zeman, W., Mealey, J., Jr.: Subacute Sclerosing Panencephalitis: Propagation of Measles Virus from Brain Biopsy in Tissue Culture. Science 163:1193-1194, 1969.

13. Cunningham-Rundles, S., DuPont, B., Posner, J.B., Hansen, J.A., Good, R.A.: *In Vitro* Lymphocyte Transformation of M.S. Patients to Paramyxovirus Antigens. Acta Neurol. Scand. 55: (Suppl. 63), 145-154, 1977.

14. Dawson, J.R.: Cellular Inclusions in Cerebral Lesions of Lethargic Encephalitis. Am. J. Pathol. 9:7-19, 1933.

15. Degos, L., Dausset, J.: Histocompatibility Determinants in Multiple Sclerosis. Lancet I:307-308, 1974.

16. Drachman, D.A., Davison, W.C., Mittal, K.K.: Histocompatibility (HL-A) Factors in Familial Multiple Sclerosis. Arch. Neurol. 33:406-413, 1976.

17. Fraser, K.B., Haire, M., Millar, J.H.D.: Measles Antigen in Jejunal Mucosa in Multiple Sclerosis. Lancet I:1313-1314, 1977.

18. Freeman, J.O.: The Clinical Spectrum and Early Diagnosis of Dawson's Encephalitis. J. Pediatr. 75:590-603, 1969.

19. Gajdusek, D.C.: Unconventional Virus and the Origin and Disappearance of Kuru. Science 197:943-960, 1977.

20. Gajdusek, D.C., Gibbs, C.J., Alpers, M., (Eds.): *Slow, Latent, and Temperate Virus Infections.* U.S. Dept. of Health, Education and Welfare, NINDB Monograph No. 2, Washington, D.C., 1965.

21. Gajdusek, D.C., Gibbs. C.J., Alpers, M.: Experimental Transmission of a Kuru-Like Syndrome to Chimpanzees. Nature 209:794-796, 1966.

22. Gajdusek, D.C., Gibbs, C.J.: Survival of Creutzfeldt-Jakob Disease Virus in Formol-Fixed Brain Tissue. N. Engl. J. Med. 294:553, 1976.

23. Gajdusek, D.C., Zigas, V.: Degenerative Disease of the Central Nervous System in New Guinea. N. Engl. J. Med. 257:974-978, 1957.

24. Gibbs, C.J., Gajdusek, D.C.: Attempt to Demonstrate a Transmissible Agent in Kuru, Amyotrophic Lateral Sclerosis and Other Sub-

acute and Chronic Progressive Nervous System Degenerations of Man. In: *Slow, Latent, and Temperate Virus Infections.* U.S. Dept. of Health, Education and Welfare, NINDB Monograph No. 2, Washington, D.C., 1965.

25. *Ibid.,* p. 46.
26. Hadlow, W.J.: Scrapie and Kuru. Lancet II:289–290, 1959.
27. Haire, M.: Significance of Virus Antibodies in Multiple Sclerosis. Br. Med. Bull. 33:40–44, 1977.
28. Henson, T.E., Brody, J.A., Sever, J.L., Dyken, M.L., Cannon, J.: Measles Antibody Titers in Multiple Sclerosis Patients, Siblings, and Controls. J.A.M.A. 211:1985–1988, 1970.
29. Horta-Barbosa, L., Fuccillo, D.A., London, W.T., Jabbour J.T., Zeman, W., Sever, J.L.: Isolation of Measles Virus from Brain Cell Cultures of Two Patients with Subacute Sclerosing Panencephalitis. Proc. Soc. Exp. Biol. Med. 132:272–277, 1969.
30. Hotchin, J., Buckley, R.: Latent Form of Scrapie Virus: A New Factor in Slow-Virus Disease. Science 196:668–671, 1977.
31. Hull, R.N., Minner, J.R., Smith, J.W.: New Viral Agents Recovered from Tissue Cultures of Monkey Kidney Cells. Am. J. Hyg. 63:204–215, 1956.
32. Hunter, G.D., Collis, S.C., Millson, G.C., Kimberlin, R.H.: Search for Scrapie-Specific RNA and Attempts to Detect an Infectious DNA or RNA. J. Gen. Virol. 32:157–162, 1976.
33. Jersild, C., DuPont, B., Fog, T., Hansen, G.S., Nielsen, L.S., Thomsen, M., Svejgaard, A.: Histocompatibility-Linked Immune-Response Determinants in Multiple Sclerosis. Transpl. Proc. 5:1791–1796, 1973.
34. Källen, B., Löw, B., Nilsson, O.: Mixed Leukocyte Reaction and HL-A Specificity at Multiple Sclerosis. Acta Neurol. Scand. 51:184–192, 1975.
35. Katz, M., Rorke, L.B., Masland, W.S., Koprowski, H., Tucker, S.H.: Transmission of an Encephalitogenic Agent from Brains of Patients with Subacute Sclerosing Panencephalitis to Ferrets. N. Engl. J. Med. 279:793–798, 1968.
36. Kingston, D., Shiner, M., Lange, L.S., Mertin, J., Meade, C.: Measles Antigen in Jejunal Mucosa in Multiple Sclerosis. Lancet I:1313, 1977.
37. Kreth, H.W., terMeulen, V.: Cell-Mediated Cytotoxicity Against Measles Virus in S.S.P.E. I. Enhancement by Antibody. J. Immunol. 118:291–295, 1977.
38. Kreth, H.W., Wiegand, G.: Cell-Mediated Cytotoxicity Against Measles Virus in S.S.P.E. II. Analysis of Cytotoxic Effector Cells. J. Immunol. 118:296–301, 1977.
39. Kurent, J.E., Terasaki, P.I., Sever, J.L.: Association of HL-A Histo-

compatibility Antigen W29 with S.S.P.E. Arch. Neurol. 32:494, 1975.

40. Kurland, L.T., Reed, D.: Geographic and Climatic Aspects of Multiple Sclerosis. Am.J.Public Health 54:588–597, 1964.
41. Kurland, L.T., Westlund, K.B.: Epidemiologic Factors in the Etiology and Prognosis of Multiple Sclerosis. Ann. N.Y. Acad. Sci. 58:682–701, 1954.
42. Kuwert, E.K.: Genetical Aspects of Multiple Sclerosis with Special Regard to Histocompatability Determinants. Acta Neurol. Scand. 55:(Suppl. 63), 23–41, 1977.
43. Lehrich, J.R., Arnason, B.G.W.: Histocompatability Types and Viral Antibodies. Arch. Neurol. 33:404–405, 1976.
44. Leibowitz, U., Antonovsky, A., Medalie, J.M., Smith, H.A., Halpern, L., Alter, M.: Epidemiological Study of Multiple Sclerosis in Israel. Part II. Multiple Sclerosis and Level of Sanitation. J. Neurol. Neurosurg. Psychiatr. 29:60–68, 1966.
45. Link, H.: Immunoglobulin Abnormalities in Multiple Sclerosis. Ann. Clin. Res. 5:330–336, 1973.
46. Manuelidis, E.E., Angelo, J.N., Gorgacz, E.J., Kim, J.H., Manuelidis, L.: Experimental Creutzfeldt-Jakob Disease Transmitted via the Eye with Infected Cornea. N.Engl.J.Med. 296: 1334–1336, 1977.
47. McDonald, R.: S.S.P.E. (Subacute Sclerosing Panencephalitis): Is Measles Vaccination Promotive or Preventive? Clin. Pediatr. 16:124–127, 1977.
48. Modlin, J.F., Jabbour, J.T., Witte, J.J., Halsey, N.A.: Epidemiologic Studies of Measles, Measles Vaccine, and Subacute Sclerosing Panencephalitis. Pediatrics 59:505–512, 1977.
49. Norrby, E., Link, H.: Immunological Parameters in the Spinal Fluid. Acta Neurol. Scand. 55:(Suppl. 63), 161-171, 1977.
50. Padgett, B.L., Walker, .L.: Prevalence of Antibodies in Human Sera Against J.C. Virus, and Isolate from a Case of Progressive Multifocal Leukoencephalopathy. J. Infect. Dis. 127:467–470, 1973.
51. Padgett, B.L., Walker, D.L., Zu Rhein, G.M., Eckroade, R.J.: Cultivation of Papova-Like Virus from Human Brain with Progressive Multifocal Leukoencephalopathy. Lancet I:1257–1260, 1971.
52. Paty, D.W., Furesz, J., Boucher, D.W., Rand, C.G., Stiller, C.R.: Measles Antibodies as Related to HL-A Types in Multiple Sclerosis. Neurology 26:651–655, 1976.
53. Payne, F.E., Baublis, J.V., Itabashi, H.H.: Isolation of Measles Virus from Cell Cultures of a Brain from a Patient with Subacute Sclerosing Panencephalitis. N.Engl.J.Med. 281:585–589, 1969.
54. Pertschuk, L.P., Cook, A.W., Gupta, J.: Measles Antigen in Multiple Sclerosis: Identification in the Jejunum by Immunofluorescence. Life Sci. 19:1603–1608, 1976.

55. Pertschuk, L.P., Nook, A.W., Gupta, J.K., Broome, J.D., Vuletin, J.C., Kim, D.S., Brigati, D.J., Rainford, E.A., Nidsgorski, F.: Jejunal Immunopathology in Amyotrophic Lateral Sclerosis and Multiple Sclerosis. Lancet I:1119–1123, 1977.

56. Petrányi, G. Gy., Benczur, M., Ónody, C.E., Hollán, S.R.: HL-A 3, 7 and Lymphocyte Cytotoxic Activity. Lancet I:736, 1974.

57. Poskanzer, D.C., Schapira, K., Miller, H.: Multiple Sclerosis and Poliomyelitis. Lancet II:917–921, 1963.

58. Prasad, I., Broome, J.D., Pertschuk, L.P., Gupta, J., Cook, A.W.: Recovery of Paramyxoma Virus from the Jejunum of Patients with Multiple Sclerosis. Lancet I:1117–1119, 1977.

59. Prineas, J.: Paramyxoma Virus-Like Particles Associated with Acute Demyelination in Chronic Relapsing Multiple Sclerosis. Science 178:760–762, 1972.

60. Raine, C.S., Powers, J.N., Suzuki, K.: Acute Multiple Sclerosis: Confirmation of "Paramyxoma-Like" Intranuclear Inclusions. Arch. Neurol. 30:39–46, 1974.

61. Sigurdsson, B.: Observations on Maedi, Paratuberculosis, and Rida, Three Slow Infections of Sheep. Br. Vet. J. 110:255–270, 307–322, 341–354, 1954.

62. Terasaki, P.I., Mickey, M.R.: A Single Mutation Hypothesis for Multiple Sclerosis Based on the HL-A System. Neurology 26:56–58, 1976.

63. Terasaki, P.I., Park, M.S., Opelz, G., Ting, A.: Multiple Sclerosis and High Incidence of a B Lymphocyte Antigen. Science 193:1245–1247, 1976.

64. Tourtellotte, W.W.: Multiple Sclerosis—The Hunt for Etiology. Hosp. Pract. 4:7:29–33, 1969.

65. Tourtellotte, W.W.: Cerebrospinal Fluid Immunoglobulins and the Central Nervous System as an Immunological Organ Particularly in Multiple Sclerosis and Subacute Sclerosing Panencephalitis. Res. Publ. Assoc. Nerv. Ment. Dis. 49:112–155, 1971.

66. Tower, D.B.: D. Carleton Gajdusek, M.D.—Nobel Laureate in Medicine for 1976. Editorial. Arch. Neurol. 34:205–208, 1977.

67. Utermohlen, V., Winfield, J.B., Kulisek, E., Zabriskie, J.B.: Cell-Mediated Immunity to Viral Antigens in Multiple Sclerosis and Other Disorders. In: The Role of Immunological Factors in Infectious, Allergic and Autoimmune Processes, Beers, R.F. and Basset, E.G., (Eds.) Raven Press, New York, 1976. pp. 151–161.

68. Weiner, L.P., Herndon, R.M., Narayan, O., Johnson, R.T., Shah, K., Rubinstein, L.J., Preziosi, T.J., Conlet, F.K.: Isolation of Virus Related to SV40 from Patients with Progressive Multifocal Leukoencephalopathy. N. Engl. J. Med. 286:385–390, 1972.

69. Zu Rhein, G.M., Chou, S.-M.: Particles Resembling Papova Viruses

in Human Cerebral Demyelinating Disease. Science 148:1477–1479, 1965.

ADDENDUM

While this volume has been in production, new evidence has appeared that supports the contention of Cook, Pertschuk, et al that multiple sclerosis and amyotrophic lateral sclerosis may be caused by an incompetent immune system that allows a viral infection to persist.

Even though Woyciechowska, et al failed,[4] Ebina, et al most recently reported the isolation of measles virus from multiple sclerosis jejunal biopsies, using techniques quite different from those of Cook, Pertschuk, et al[2]. Mitchell, et al have found an infectious agent that may be a paramyxovirus in the bone marrow of multiple sclerosis patients.[3] Behan, et al have demonstrated impaired T-cell function and evidence of chronic poliomyelitis in the jejunum of amyotrophic lateral sclerosis patients.

These exciting lines of inquiry are not yet conclusive. They provide early confirmation of chronic viral infection using techniques that are not yet generally accepted. They still fail to provide a *mechanism* that describes how these agents living in the jejunum, bone marrow, and perhaps elsewhere, cause central nervous system demyelination and death of central nervous system motor neuron cells.

The reader must remain alert to this rapidly developing area of research and recognize that controversy eventually generates answers. Once we can find answers to the mechanisms of these diseases, then perhaps we can generate controversy about the effectiveness of truly rational therapies.

REFERENCES

1. Behan, P.O., et al.: Persistent Virus in Motor-Neuron Disease. Lancet II:1176, 1977.
2. Ebina, T., et al.: Measles Virus in Jejunum of Patients with Multiple Sclerosis. Lancet I:99, 1979.
3. Mitchell, D.N., et al.: Isolation of an Infectious Agent from Bone Marrows of Patients with Multiple Sclerosis. Lancet II:387–391, 1978.
4. Woyciechowska, J.L., Madden, D.L., Sever, J.L.: Absence of Measles-Virus Antigen in Jejunum of Multiple Sclerosis Patients. Lancet II:1046–1049, 1977.

CHAPTER 13

Diagnosis and Management
of Multiple Sclerosis

INTRODUCTION

Multiple sclerosis patients now live longer than they used to because there is more effective treatment for urinary tract infections and pneumonia. The pharmaceutical industry has discovered medications that relieve spasticity and help to maintain control of bowel and bladder function. Physical disability is delayed through the application of modern technology to lighter braces, walkers, and wheelchairs, and to motorized vehicles of many kinds that allow a disabled person to remain mobile and even employed, despite increasing paralysis. Various resources for physical and occupational therapy, home nursing care, and transportation are available to disabled people. While these are important to the person who faces increasingly severe disability, he would still rather have an effective treatment for the MS itself.

Despite an improved understanding of the pathogenesis of MS, which was discussed in the previous chapter, there is still no way to establish the diagnosis unequivocally during life, and effective treatment of the disease itself eludes us. Until diagnostic laboratory abnormalities are discovered and effective treatments become available, patient and physician must depend upon their resourcefulness to be certain that treatable diseases are not misdiagnosed as MS and to tap all available resources so that life may be as normal as possible despite the disease.

DIAGNOSIS OF MULTIPLE SCLEROSIS

History

Throughout earlier sections of this volume, we have stressed the significance of accurate history and of careful, planned neurological examinations. These are especially important to the diagnosis of MS because accurate diagnosis depends directly upon the history and physical examination; laboratory and radiographic aids are of only limited assistance.

The significant pathology of multiple sclerosis is confined to discrete "plaques" of demyelination within the central nervous system that prevent or delay transmission of nerve impulses. The clinician may identify the location of some of these placques through analysis of the neurological deficits they cause by demyelination in specific fiber bundles. The performance of a skilled neurological examination is rewarded by the discovery of more definitive signs of *multifocal* lesions in MS patients, and by more certainty that the diagnosis is accurate.

This is important, because the clinical *hallmark* of MS is the *sequential development of discrete lesions within the central nervous system.* All other diagnostic considerations are of secondary importance.

The first symptoms of MS usually appear in early adult life, rarely before 15, and uncommonly after 40. Although exceptions do occur,[2] it is dangerous to make a diagnosis of MS in a patient who develops his first symptoms outside that limited range, because MS will usually be the wrong diagnosis.

When MS begins in early life, it is often characterized by acute exacerbations, lasting days or months, and later remissions. Each exacerbation is followed by less complete remission, so the progressive nature of the disease is determined by following the course of disability during remission. Some patients who develop severe exacerbations make nearly complete recoveries, even after many months of disability. This characteristic is important in planning for physical assistance for the patient during his exacerbations. If he can remain mobile, despite disability, he may be able to keep his job. If he cannot, he will be fired long before the severity of his baseline disease warrants early retirement.

Patients who develop their disease after age 35 more commonly display a relentlessly progressive course, and the diagnosis must be based on the multiplicity of lesions and the absence of physical and laboratory evidence of other disease.

The course of MS depends upon the specific location of lesions and the cadence of the disease. Frequently, there are symptoms only from the spinal cord and few signs of involvement above the foramen magnum. Other patients develop localizing symptoms from many parts of the brain, brainstem, cerebellum, and spinal cord. "Malignant" MS progresses rapidly to total disability and leads to death in a few years. Other patients follow a much more benign course and do not develop disabling symptoms for many years. Usually, MS patients have significant disability within five years of first symptoms, especially if they have frequent exacerbations. Even partially disabled people may still be fully employed for many years despite increasing disability, but they need help in finding aids to mobility.

Physical Examination

There are no pathognomonic signs of multiple sclerosis, but there are symptoms that occur commonly in multiple sclerosis patients. *Bilateral* internuclear ophthalmoplegia (pp. 89-90) is the most certain sign of demyelinating diseases in general. Unilateral optic- or retrobulbar neuritis in MS frequently causes unilateral central scotoma, optic atrophy, and an afferent pupil (pp. 72-73). Patients with lesions in the cervical spinal cord may complain of an electrical sensation that shoots down the back into the legs or into the arms, unilaterally or bilaterally. Usually this occurs when they bend their neck forward, and the electric tingle lasts only a moment. This is called Lhermitte's sign. Its occurrence is most frequent in MS but is not limited to MS patients. Except in its earliest stages, MS is a *bilateral* disease of the nervous system, so neurological abnormalities are found on both sides of the body.

Apart from these brief guidelines, the physician must search carefully for evidence of localized involvement of the motor system, sensory systems, cerebellum, and brainstem as we have outlined in other sections. Once he has identified neurological abnormalities, he must decide for himself how he *knows that the symptoms derive from lesions of discrete portions of the central nervous system and how he is certain* that they have developed at different times during the disease.

Pitfalls in the Diagnosis of Multiple Sclerosis

Slowly growing gliomas and meningiomas in the parasagittal region, the posterior fossa, and the region around the optic chiasm are especially likely to be misdiagnosed. Spinal tumors are also misdiagnosed as MS on occasion, but this is less common because myelography is widely available.

Parasagittal Tumor

Slowly progressive paraparesis occurs in some patients with MS and in patients with bilateral involvement of brain structures caused by a parasagittal meningioma, or midline glioma (p. 52). The MS patient with spinal cord involvement usually displays distinct sensory levels or other definite signs of segmental spinal cord involvement, while the patient with parasagittal tumor has a more graded deficit between the lower and upper extremities. Parasagittal lesions may also be accompanied by generalized hyperreflexia and a positive jaw jerk, and these may be mistaken for signs of disseminated disease. A good rule for the evaluation of a patient with quadriparesis or apparent paraparesis is that he does *not* have MS unless there is, in addition, a distinct segmental finding that cannot be related to the general paraparesis.

Posterior Fossa Tumor

Posterior fossa meningioma, acoustic neuroma, or pontine glioma is especially apt to be misdiagnosed as MS because each causes many combinations of asymmetrical quadriparesis, sensory loss, double vision, and cerebellar dyssynergia. The symptoms occur in widely separated parts of the *body* so they may be mistaken for disseminated lesions in the CNS. The CT and nuclear brain scans are not as sensitive in this region as they are in the brain itself. Posterior fossa myelography and arteriography are more difficult procedures, but more accurate, especially if metrizamide posterior fossa myelography is performed using the CT scan (p. 23). If they are not ordered initially, the physician may discover later that he has missed the diagnosis of a potentially treatable disease. Again, it is important to remember that *all* motor, sensory, and cranial nerve functions travel through the posterior fossa. Without segmental findings definitely originating outside the posterior fossa, a diagnosis of MS *cannot* be made until definitive radiographic visualization of this area has been accomplished.

Tumor Near the Optic Chiasm

Pituitary tumors and meningiomas in the region of the optic chiasm cause gradually failing vision and may also cause progressive quadriparesis. If, in addition, they invade the cavernous sinus, there may be cranial nerve dysfunction as well. Unless the clinician is knowledgeable, he may use these findings incorrectly and conclude that the disease is disseminated.

These cautions may lead the reader to believe that most cases of MS actually represent disguised brain tumors. This does not happen if the clinician has taken a careful history and analyzed the significance of current and previous symptoms, has looked for localizing neurological abnormalities in body regions of specific complaints, and has demanded that current and past symptoms have an anatomical explanation, but the possibility must always be kept in mind, and the clinician must never let down his guard if there is the slightest clinical doubt about a mistaken diagnosis.

Hysterical Symptoms vs. Multiple Sclerosis

Multiple sclerosis is common in northern cities. It is known as a crippling disease that produces symptoms of shifting numbness, weakness, double vision, and staggering. Nervous people develop such symptoms too. They focus on them, magnify them, and frequently they wonder whether they have multiple sclerosis. Some of them even have thought so much about multiple sclerosis that their history nearly duplicates the history of actual MS patients. However, nervous people do not develop unequivocal abnormalities of their neurological examination; MS patients do. Remember that each exacerbation of MS is followed by less complete remission. MS is a progressive crippling disease, and the crippling is caused by discoverable abnormalities of coordination, power, and sensation whose distribution is related to neuroanatomy. The diagnosis of MS does not depend upon the history alone, but upon the history *documented* by related abnormalities in the neurological examination.

It is a most tragic mistake for the physician to listen to his patient's history and decide that the diagnosis "could be MS;" then after the examination is over to tell the patient that the examination is normal, but he "could have multiple sclerosis." The neurological examination may be completely normal during a remission early in the course of the disease, but if the patient has disability and a long history of symptoms, *he cannot have MS without an abnormal neurological examination that explains the disability.*

A wrong diagnosis of MS allows the nervous person to fixate on his symptoms. It saps his strength and allows continuing concern about his physical symptoms, while he continues to avoid attacking whatever problems generated his physical complaints in the first place. It strains relations within the family and deprives the nervous person of proper emotional counseling if this is indicated. Worst of all, once a doctor has said, "It could be MS," subsequent examiners are more likely to say the same thing, and a mistaken diagnosis may be perpetuated for years.

On the other hand, actual symptoms of MS may be mistaken for hysteria. Many people with nervous dispositions are shunted away when they complain of numbness and staggering. One example of such an error: A patient who was paraplegic and incontinent for weeks while hospital personnel wrote that they were leaving food outside his door to "motivate him to walk." When he finally regained his feet, they were gratified that their treatment had been so successful. However, a psychiatrist who subsequently examined him found that he did not have serious psychopathology but that he did have bilaterally present Babinski's signs!

Laboratory Examinations

If the recent discovery by Pertschuk et al of measles antigen in the jejunal biopsies of 100 percent of MS patients becomes an easily reproducible examination, it would represent the most accurate test yet described. However, as we mentioned in the previous chapter, this work is still under controversial scrutiny. Other laboratory tests depend upon the unusual reactivity of lymphocytes from MS patients to measles virus-infected human epithelial cells,[6] on the altered reaction of MS macrophages when they are exposed to small concentrations of linoleic acid,[5] or on the decreased lymphocytic reaction to specific viral antigens.[9] These are difficult tests to perform, do not provide an unequivocal distinction between MS patients and controls, and are not available for routine hospital use.

Examination of the spinal fluid may support a diagnosis of multiple sclerosis. If agar gel electrophoresis is available, oligoclonal IgG may be identified.[7] If it is not, the simple determination of spinal fluid gamma globulin is routinely performed by most hospital laboratories. The normal value is less than 10 percent of the total spinal fluid protein. If the gamma globulin rises above 15 percent of total spinal fluid protein, it is clearly abnormal. But abnormalities of CSF gamma globulin are not specific for multiple sclerosis, because other diseases may also elevate the spinal fluid gamma globulin and produce oligoclonal IgG.

There may also be a modest elevation of spinal fluid protein, and during an acute exacerbation, there may be a lymphocytic pleocytosis in the spinal fluid. If these abnormalities occur during the first attack, MS cannot be clearly distinguished from acute disseminated encephalomyelitis. Patient and physician must wait to determine whether the symptoms return during subsequent years in order to make an accurate diagnosis.

The CT scan has proved its value in the diagnosis of MS as well as of structural lesions. Aita et al[1] reported the visualization of acute enhancing plaques during an MS exacerbation. If this result occurs and is accompanied by a consistent history and physical examination, it would confirm the diagnosis of MS more strongly than any other test, because it simultaneously discloses multiple discrete lesions and rules out the presence of structural disease (See Fig. 13-1).

LONG-TERM MANAGEMENT OF MULTIPLE SCLEROSIS

Available medicinal treatments do not alter the long-term course of MS, but the long-term welfare of MS patients is an area of proper concern for many kinds of health professionals. We may be instrumental in providing marked improvement for our patient's life if we are willing to invest time and effort in the project.

The most important aspect of the management of MS is education of patient and family. When the diagnosis of MS is made, it must be communicated to the patient. If necessary, consultation should be recommended to confirm the initial conclusions. This is frequently a difficult time for patient, family, and physician, but

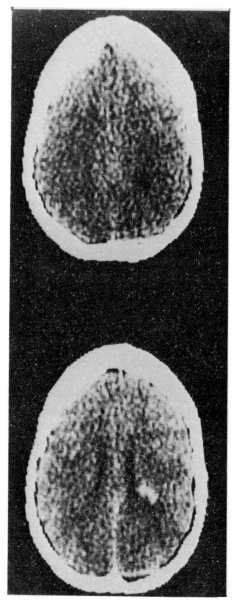

Figure 13-1. *Acute lesion of multiple sclerosis. The area of radiolucency is seen before enhancement (upper figure), but after enhancement (lower figure) the same area shows in marked contrast to the rest of the brain.*

direct, honest communication must occur at the beginning of the illness or it cannot develop later when the patient learns the truth. The course of MS, like the course of many diseases, is not under our control, but we can prepare ourselves to meet the challenges of disability if we know in advance what they are. We can be relieved of some of the bitterness of being sick if we are consistently told the truth. Multiple sclerosis is a chronic disease that usually produces no dementia, so patient and physician can expect to meet each other over a period of many years. The physician who begins his relationship with medical competence and honesty can lead his patient through the needed treatments and the stresses of illness with friendship, despite increasing disability.

Frequently, through inquiry or examination, the examiner can detect early symptoms of disability weeks or months before it becomes evident to the patient. He can discuss his findings with patient and family and examine with them the various options available for preventive exercises now, and corrective treatments or appliances when things get worse. If information passes between them in this manner, both clinician and patient have time to adjust to changing circumstances and to investigate their various choices so they can make decisions together. A number of common complications of MS need attention at regular intervals, or from time to time as they develop. These include the effects of spasticity, gait disturbance, loss of bowel and bladder control, changing sexual adjustments, management of heat intolerance, tremor, and the treatment of intercurrent infections. Available community resources may be called upon for homebound patients as well as those in the hospital; and finally, acute exacerbations may be treated with ACTH or prednisone.

Evaluation and Treatment of Spasticity

Increasing spasticity often affects the peronei and anterior tibial muscles more than the proximal muscles in the lower extremities. This causes a dropped foot, so the patient stumbles and falls over small obstacles like rugs, curbs, and steps. If the ankle becomes weak, he may sprain or fracture it as he falls. Regular examination of the strength of dorsiflexion and external rotation of the ankle is important. This allows the examiner to detect paresis as it develops and to prescribe regular muscle strengthening exercises. He can teach these exercises himself or he can ask the physical therapist to instruct the patient and family. Recently, a light ankle dorsiflexion orthosis made of plastic has become available, which does not require special shoes and is almost invisible, even under a woman's nylon stockings. When the clinician detects early signs of a dropped foot, he need not prescribe the brace, but the patient can know of its existence and can know that the brace will be available later if exercise does not continue to help his strength.

Gait becomes of increasing concern when strength and balance fail. There is no need for physical therapy until the patient's gait begins to deteriorate, but once this happens, gait training and balance exercises, done regularly, and coupled with regular exercises to strengthen muscles of the lower extremities, can delay significantly the use of physical aids to walking. When the patient begins physical therapy, he has the opportunity to examine the canes, Lofstrand crutches with elbow supports, walkers and wheelchair options that will be available to him as his condition worsens. If he has time to examine these options before he needs them, he will make better choices with less emotional turmoil when eventually he must use them.

The prescription of wheelchairs is a specialized art that should not be undertaken by the physician without study. There are many types, weights, qualities of and accessories for the wheelchair. Some are especially designed for competition basketball among paraplegics, while others are designed for the total care of a completely disabled person for many years. There are many styles of tires and several manual drive options. Some electric powered chairs move as fast as a man can walk, and can maneuver accurately through the obstacle course of a normal day's work.

The proper prescription of a wheelchair involves an assessment of the duration and kind of disability the patient can expect. There is no reason to prescribe an expensive electric wheelchair for a patient with rapidly progressing disease, who will soon be totally bedridden or who may be dead in a few months. On the other hand, the patient with early MS, whose symptoms fluctuate wildly between exacerbation and remission, may need an electric wheelchair for his initial purchase in order to keep his job. Patients with slowly progressive disease may need several chairs for their various activities at home and at work. If the clinician is uninformed about the modern accessories and brands, his patient may receive good advice from a trained physical or occupational therapist or from various manufacturers representatives, so that he can compare products and decide what chair and accessories best suit his needs.

Patients with early stages of spasticity may benefit from the use of baclofen (Lioresal®) or dantrolene (Dantrium®). Either may provide marked relief of spasticity, and should be offered in addition to other measures as spasticity becomes disabling. The strategy of treatment is to increase the dose gradually to a point of least spasticity with fewest medication side effects. The patient should determine his own dose within the limits of safety.

Dantrolene is supplied in capsules of 25 mg, 50 mg, 75 mg, and 100 mg The starting dose is approximately 50 mg per day with planned increments at weekly intervals of 25-50 mg each day. The usual therapeutic dose is about 150-250 mg per day in 2-4 divided doses, but some patients achieve maximum benefit at lower or much higher doses. The usual side effect of dantrolene overdose is generalized flaccid weakness. It is a sign for the patient to decrease the dose and find "his dose" below that level. Dantrolene has caused fatal toxic hepatitis, so it should be discontinued if there is no benefit after 4-6 weeks of treatment, and should not be prescribed unless the patient has significant disability due to his spasticity.

Baclofen is a much newer medication. It is specific for the treatment of spasticity due to multiple sclerosis and spinal cord injury. Baclofen is supplied in 10 mg tablets only. The dose of baclofen is increased gradually from 15 mg per day, in three divided doses, to a maximum of 80 mg per day. Both baclofen and dantrolene are relatively new medications, so their long-term side effects are not known.

Bladder Control

Bladder tone is mildly diminished by baclofen and dantrolene. Many patients need medications that specifically increase or decrease bladder smooth muscle tone. Pyramidal tract lesions above the lumbar spinal cord result in a tight spastic bladder that does not permit adequate filling. Bladder muscle spasm, urgency, and involuntary urination occur at small bladder volumes. On the other hand, lesions of the sensory pathways from the bladder, or the sacral cord, produce a flaccid bladder with few contractions and large residual urine volume. There is frequent overflow dribbling of urine.

Because of the multiplicity of their lesions, MS patients usually have a combination of the two symptoms, so an accurate diagnosis of the predominant bladder malfunction is best made by the use of a cystometrogram. If the physician does not have a cystometrics easily available to him, he and his patient may engage in a controlled experimental trial.

If the physician predicts that his patient's primary malfunction is caused by bladder spasticity, he may prescribe oxybutynin chloride (Ditropan®), which is supplied in 5 mg tablets. This medication reduces bladder spasticity, and while it acts it promotes bladder filling. The patient takes one tablet at intervals during the day, allowing the medication effect to decrease between doses so he can empty his bladder. He takes the medication before he retires for the night to allow bladder filling so he can sleep through the night without urinating. The maximum dose is 20 mg per day. Oxybutynin should be used advisedly if there is associated gastrointestinal disease. It is contraindicated if the patient also has glaucoma.

If bladder flaccidity is the primary problem, bethanechol chloride (Urecholine®) may effectively increase detrusor tone and promote bladder emptying. It is supplied in 5 mg, 10 mg, and 25 mg tablets. Recommended dose is up to 120 mg per day in divided doses. The patient takes 5 to 30 mg of bethanechol on arising and urinates 30 to 60 minutes later, attempting to empty his bladder as completely as possible. As the medication effect wears off, the bladder fills, and the patient takes another dose at noon, and again in late afternoon in order to urinate each time. He does not take bethanechol before going to bed in order to allow his bladder to fill so he can sleep through the night.

If doctor and patient do not have cystometrics to guide them, they must evaluate the results of one medication first. Should his bladder control improve, the patient must then search for an optimal dosage schedule; if he worsens, the clinician will switch to the other medication, and start again. Unfortunately, treatment regimens for bladder control are never as easy and clear-cut as we have indicated above, but these medications can provide a significant measure of relief for the patient who is willing to learn to use them and to accept their limitations.

Eventually, most patients with MS need either intermittent or continuous catheter drainage. Male and female patients can learn to catheterize themselves intermittently if they have unimpaired coordination of the upper extremities. This is more difficult for a female patient, but by no means impossible, and if the patient is employed, an indwelling catheter and leg bag are an unwanted nuisance. Intermittent self-catheterization is therefore preferable in some cases.

Indwelling catheters promote bladder infection, but they are preferable to the constant wetness and odor associated with incontinence. Decubitus ulcers develop more readily if the patient is constantly wet, and friends do not visit, nor can the patient leave home if he smells of urine. Bladder irrigation, acidification of the urine with at least two grams of vitamin C per day, high fluid intake, especially cranberry juice, and prompt treatment of febrile urinary tract infections are central to catheter management. Silastic catheters do not need as frequent changing as the rubber ones, but each kind needs a regular replacement program designed for the patient's rate of catheter encrustation. Patients with indwelling catheters may find that their catheter crusts less severely if they avoid milk products.

The clinician must *ask* about bladder control, or he will not hear about disorders until they are far advanced. Some patients are even willing to urinate every hour without mentioning it, but they appreciate the benefits of Ditropan® and Urecholine®, and they appreciate the care taken by their clinician in asking about troublesome symptoms.

Bowel Control

Of all disabilities, incontinence of stool is the most disconcerting. A person cannot leave home unless he can plan the timing of bowel movements. This may be achieved sometimes by the addition of bulk with Metamucil® or bran, often through a combination of bulk and peristaltic stimulants like Doxidan® or Peri-Colace®. Some patients find that direct stimulation of the rectum with glycerin suppositories, or reflex stimulation by scratching the skin over the lower coccyx, produces bowel movements on demand. Regular cleansing enemas once or twice a week with manual disimpaction are a last resort, frequently needed if there is severe bowel dysfunction. Each patient must discover a regimen for himself, which should aim toward planned bowel movements. People sometimes give up on this goal. They need encouragement and permission to experiment with various medications and dietary regimens, but a good result is worth the effort.

Adjustment to Changing Sexual Response

Multiple sclerosis is a disease of young adults. Changing sexual response is of frequent concern to men who become impotent, and to women who lose sensation in the perineal region. Couples are frequently able to discover ways to satisfy each other's sexual needs if they are encouraged to talk and to experiment. Occasionally, the situation becomes so difficult that they need sexual counseling by an expert, but this is usually not the case if the clinician anticipates that sexual problems will develop and starts the discussion between the couple before the problems become too large to handle.

Husbands are frequently concerned about intercourse after the wife has indwelling catheter drainage. This concern may unnecessarily delay the use of an indwelling catheter when it is needed. There is no reason to forbid sexual intercourse simply because the woman is catheterized. Intercourse is one risk factor in the production of urinary tract infection, but a couple can maintain excellent catheter care by acidifying the urine with vitamin C and cranberry juice, high fluid intake, and immediate treatment of any symptomatic infection. When the clinician begins to consider a recommendation for chronic catheterization of a female patient, he can bring up this problem himself and allay anxiety on that point.

Treatment of Intercurrent Infection

Viral upper respiratory infections, pneumonia, bladder infection, or any other intercurrent infection may worsen the disability of MS patients. Part of this may be related to the MS patient's intolerance to fever, part may simply be an accentuation of the normally increased disability of being sick, made worse by the presence of neurological disease. If the patient is not already badly disabled, he may recover adequately at home. More severely disabled patients become prostrate, and need hospital care, intravenous therapy, antibiotics if indicated, and strict bed rest. If families have had a previous discussion of alternative plans for acute care during some previous office visit, they do not wait to contact the physician until their patient has become totally bedridden by an infection, so disability can be minimized by appropriate action.

Heat Intolerance

Multiple sclerosis patients become dramatically worse when their body temperature is raised. This characteristic of MS is occasionally used as a diagnostic test, but it must be used with extreme caution, because, in addition to diplopia and nystagmus, the patient may rapidly become paralyzed and drown in the hot water bath, or become dyspneic and suffocate from weakness of respiratory muscles. If this test is used and the patient does become rapidly worse, treatment is directed toward immediate lowering of body temperature with cold water in the bath, and life support measures if necessary. The test should not be taken lightly, and the patient must not be left alone!

MS patients are worse in summer unless they have air conditioning at home and in the car. A swimming pool is useful for physical therapy and for prevention of overheating. These are expensive, but like other treatments and appliances, they are part of a therapeutic regimen and as such, are tax deductible medical expenses, if the physician writes a prescription for them when they become needed. Such a tax "advantage" is small recompense for disability.

Tremor and Dyssynergia

Most patients with MS never need a thalamotomy, usually because their tremor never becomes so severe that surgery is warranted, or because the patient's general medical condition is so bad that the surgical risk is unacceptable. But should the clinician encounter a patient with slowly progressive MS who develops severe tremor, he should ask for a neurosurgical consultation at a center where thalmotomy is performed, to determine whether the patient might become a candidate for this procedure (p. 154).

Community Resources

Each city and county has at least some resources for the outpatient care of partially disabled people. The clinician may investigate these for himself or ask for help from other community agencies. Outpatient occupational and physical therapy, public transportation for the disabled, and various hospital and home nursing programs are available. The Public Library has "Talking Books" free of charge to the blind and physically handicapped. This provides a wide selection of classical literature and current magazine selections on long-playing records. The National Multiple Sclerosis Society has local chapters in most large cities. Each chapter is available to provide emotional support on the phone, or to introduce to each other patients and families similarly affected. The MS chapter can become a center of social activities for even badly disabled patients. Some chapters have wheelchairs and other appliances in "loan closets," and may supply transportation to clinic or to the hospital.

Medicinal Therapy for Acute Exacerbations

ACTH-gel for intramuscular injection is available in 40 unit/cc and 80 unit/cc strength. Prednisone tablets are available in 5 mg and 20 mg tablets. These may be used for the treatment of the MS patient with an acute disabling exacerbation of symptoms. They should not be used for every daily fluctuation of disability, nor for every mild exacerbation, but only if disability changes in such a way that it interferes with daily activities.

Neither ACTH-gel nor prednisone should be used for long-term therapy of multiple sclerosis, but ACTH-gel has been shown in a double-blind prospective study to shorten the duration of an acute exacerbation and to help prevent immediate worsening of symptoms once treatment has begun.[8] Treatment regimens vary. The Cooperative Study regimen used 80 units per day for seven days, 40 units per day for four days, and 20 units per day for three days. If a patient responds dramatically within several days, the injections may be terminated earlier than this. ACTH injections should not be prolonged beyond 14-21 days. Some patients who do not respond to IM ACTH-gel seem to improve during hospitalization, where intravenous ACTH, 100 units per day, may be delivered over an 8-12 hour period in 500-1000 cc of five percent dextrose in water. Some patients do not respond to ACTH in any form. If they fail to respond to several individual courses, doctor and patient may decide not to reorder it. While the Cooperative Study found IM ACTH-gel to be more effective than placebo injections over a short period of evaluation, the effects of IV ACTH and prednisone have not been evaluated in a controlled study.

There is a psychological advantage to the use of ACTH-gel

injections. The patient can do little enough for himself medically. Shots are perceived to be more effective than pills, and the patient can learn to deliver the shots himself to the muscle of the anterior thigh. This site is immediately available to him as he sits, and is a safe injection site for intramusclular medications. The self-administration of ACTH-gel is an important service he can perform himself, instead of depending always upon other people.

Experimental treatments for MS are based on the immunological abnormalities mentioned in the previous chapter. 1) *Immunosuppression therapy* with drugs, antilymphocytic globulin, and thoracic duct drainage is designed to suppress the immune response which causes excessive IgG production within the brain and perhaps elsewhere. 2) *Immunostimulation therapy* with transfer factor [4,9] is designed to correct the specific inability of MS lymphocytes to recognize measles antigen *in vitro*. Currently, transfer factor therapy is receiving the most intense interest.

There are immense problems associated with the clinical evaluation of treatments for multiple sclerosis. Patients differ in their age, sex, clinical stage, rate of progression, as well as in their genetic makeup. Transfer factor is difficult to make in quantity, so trials have been confined to small numbers of patients serving as their own control. After two years of transfer factor therapy in 12 patients, Fog[3] was able to state with certainty only that he had not shown the treatment to be without value.

SUMMARY

The diagnosis and management of multiple sclerosis still depends upon an astute clinician who is able to examine his patients, rule out treatable disease, and recognize constellations of symptoms that document disseminated discrete lesions. Laboratory assistance is available from the CT scan and the spinal fluid gamma globulin, but neither of these alone can *make* a diagnosis of multiple sclerosis; they can only *confirm* it.

Management, too, depends upon cooperation between doctor and patient. The patient needs to learn from his doctor what to expect in the future and what he can do about progressive disability as it appears. Then he needs to communicate his progress so that he can manage new symptoms as they appear. Except for the antibiotic treatment of infection, medicinal treatment is of secondary importance.

We still need more information about pathogenesis before we can approach the treatment of multiple sclerosis rationally, but knowledge is advancing so rapidly that the information may be available when the reader reaches this chapter.

REFERENCES

1. Aita, J.F., Bennett, D.R., Anderson, R.E., Ziter, F.: Cranial C.T. Appearance of Acute Multiple Sclerosis. Neurology 28:251–255, 1978.
2. Alter, M., Kurtzke J.F., (eds): *The Epidemiology of Multiple Sclerosis.* Charles C Thomas, Springfield, Ill., 1968, p. 67.
3. Fog., T., et al.: Transfer Factor Treatment of Multiple Sclerosis. A Pilot Study. Acta Neurol. Scand. 55:(Suppl. 63) 253–259, 1977.
4. Grob, P.J.: Transfer Factor. General Aspects. Acta Neurol. Scand. 55:(Suppl. 63) 217–225, 1977.
5. Jenssen, H.L., Meyer-Rienecker, H.J., Köhler, H., Günther, J.K.: The Linoleic Acid Depression (LAD) Test for Multiple Sclerosis Using the Macrophage Electrophoretic Mobility (MEM) Test. Acta Neurol. Scand. 53:51–60, 1976.
6. Levy, N.L., Auerbach, P.S., Hayes, E.C.: A Blood Test for Multiple Sclerosis Based on the Adherence of Lymphocytes to Measles-Infected Cells. N. Eng. J. Med. 294:1423–1427, 1976.
7. Link, H.: Immunoglobulin Abnormalities in Multiple Sclerosis. Ann. Clin. Res. 5:330–336, 1973.
8. Rose, A.S., et al.: Cooperative Study in the Evaluation of Therapy in Multiple Sclerosis: ACTH vs. Placebo. Neurology 20-Part 2:1–59, 1970.
9. Zabriskie, J.B., Espinoza, L.R., Plank, C.R., Collins, R.C.: Cell-Mediated Immunity to Viral Antigens in Multiple Sclerosis. Acta Neurol. Scand. 55:(Suppl. 63) 239–251, 1977.

CHAPTER 14.

Migraine and Other Headaches

INTRODUCTION

Headache is a highly subjective topic. A factual basis for discussion of headache does exist, and there is clinical information about diagnosis, but there is usually no discoverable pathologic substrate for the patient's pain.

Harold G. Wolff spent his entire professional life on the study of headache, with special interest in the migraine syndrome. He established early that there are specific pain-sensitive structures in the head and that headache originates from one or more of these. They include: the scalp and scalp vessels on the outside of the clavarium, dura at the base of the skull, the middle meningeal arteries but not the adjacent dura over the convexities, major branches of the internal carotid artery within 2 cm of the circle of Willis, the specific cranial nerves which carry pain fibers, the transverse and sigmoid sinuses, and parts of the superior sagittal sinus. The skull itself is not pain-sensitive and neither are the brain and small vessels feeding the brain. Pain is perceived if there is pressure, stretching, or inflammation of pain-sensitive structures, or dilatation of pain-sensitive arteries. Headaches originating in scalp vasculature are by far the most common, and we shall discuss these first, beginning with the migraine syndrome.

MIGRAINE HEADACHE

Physical and Chemical Basis of Migraine

Harold Wolff and his co-workers are responsible for a large amount of basic information concerning migraine. The reader will find that the most recent edition of his book provides a fascinating education in the topic of headache.[7] It still contains large portions of Wolff's original work, coupled with more modern information.

Wolff described the migraine attack in terms of the stages of its development. He found that the initial stage consists of vasoconstriction. He studied the effects of vasodilator agents like amyl nitrite and carbon dioxide on this stage and showed that he could alter the prodromal symptoms with these agents but could not reliably prevent the headache itself.

Wolff and his collaborators showed clearly that the second, painful, stage of a migraine attack is caused by vasodilatation of arteries in the painful area. Not all arteries in the head, or even all those on one side, participate at once. Certain branches of the external carotid artery dilate painfully during the attack, while other branches may join the first only later in the headache. Sometimes, painful arterial dilatation extends to vessels in the neck, shoulders, or face and sinus areas. Migraine is *not* simply a painful affliction of the top of the head!

Wolff examined the actions of ergotamine tartrate. This agent acts as a vasoconstrictor to branches of the *external* carotid artery. It has little effect on the internal carotid artery circulation, which helps to explain the infrequency of serious cerebral ischemic side effects during therapy with ergotamine tartrate.

He showed that scalp vessels remain responsive to ergotamine tartrate only during the early portions of a migraine attack. As the attack progresses, migrainous vessels become partially paralzyed and do not regain their full responsiveness to ergotamine tartrate until after the attack has passed. This fact is *central* to the strategy for treatment of the acute migraine attack.

During a migraine attack, the scalp may become edematous and tender. Wolff showed that the edematous fluid contained "headache stuff," which he thought probably consisted of short-chain polypeptides related to neurokinin or bradykinin. He extracted "headache stuff" from the boggy scalp of migraineurs and injected it into the scalp of control subjects. The subjects developed scalp tenderness in the site of injection which did not appear after the injection of saline. Scalp tenderness is an important clinical sign because it helps to distinguish the *extracranial* origin of a migraine attack from headaches due to serious intracranial disease, which are not usually accompanied by scalp tenderness.

Wolff and his group investigated aspects of abnormal fluid and electrolyte metabolism in migraine. They described marked fluctuations in body weight and discussed the influence of premenstrual edema on migraine. On the basis of direct experiments, they concluded that edema itself was not the cause of a migraine attack, but merely a concomitant symptom, related somehow to the basic migraine mechanism.

Recently, new details about the chemical nature of migraine have come to light. It appears that Wolff was right about neurokinin.[8] Lance and his co-workers[2,6] and Rydzewski[16] and others have begun to unravel the problem of vasoconstriction by disclosing a precipitous drop in blood serotonin levels at the onset of migraine attack. These levels remain low until after the attack passes. Serotonin is active in the control of vascular tone by virtue of its various known metabolic and chemical abnormalities.

Wolff used methysergide (Sansert®) as an experimental agent. This medication and cyproheptadine (Periactin®) are both serotonin antagonists and stabilize the migraine syndrome, perhaps by reason of their ability to occupy serotonin-active sites. We shall discuss these two agents later when we consider the prophylactic treatment of the migraine syndrome.

Prevalence of Migraine

It has always been known that migraine runs in families, but its mode of inheritance is not certain even now. The migraine syndrome is probably permitted by the presence of a single autosomal dominant gene with incomplete penetrance and extremely variable expressivity. This variability makes prevalence studies difficult. Some carriers of the migraine trait are disabled throughout their lives, while others have only occasional mild headache – or none.

Early estimates of migraine prevalence in the population ranged from 5-15 percent. Recently, Waters[19] and Waters and O'Connor[20] completed studies of three different populations and found that up to 30 percent of women and somewhat fewer men had had migraine attacks during the previous one year. These data were compiled from written questionnaires sent by mail to members of the study population. Many mild headaches may have gone unreported under these circumstances, so the figures must be below the true incidence. We cannot know the actual gene frequency of migraine, but it is probably very high!

Migraine Syndromes

With this factual background in mind, let us consider the migraine syndromes. Two important kinds of migraine are recognized: classic migraine and common migraine.

Classic Migraine

Classic migraine is less prevalent than common migraine. It is a predominantly unilateral headache, preceded by an aura and accompanied by numerous associated symptoms. The aura develops gradually over a 10-30 minute period. This slow development of the migraine aura is an important diagnostic point which helps to distinguish the symptoms of migraine from the more rapid onset of transient ischemic attacks and ischemic stroke.

The nature of the migraine aura depends upon the area of brain involved. Most frequently the aura originates in occipital cortex with an indefinite aberration of vision. This quickly develops into lines and dots of shimmering brightness, sometimes colored. These are *scintillations*. They flash and move in the visual field, gradually growing in area. As the scintillations progress, the person becomes aware that he cannot see through them. At this point, he has a scintillating *scotoma*. The scotoma may remain localized to one portion of the visual field, but frequently it progresses and becomes a scintillating homonymous hemianopsia. If hemianoptic fields are involved bilaterally, there is temporary blindness filled with scintillations. Visual loss in stroke and transient ischemic attack appears rapidly or suddenly and only the *deficit* symptom of blindness occurs in most cases. Scintillations may be considered an *irritative* phenomenon. Certainly, the occipital cortex is functioning in order to produce the flashes, but it is not registering outside stimuli.

Other more-or-less common neurological complaints associated with a migraine headache originate from other parts of the brain: migrating prickling numbness, heaviness or paralysis of a hand or an entire side of the body, aphasia, confusional syndromes, cranial nerve paralysis, and double vision may all represent the aura of a migraine attack or appear during the attack itself. When patients have these localizing symptoms, especially when they have cranial nerve palsies, the clinician should be especially careful to establish that there is no structural disease. "Ophthalmoplegic migraine"or "hemiplegic migraine" may actually represent symptoms from a carotid artery aneurysm, a tumor in the pituitary fossa, or an arteriovenous malformation!

The aura clears more rapidly than it develops and shortly thereafter the headache begins. The headache frequently appears on the same side of the head which originated the aura, but this is by no means universal. Sometimes the headache strikes rapidly. At other times, or in other patients, it develops over a period of minutes or hours to a peak, then falls away and disappears. If the patient can only fall asleep early in the attack, he frequently can abort much of the syndrome. At other times it disappears spontaneously during the day or quietly during the night. The total length of a given headache may be only a few minutes, or it may last many days.

During a prolonged attack, the headache begins in one area, but later moves to other portions of the head and neck. Individuals with migraine recognize similar patterns in their own headaches, but there is no fixed pattern characteristic of migraine in general. Most migraines do shift sides either during an individual attack or from time to time over the years. This is an important diagnostic point, since the usual pain of aneurysm, arteriovenous malformation, or brain tumor remains on the same side indefinitely. Unfortunately for the diagnostician, some migraineurs also have strictly unilateral headache.

Associated symptoms usually develop during an attack of classic migraine. Anorexia is almost universal and may progress to nausea and eventual vomiting. Constipation may warn the sufferer that a headache is approaching. Diarrhea may develop with the headache, or a normal bowel movement may signal the approaching termination of the attack. Patients frequently blame the headache on bowel irregularity, but it is probable that this is simply one more systemic manifestation of the migraine syndrome. Blurred vision, photophobia, and recurrent scintillations are common. Noises appear abnormally loud and irritating. Frequently the sufferer is restricted to a darkened room hoping for total silence in the house, praying for an end to pain and the revolution in his gastrointestinal system.

Two more associated signs of migraine are of special diagnostic importance. These are diuresis and scalp tenderness. Diuresis documents that the headache is part of a *systemic* process; scalp tenderness shows that the headache originates in the scalp, not inside the head itself. Both are important symptoms and help to eliminate considerations of serious intracranial disease. The author was embarrassed once by getting the history of scalp tenderness in a young man and concluding that he had migraine. He actually had a chronic subdural hematoma! This experience has shaken my confidence in the diagnostic infallibility of the symptom, but it is nonetheless, a common complaint in migraine and an unusual one in intracranial disease.

Diuresis *occurs* frequently, but it is not a common *complaint*. Patients frequently have not recognized it as a symptom of their migraine, but once they have been questioned on the point, they report its presence after a subsequent attack.

Both classic and common migraine may occur in relation to the menses, usually on the day before or the first day of the menstrual flow, but sometimes toward the end of the menses or even regularly at the middle of the cycle.

Common Migraine

Common migraine is a bilateral headache located behind the eyes, in the temples, at the back of the head. It is usually not preceded by an aura and is usually less severe than a classic migraine attack. Nausea and vomiting may occur if the headache is severe, but are less frequent in common migraine than in classic migraine. The common migraine patient may have daily headaches for years, while the classic migraine sufferer is frequently pain-free between his attacks. Even so, patients with predominantly common migraine usually have had one or more severe unilateral headaches of the classic migraine type.

Common migraine frequently awakens the patient in the small-hours of the morning or develops within minutes of waking in the morning. Blurred vision is common, but scintillations are not as prominent as they are in classic migraine. Vasomotor instability appears to be more prominent in common migraine, perhaps because, in common migraine, the migraine syndrome is more constantly active. Dizzy spells on rising rapidly from bed or sitting and occasional fainting spells are frequently reported, which are worse when the headaches are more frequent or more severe. Focal neurological complaints are not part of the common migraine syndrome.

Treatment of the Migraine Syndrome

We have progressed from well-established facts about

pathogenesis of migraine to clinical lore about its symptomatology. Now we continue to the much more subjective topic of treatment. People do not die of migraine. There is no treatable pathologic anatomy to establish criteria for treatment success. Most doctors and patients believe that emotional factors are important in the initiation of a migraine headache. Doctors tend to advise their patients on the basis of that belief, and patients tend to be ashamed that they have headaches on the same basis. Headache "means" serious illness, disability, and death to the sufferer even if he really knows he only has migraine.

Put a physician and his prescriptions into this situation and the results are not predictable. There are pharmacologically effective medications for the treatment of migraine, but the pharmacology of doctoring is an important factor in the results of treatment and probably accounts for the wide divergence of preference, by various doctors, for one or another medication. This discussion of treatment is of necessity, then, a combination of pharmacology and prejudice. We shall attempt to distinguish them from each other in the text.

Psychological Management of Migraine

The most important aspect of migraine management is to establish that the diagnosis is really right. If patient and doctor are not absolutely certain that they are treating migraine instead of serious neurological disease, they should have further studies or consultation. But if the history is typical, and careful neurological examination is normal, treatment may begin with a discussion of those facts, coupled with further statements that the response to treatment will serve to strengthen the diagnosis over the next few weeks. Such care, taken during the initial interview, removes some of the "meaning" of head pain and removes the aggravation of some of its associated anxiety. This alone is worth several prescriptions.

Some texts discuss detailed suggestions for the fundamental alteration of a patient's life-style, based on ideas about the migraine personality, and the psychopathology associated with migraine. The migraine personality may be a reality, but we have already discussed the probable genetic background of migraine and biochemical correlates with individual headaches. The author has found that most of his migraine patients are otherwise normal people who have headaches. True, they are caught up in their life stresses, but they have not come to the physician for advice about their life-styles, and they are extremely unlikely to accept his advice, although they may listen politely as it is given. They want relief from headache. If the physician finds that the patient's life is *overwhelmingly disrupted* by emotional or physical stress and that the headaches are directly related to these and to depression, he can perform his best service by discussing these findings with the patient and referring him for counseling or psychiatric help. Otherwise, he should begin to think about effective *medicinal* management.

Medicinal Management of Migraine

Two basically different groups of medication are used to treat migraine. The first are for treatment of an acute migraine attack, and consist of various preparations of ergotamine tartrate and adjunctive medications to assist vasocontriction, control vomiting, or to provide sedation. The second are a group of widely different medications which are effective in the prevention of future attacks.

Treatment of the Acute Migraine Attack

Because vasomotor paralysis develops as the attack progresses, an attack of migraine is less and less responsive to ergotamine tartrate after it has begun. Therefore, treatment begins as *early in the attack* as possible, preferably before there is any vasodilation at all. Patients with a long aura, and patients whose headaches develop slowly, can use this strategy successfully in most instances. Patients whose headaches strike suddenly, and those who awaken with headache already in progress, may have better success with a rapidly acting preparation like the Ergotamine Medihaler® (Riker Laboratories, Inc.), but even this may not be fast enough.

The author prefers to use Cafergot tablets and the Ergotamine Medíhaler®. If parenteral treatment is needed, intramuscular or subcutaneous ergotamine tartrate (Gynergen®) is more reliable than other ergot preparations. Cafergot® has the disadvantages of relatively slow release and frequent aggravation of nausea and vomiting, but it is relatively cheap and the tablet is virtually indestructible. This means that Cafergot® tablets may be left in the office, in the car, at home, and even in the fishing box, and they will always be there when the headache starts. If the patient has a long enough warning, Cafergot® is an extremely effective antimigraine preparation. "The dose" is usually 2-4 tablets at the *onset* of headache. A new migraine patient is instructed to experiment with the medication, taking one or two when he has no headache to familiarize himself with its side effects, and then again when he *first knows* that he is about to have a headache. The dose may be repeated in 20 minutes, and he should keep track of side effects and effectiveness of headache suppression. Next time, he will know whether he needs three or perhaps four tablets at the onset of headache. He will learn to concentrate on taking the total effective dose as early as side effects allow during the *initial* stages of his attack. Should pain return in several hours, an additional tablet may easily suppress it. Limits are six tablets per day, not more that 10 per week. Larger doses cannot be recommended, but there are patients who take 50 or more tablets per week to control prolonged severe status migrainosus. Such patients might find relief from preparations designed to prevent migraine, but if preventative medications do not work, they sometimes elect to take the chance of later ergotism in return for headache relief now.

If Cafergot® is not fast enough or if it causes too much nausea, the Ergotamine Medihaler® (Riker) is highly effective because it delivers a fine mist of ergotamine tartrate *directly* to the circulation via the lungs. Patients need careful instruction on the use of the Medihaler® so they are certain to get the dose deep into the lungs. Ergotamine tartrate spray on the teeth is ineffective. The Medihaler® needs to be shaken before use, and if it has lain idle, the first puff may have lost its pressure and not be effective. The Medihaler® is relatively expensive, and unless the patient buys several, he has only one of them so it cannot be spread around as tablets can. Men, who carry no purse, may find this difficult. Nonetheless, if the person keeps his Medihaler® with him, its great speed of action and invulnerability even to frequent vomiting, make this preparation an excellent choice in special circumstances. The dose, like that of Cafergot®, is 2-4 whiffs at the onset of headache, not more than six per day nor 10-15 per week. If needed, an initial dose may be repeated in 5-10 minutes. Contraindications to ergotamine tartrate preparations include pregnancy, uncontrolled hypertension, peripheral vascular disease, coronary artery disease, and liver or kidney disease.

Parenteral treatment of the acute migraine attack should be reserved for the emergency room except under unusual circumstances. The preferred emergency treatment is subcutaneous or intramuscular ergotamine tartrate (Gynergen®) 0.5 mg *once*. Usually after about 30 minutes, the patient begins to vomit and retch. The

TABLE 14-1

Medications for the Treatment of an Acute Migraine Attack

Trade Name	Ingredients	Dosage
Gynergen Tablet	Ergotamine tartrate 1.0 mg	
Cafergot Tablet	Ergotamine tartrate 1.0 mg Caffeine 100 mg	
Cafergot-PB Tablet	Ergotamine tartrate 1.0 mg Caffeine 100 mg Belladonna Alkaloids 0.125 mg Phenobarbital 30 mg	1-4 tablets at onset; repeat in 15-20 minutes; maximum of 6/day, 10/week
Migral Tablet	Ergotamine tartrate 1.0 mg Caffeine 50 mg Cyclizing HCL (antinausea) 25 mg	
Wigraine Tablets	Ergotamine tartrate 1.0 mg Caffeine 100 mg	
Wigraine Suppositories	Belladonna Alkaloids 0.1 mg Phenacetin 130 mg	
Cafergot Suppository	Ergotamine tartrate 2.0 mg Caffeine 100 mg	1 suppository at the onset of attack; repeat in one hour; maximum of 2/day, 5/week
Cafergot-PB Suppository	Ergotamine tartrate 2.0 mg Caffeine 100 mg Belladonna Alkaloids 0.25 mg Phenobarbital 60 mg	
Ergomar Sublingual Tablets	Ergotamine tartrate 2.0 mg	1 tablet at onset; repeat in 30 minutes; maximum 3/day, 5/week
Ergostat Sublingual Tablets	Ergotamine tartrate 2.0 mg	
Ergotamine Medihaler	Ergotamine tartrate 0.3 mg/whiff	2-4 whiffs at onset; repeat in 10 minutes; maximum 6/day, 20/week (see package insert for instructions)
Gynergen Injection	Ergotamine tartrate 0.5 mg/ml	0.5-1 ml sc or IM *once*; not more than 2 ml/week

headache frequently clears during the vomiting. Often, emergency room treatment is ineffective. Either the headache is unabated or it stops long enough for the sufferer to get home to bed, where it returns to run its course. The most effective part of an emergency room visit is planning for an office visit after the attack, so the patient can begin his education into the management of migraine and avoid future visits to the emergency room.

Codeine and even meperidine (Demerol®) have their place in the treatment of unappeased migraine. They carry the risk of addiction in a patient with frequent attacks and should be avoided if possible.

Aspirin, too, can help abort some migraines if it is taken early in the attack, but aspirin and the myriad aspirin-containing analgesics cannot be central to the treatment of severe migraine.

Prevention of Future Migraine Attacks

The patient with frequent disabling head pain may find that it is worth his while to take medication *every single day* to prevent future attacks. This is especially true when headaches are so frequent that he would be using more than the proper doses of ergotamine tartrate or if headaches are interfering with normal life activities.

Table 14-2 lists a number of medications of diverse nature. The author prefers Bellergal tablets for treatment of frequent common migraine headache with dizzy spells. Cyproheptadine (Periactin®) is highly effective. Usually there are no side effects from cyproheptadine. An occasional patient cannot take this medication at all because it causes overwhelming sedation. Most commonly, the patient can start with four tablets a day and quickly go to five. If headache is unrelieved in 10 days, he is directed to increase the dose gradually to a total of eight tablets per day. Many patients need this maximum dose to bring their migraines under control. If the headaches stop at a given dose, the patient continues that dose for several weeks before decreasing it step-wise to discover the lowest effective dose. During a later period of exacerbation, he may need to increase his dose again. If he tests periodically to find his lowest effective dose, he may find that he can even discontinue the medication completely for a time, but he should plan to use it again during the next period of migraine activity.

Tricyclic antidepressants are occasionally useful. It is not clear whether their effectiveness is based directly on biochemistry, or on the effective treatment of depression. Monoamine oxidase inhibitors are another class of antidepressant medications which are effective in the treatment of migraine, but these agents are dangerous and should not be prescribed by the clinician who is not used to instructing his patients about precautions and following their responses to it.

Controlled studies have shown propranolol (Inderal®) to be an antimigraine preparation in doses of 80-160 mg per day.[5,10,21] However, even though it is perhaps statistically better than placebo, the author has not found propranolol to be a highly effective antimigraine agent.

Methysergide (Sansert®) is in a class by itself because it is at once the most highly effective antimigraine agent available, and the most dangerous. Patients who do not respond to any of the other antimigraine regimens, and who are disabled by headache, may become candidates for methysergide, and it may stop their headaches when all else has failed. Methysergide has rare but potentially fatal side effects. Complications include fibrosis in the retroperitoneal space, the pleural space, and on heart valves; ischemic necrosis distally in the limbs, thrombophlebitis, and peripheral edema.

TABLE 14-2

Medications Used to Prevent Future Migraine Attacks

Trade Name	Ingredients	Dosage
Bellergal Tablets	Ergotamine tartrate (0.3 mg) Phenobarbital 20 mg Belladonna Alkaloids 0.1 mg	2-4 tablets/day
Oxoids	Ergotamine tartrate 0.3 mg Phenobarbital 20 mg Belladonna extract 0.8 mg	
Periactin	Cyproheptadine tablets 4 mg	4-32 mg/day
Inderal	Propranolol tablets 10 mg, 40 mg, 80 mg	40-160 mg/day
Elavil Endep	Amitriptyline tablets 10 mg, 25 mg, 50 mg, 75 mg 100 mg, 150 mg	75-150 mg/day
Sansert	Methysergide tablets 2 mg	4-8 mg/day

The patient who is disabled by migraine but can respond well to other medications should avoid methysergide. If the patient is not disabled, he should consider the possible complications of methysergide and avoid it. If the patient arrives at a point in treatment where the clinician thinks he needs methysergide, referral to a neurologist would be appropriate so the consultant and patient can also assess the problem together before the drug is prescribed.

Treatment of Exertion Migraine

Prevention of "gym headache" is an easy and special case. Some people develop a migraine when they do heavy physical exercise. One or two Cafergot® tablets taken 30 minutes before heavy exertion prevents this.

Migraine and Birth Control Pills

There is no question now that many migraineurs develop their headaches for the first time, or develop worse, more frequent or more complicated migraines when they are on "the pill."[9,15] Permanent ischemic stroke occurs in migrainous women on the pill and the impression is that the pill was the cause. Patients with severe migraine should use other forms of contraception. Those whose migraines are aggravated when they start taking birth control pills should discontinue their use.

Common Migraine vs. Muscle Tension Headache

It is traditional to distinguish between common migraine and muscle tension headache, although emotional and physical tension are recognized as causative factors in each. The author is aware of the distinction, but is unable to help the reader to make it, because the history of chronic recurrent headache in his patients nearly always sounds like common migraine. The Ad Hoc Committee on Classification of Headache does not offer a clear clinical distinction, except to state that one is caused by muscle tension and the other is a vascular headache.[1] In his study of headache and life stress, Stenback defines muscle tension headache as one which does not throb,[17] and this is a commonly used distinction. Friedman[13] describes bright spots in front of the eyes (scintillations?) and distribution into frontal and face regions. He says that some patients with muscle tension headache have pulsation which may be confused with migraine.

In this author's practice, headache patients nearly always complain of symptoms which should not originate with muscle tension. They wake from sleep with headache in the small hours of the morning or develop a headache within minutes of waking. They have blurred vision, photophobia, nausea, occasional vomiting, scalp tenderness, dizzy spells and syncopal attacks. They do occasionally have scintillating scotoma. These symptoms do not have a neurological explanation on the basis of muscle contraction in the neck or anywhere else. Additionally, many of these patients have a history of one or more classic migraine attacks and frequently a family history of recurrent headaches or frank migraine. Not every headache in a patient's past has all, or even some, of these characteristics, but if the clinician asks, he will find that the symptoms are present in various headaches during life.

We have discussed the wide variability of migraine symptoms; the fact that a migraine may move to various places during a single headache, and from headache to headache; that some patients with migrainous heredity are sorely afflicted with headaches of varying severity and location, while others have fewer headaches or no headaches at all. The author believes that most patients with tension headache suffer from common migraine, not muscle tension. It is a prejudice based on personal experience and on frustration with a distinction he has not been able to make. The clinician who is able to make the distinction may continue to do so. The clinician who cannot, may benefit by reading other descriptions and by examining his own practice; then he can come to his own conclusions about the question.

There *are* headache patients whose history clearly *does* point to muscle spasm, but these headaches are not related to nervous tension. The farmer with cervical spondylosis, who develops neck and occipital ache when he does heavy lifting and throwing, or the truck driver with a normal neck, who has pain after he drives on a bumpy road, both complain of muscle spasm. These are the history of normally severe stresses upon abnormal anatomy, or of unusual stresses on normal anatomy, and they produce spasm and pain in the neck just as they do elsewhere in the body.

Eye Strain Headache and Sinus Headache vs. Tension Headache

It is true that some people who have astigmatism or glaucoma develop aching eyes and pain in the orbits. It is not true that these are common causes of chronic recurrent headache.

It is also true that acute sinusitis is extremely painful, but chronic sinusitis is accompanied by chronic nasal discharge, breath odor, local tenderness, brain abscess; not by history of chronic recurrent headache.

Spare the headache patient his initial consultations with the ophthalmologist and otolaryngologist unless there is indication by history or examination that the cause lies within the province of one of these specialities. Most patients who complain of "eye strain headache" because they have blurred vision and photophobia, or "sinus headache" because they have pain behind the eyes, or "normal headache" because everyone in the family has it too, really have "tension headache" and respond to treatment for common migraine syndrome.

CLUSTER HEADACHE

Cluster headache is a vascular headache, but it is usually limited to the eye and the lower half of the face. Prominent autonomic signs accompany an attack of cluster headache including tearing of the eye, stuffy nose, and red face all on the same side as the head pain. Pupillary constriction on the side of the pain occurs regularly. During a cluster of recurrent headaches, this constriction may be present between individual attacks and may eventually become a permanent residuum.

Between a cluster, the patient is usually headache-free. During a cluster, which may last for weeks or months, he has predictable, daily headaches, always on the same side, which occur up to 6-8 times a day almost as though on schedule. There is no aura. Suddenly is he struck with searing, agonizing pain, lasting for 20 minutes to somewhat over an hour. During the headache he paces the floor in agony. Then the pain leaves as quickly as it had appeared, and it is gone until the next attack.

The pain of cluster headache must rank with that of trigeminal neuralgia. Patients sell their firearms because they are afraid they will kill themselves during an attack. Physicians turn in their narcotics licenses for fear of addiction. Scheduled attacks during the day and subsequent clusters in the future are awaited with dread. The physician who finds relief for his patient has performed miraculous service.

Cluster headache is a different disease from migraine, but in some patients the clinicial distinction is difficult. The headache may concentrate on the eye and the forehead, last up to five hours, or be accompanied by nausea and vomiting. Occasionally there is an aura; but occasional similarities between cluster headache and migraine should not blur the usually easy clinical distinction between the two types of headache.

Chemical indications of the distinction between migraine and cluster headaches are based on the serotonin studies. Lance and his co-workers[2] have shown that the change in blood serotonin, characteristic of migraine, does not occur in cluster headache and that there is a significant rise in blood histamine during a cluster headache, which is minimal in migraine.

Treatment of Cluster Headache

A headache which starts suddenly without warning, lasts 30 minutes, and is scheduled to stop at that time is not amenable to oral medications taken at the onset of headache. If intravenous treatment were practicable, it might work, but self-administration of intravenous medication is difficult for the average lay person in agony. Even the Ergotamine Medihaler® usually fails to bring relief. The best treatment is prevention and even this frequently fails.

Probably the most effective treatment is that described by Symonds[18] and detailed by Bickerstaff.[4] They recommended regular prophylactic injections of ergotamine tartrate, 0.25 mg three times each day during five days of each week. Two days per week are spent off ergotamine to prevent cumulative side effects of the drug and to allow the patient to detect the end of his cluster.

This regimen is dramatically effective in some cases, but on other occasions after initial success, the cluster changes its cadence and continues despite the medication. On these occasions, the patient takes larger and larger doses in an attempt to keep even partial control of his disease. Methysergide and cyproheptadine have been reported as efficacious in treatment of cluster headache, but the author has had disappointing results with these agents when ergotamine tartrate injections have failed. The clinician who does not regularly care for headache patients would be well advised to consider prompt referral of his cluster headache patient if prophylactic ergotamine tartrate injections are ineffective.

TEMPORAL ARTERITIS

Temporal arteritis is totally different from other vascular headaches because it is recognized pathologically as a variant of giant cell arteritis occurring in old age. Patients with temporal arteritis are usually over 65 years old, almost never under 50. They frequently complain of neurological symptoms resembling transient ischemic attacks or ischemic stroke, and for this reason, the diagnosis may be missed. Usually, headache is a prominent symptom, associated with general malaise, fatigue, lassitude, and weakness. Claudication of jaw muscles during meals, and angina pectoris, may appear as the disease develops. If the disease is not recognized and properly treated, the patient may die from a heart attack or stroke. This is a *new* headache, different from all others the patient has had in the past. It is a continuous burning in the temple, associated with tenderness, specifically located over the temporal artery or other scalp arteries. If giant cell nodules are present, they are points of special tenderness.

Prompt diagnosis and treatment of temporal arteritis ranks as one of the few neurological emergencies. Common complications, like retinal artery thrombosis and blindness, multiple small strokes, or a single massive one, coronary occlusion, and death can be averted by proper treatment with prednisone. For this reason, treatment must be started immediately when the diagnosis is established, because there is no way to predict the occurence af serious occlusive vascular symptoms.

The diagnosis is based first upon the history of recent onset of headache in an elderly person with or without systemic symptoms. Examination reveals tenderness of the scalp over the temporal artery or of other scalp arteries. If the disease has been present for some time, the scalp may be edematous, and the observer may be able to see or palpate one or more 2-5-mm exquisitely tender nodules on a scalp artery. If the disease is of recent onset, such nodules may not be visible even during the biopsy procedure. In this case, a 4-6-cm long segment of artery must be removed to give the pathologist his best chance of finding a segment with characteristic pathological changes in it.

Laboratory examinations disclose an elevated Westergren sedimentation rate. Initially the Westergren ESR may be in the range of 100 mm per hour but may be as low as 30-50 mm/hr. There may be mild anemia, and the WBC may be moderately elevated. Examination of the in-patient chart sometimes reveals low-grade fever, but all these indications may be absent except the elevated ESR, and there are reported cases of temporal arteritis with a normal ESR! Such patients must receive their diagnosis on the basis of a characteristic history and biopsy proof.

The clinician is at a disadvantage in his diagnosis of temporal arteritis. Biopsy information is the only absolutely diagnostic finding. He must diagnose and treat temporal arteritis promptly, but he must avoid biopsies of patients with migraine, nervous people, or patients with toothache. The author cannot give information guaranteed to prevent errors, except that if the case is not typical and if the ESR and biopsy information are equivocal, both patient and doctor will benefit from a period of further observation before launching into long-term high-dose prednisone therapy for a diagnosis that may be wrong.

Treatment of Temporal Arteritis

The treatment of temporal arteritis is not benign. It consists initially of very high-dose daily prednisone, 80-100 mg or more each morning. Temporal arteritis does not respond well to alternate-day steroid regimens.[14] The ESR is followed daily and begins to fall after 4-10 days of treatment. The large doses of prednisone are continued until the ESR approaches normal, usually after 2-3 weeks. Thereafter, the ESR and the clinical symptoms determine the dose.

The strategy of treatment is to find the smallest dose which controls both ESR and symptoms. During the first months of treatment, the ESR is taken weekly and the dose of prednisone is reduced each ten days to two weeks by 5-10 mg/day as long as the ESR remains below 15 mm/hour. At some point in the regimen, usually around a dose of 30 mg per day, the ESR rises into the high teens or headache reappears. The dose has been reduced rapidly, and the patient probably needs much more than 30 mg per day to control the disease, so the dose is increased sharply to 50-60 mg per day, and patient and clinician wait till the ESR falls again below 15 mm/hour. Then the dose is again reduced, but this time more slowly, at 3-4 week intervals, and at 2.5-5 mg per day decrements. When symptoms reappear or the ESR rises again, the dose is again raised, but not as sharply; then, even more slowly, it is returned toward the therapeutic threshold.

This procedure assures patient and physician that they are constantly approaching the smallest therapeutic dose of a toxic medication. As the disease runs its course, less prednisone is usually needed to control it, and the dose automatically follows the disease. This constant testing assures the participants that they will encounter the fewest side effects over the long term, both from the disease and from the medication.

In some patients, the disease is so aggressive that it demands toxic doses for long periods. If this is the case, the patient may die anyway because of muscle weakness or broken bones due to side effects of his treatment, or because of heart attack or stroke caused directly by his disease.

Temporal arteritis is often said to run its course over a period of months or a few years. Certainly, patients require less and less prednisone over this time, and some may eventually be able to stop the medication completely, but doctor and patient should plan for long-term treatment at the outset because many patients with the disease can never stop prednisone without recurrent symptoms.[3]

Temporal arteritis is usually a rewarding disease to treat if the physician has a well-developed sense of catastrophe. He must be able to respond promptly to changes in either the laboratory results or his patient's symptoms with generous increases in prednisone dosage when this is indicated. If the patient is intelligent and able to participate in the plan of management, there is no need to refer him to a specialist for treatment. However, if there is any difficulty about the rapid transmission of information among the laboratory, the doctor and the patient, the case is best referred to a physician whose practice may be built around a sense of therapeutic urgency.

TRIGEMINAL NEURALGIA

Trigeminal neuralgia frequently causes diagnostic confusion, probably because the physician or dentist who first sees the patient fails to consider the diagnosis. The syndrome is uncommon, but the clinical history and the anatomical distribution of the pain are distinctive and should alert the clinician to the correct diagnosis.

Trigeminal neuralgia pains are *confined* to distribution of one (very occasionally two) division of the trigeminal nerve on one side of the face. This is usually the second division, but any of the three divisions may be involved.

The pain is extraordinarily intense, but brief. It usually lasts 2-5 seconds. Trigeminal neuralgia pain is the only one that is "truly felt" by the observer because it is so abrupt and so severe. Suddenly, the patient freezes with an intensely painful expression, usually no sound. He stops everything he is doing while he concentrates on his pain; then straightens up and continues the conversation. The pains occur infrequently if he is careful, but as he attempts to tell his story, the simple act of talking triggers paroxysms of pain, and he resorts to written or typed answers. Eating, like talking, may trigger repeated pains; and at one time, both actions resulted in emaciation. Triggering of pain is seen only with trigeminal and other neuralgias. Usually, there is a specific trigger area on the skin of the face where light touch produces a single paroxysm of pain. If the second division is involved, the trigger zone is usually on the upper lip, just lateral to the nose.

Patients discover a fatigue factor in the pain. If they first stimulate the trigger zone repeatedly and suffer repeated attacks of pain, it stops for a time, and they can eat or shave in relative comfort for a few minutes before it returns.

Trigeminal neuralgia may occur as a symptom of underlying neurological disease. Multiple sclerosis is a common cause of trigeminal neuralgia. Meningioma or other tumors in the posterior or middle fossa cause trigeminal neuralgia on occasion. Each patient with this syndrome must be examined with the question of other primary pathology in mind. Primary trigeminal neuralgia is not associated with abnormalities in the neurological examination. Multiple sclerosis and brain tumor are. The physician should search for sensory loss on the affected part of the face, unilateral weakness of muscles of mastication or of facial expression, other cranial nerve palsies and abnormalities of long tract function. If these are present, they indicate the presence of an underlying disease and call for further diagnostic evaluation.

Treatment of Trigeminal Neuralgia

The current treatment of choice for trigeminal neuralgia is carbamazepine (Tegretol®). Treatment is begun with 100 mg twice each day and increased daily to a total dose of 600-1200 mg per day. In some cases, the pain disappears after the first half tablet, and the patient can keep his pain under control indefinitely. He is instructed to use the smallest dose which controls the pain and to experiment periodically by decreasing the dose, because trigeminal neuralgia has remissions and he may not need the carbamazepine continuously. Side effects of carbamazepine are discussed in the chapter on seizure disorder (p. 199).

If carbamazepine is ineffective, injection of the hilum of the Gasserian ganglion with minute amounts of absolute alcohol may be effective in producing specific loss of pain sensation to pinprick while not interfering with touch sensation over the face or with corneal sensitivity.[11,12] Small radiofrequency lesions may be placed stereotactically in the same region with similar results. These procedures can produce immediate and permanent loss of the pains of trigeminal neuralgia. They are delicate procedures to be performed only by an experienced therapist.

HYSTERICAL FACIAL PAIN

This syndrome has many names including atypical facial neuralgia. It consists of incapacitating facial pain that does not follow the distribution of nerves, does not respond well to treatment, and is not associated with the presence of detectable organic disease. As time passes, the patient frequently becomes more and more restricted in his life activities. In contrast to the agonized expression on the faces of patients with cluster headache and trigeminal neuralgia, the patient with hysterical facial pain may appear to be fairly comfortable despite the colorful verbal descriptions of severe pain.

If there are abnormalities in the physical examination, these are distributed in an hysterical pattern; for instance, facial numbness, which stops at the hairline and extends to the angle of the jaw, but includes the entire non-neurological face (Figure 14-1).

If the patient recognizes that his pain is of an emotional origin or that he is significantly depressed or disturbed and if he wants psychiatic treatment, this kind of help is sometimes effective. Hysterical facial pain often masks depression and may respond to vigorous antidepressant therapy with medications like amitriptyline (Elavil®), but the patient must first be convinced that the treatment is better than the disease.

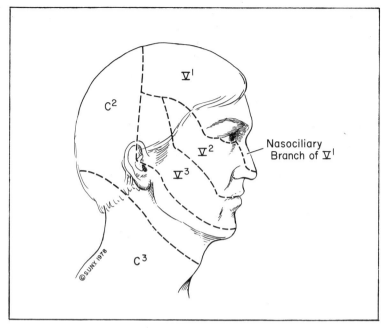

Figure 14-1. *Anatomical distribution of the three divisions of the facial nerve. Note especially that the first division does not stop at the hairline but innervates the scalp to the vertex; and that the second and third divisions do not extend to the angle of the jaw, which is innervated by branches of the sensory root of C².*

HEADACHE DUE TO SERIOUS INTRACRANIAL DISEASE

Most patients who come to medical attention for treatment of headache do not have serious intracranial disease. This is partly because diseases like brain tumor, subdural hematoma, and the like produce focal neurological complaints as well as headache, and may be diagnosed with modern techniques. Nonetheless, the physician needs to keep in mind that serious intracranial disease may be the cause of his patient's distress, so careful consideration of the headache history and the complete neurological examination are important in establishing an accurate diagnosis. Here are some characteristics which may help to identify the patient whose headache is a symptom of serious intracranial disease:

1) The history does not fit descriptions of headache syndromes described above.
2) Recent onset of headache, especially after age 40, with no previous headache history.
3) Strictly unilateral headache which *never* switches sides.
4) Progressively severe headaches over weeks or months.
5) *Sudden* onset of a headache, especially if there is also pain down the back and into the legs. (Subarachnoid hemorrhage may occasionally produce this syndrome without clouding of consciousness.)
6) Cerebral bruit. (Listen with the stethescope diaphragm over the convexities of the head and listen with the bell over the closed eyelid. The skin of the eyelid must not occlude the orifice of the bell. There should be "seashell sound" if this procedure is done correctly, but no bruit!)
7) Personality change. (Dull, apathetic, demented—aphasic!)

If the physician has doubts about the diagnosis and needs confirmation that there is no structural disease, the CT and nuclear brain scans are of immense diagnostic help. These may miss small aneurysms, but angiography is not indicated in every case of unusual headache. If the physician has the results of screening examinations and is still uneasy about the etiology of headache, neurological consultation is quite appropriate.

SUMMARY

The reader will recognize that most patients with chronic recurrent headache have no need of specialized care. Those whose headaches are especially severe, especially unresponsive to treatment, or who likely have serious neurological disease may be identified soon after they appear and are referred to a specialist for care. Most of the rest respond well to careful diagnostic procedures, education about their illness, and carefully chosen medication regimens.

REFERENCES

1. Ad Hoc Committee on Classification of Headache: Classification of Headache. Arch. Neurol. 6:173–176, 1962.
2. Anthony, M., Lance, J.W.: Histamine and Serotonin in Cluster Headache. Arch. Neurol. 25:225–231, 1971.

3. Beevers, D.G., Harpur, J.E5, Turk, K.A.D.: Giant Cell Arteritis—The Need for Prolonged Treatment. J. Chron. Dis. 26:571–584, 1973.

4. Bickerstaff, E.R.: The Periodic Migrainous Neuralgia of Wilfred Harris. Lancet 1:1069–1071, 1959.

5. Borgesen, S.E., Nielsen, J.L., Moller, C.E.: Prophylactic Treatment of Migraine with Propranolol. Acta Neurol. Scand. 50:651–656, 1974.

6. Curran, D.A., Hinterberger, H., Lance, J.W.: Total Plasma Serotonin, 5-Hydroxyindoleacetic Acid and p-Hydrooxy-m-Methoxy-mandelic Acid Excretion in Normal and Migrainous Subjects. Brain 88:997–1010, 1965.

7. Dalessio, D.J., (Ed.): *Wolff's Headache and Other Head Pain,* 3rd edition. Oxford University Press, New York, 1972.

8. Ibid., pp. 299–307.

9. Dalton, K.: Migraine and Oral Contraceptives. Headache. 16:247–251, 1976.

10. Diamond, S., Medina, J.L.: Double-Blind Study of Propranolol for Migraine Prophylaxis. Headache 16:24–27, 1976.

11. Ecker, A.: Sensory Loss and Prolonged Remission of Tic Douloureux After Selective Alcoholic Gasserian Injection. In: *Advances in Pain Research and Therapy,* Vol. I. Bonica, J.J. and Albe-Fessard, D. (Eds.) Raven Press, New York, 1976.

12. Ecker, A.: Tic Douloureux: Eight Years After Alcoholic Gasserian Injection. N.Y. State J. Med. 74:1586–1592, 1974.

13. Friedman, A.P.: Headache. In: *Clinical Neurology.* Baker, A.B. and Baker, L.H., (Eds.) Harper & Row, Pub., Hagerstown and New York, 1977, Vol. 11, Chapter 13, p. 12–13.

14. Hunder, G.G., Sheps, S.G., Allen, G.L., Joyce, J.W.: Daily and Alternate-Day Corticosteroid Regimens in Treatment of Giant Cell Arteritis. Ann. Intern Med. 82:613–618, 1975.

15. Lance, J.W.: The Pathophysiology and Treatment of Migraine. N.Z. Med. J. 79:954–960, 1974.

16. Rydzewski, W.: Serotonin (5H) in Migraine: Levels in Whole Blood in and Between Attacks. Headache 16:16–19, 1976.

17. Stenbäck, A.: Headache and Life Stress. Acta Psych. Neurol. Scand. (Suppl. 92), 1954.

18. Symonds, C.: A Particular Variety of Headache. Brain. 79:217–232, 1956.

19. Waters, W.E.: Review of the Epidemiology of Migraine in Adults. Dan. Med. Bull. 22:86–88, 1975.

20. Zaters, W.E., O'Connor, P.J.: Prevalence of Migraine. J. Neurol. Neurosurg. Psychiatr. 38:613–616, 1975.

21. Wideroe, T.-E., Vigander, T.: Propranolol in the Treatment of Migraine. Br. Med. J. 2:699–701, 1974.

CHAPTER 15

A Neurological Screening Examination

INTRODUCTION

Most sick people are neurologically intact, but it behooves the clinician to develop techniques for the rapid and complete assessment of every organ system so that he may detect abnormalities when they do occur. In this chapter, we shall consider the screening examination I use daily for neurological patients. If the patient is normal and the examiner is adept, the entire examination takes about eight minutes; and the examinations of chest and abdomen can be included while the patient is sitting up or lying down. Thus, a complete physical examination for screening purposes should take about ten minutes. If the patient has neurological disease special techniques from other portions of this volume may be utilized at appropriate points to define more precisely the cause of any abnormalities that have been discovered.

In many ways, a neurological examination resembles dance. Two people move across from each other in stereotyped fashion. As they do, they blend their neurological functions in such a way that they communicate with each other and to observers. Like dancing, this examination cannot be learned by reading a book. The student must read about moves and sequences. Then he must go out and dance for himself, honing his technique so that he receives the largest amount of accurate communication from a limited series of moves.

I shall stress technique and neuroanatomy in this discussion. Of the two, the neuroanatomy is the easier, because there is a limited amount that the clinician needs to know. But if he is not careful about his technique, he will gather inaccurate information and fail in his assessment of the situation.

The examination actually begins as your patient walks down the hall to your office, but this is not the time for a formal examination of gait. Nonetheless, you can form impressions about her and her diagnosis during this first few seconds that may later be correlated with other information you acquire (Figure 15-1). As you take the history, and consider the significant information in it, your examination of face and general body movement continues and adds to your overall impression. Then you begin the formal examination. I begin mine with an evaluation of cranial nerves, beginning with the visual fields.

EXAMINATION OF THE CRANIAL NERVES

Visual Fields

Present your fingers *symmetrically, briefly,* and *silently* first in the middle, then the lower, and finally the upper quadrant of each far peripheral visual field (Figure 15-2). Say "How many fingers did you see?" If she gives the right answer, she saw both sides. If she says "two", then ask "which side?" If she now gives the correct answer, you *know* that she saw both sides. If you had asked "both sides?" and she said "yes," your information would have been tainted by the *way* you asked the question.

If she gives accurate responses to confrontation in each of the three quadrants, then stop and go on to the next test.

Remember that the monocular portion of the visual fields is very large. The reader can define this area in his own visual field, as we demonstrate in Figure 15-3, by bringing his finger forward into the far peripheral field of one eye and holding it there. Then close that eye and bring fingers of the opposite hand forward until the opposite eye just begins to see them across the bridge of the nose.

If you examine the visual fields by keeping your fingers *back* in this monocular peripheral visual field; and if you present your fingers *silently* so that you do not test hearing as well as vision; and if your fingers are presented as *briefly* as you can move them so as to stress the function as well as you can; *and* if your patient gave accurate answers all three times, then you have learned that she does not have hemianopsia or quadrantanopsia to either side, and that she is not blind in either eye. These comprise the vast majority of undetected visual field abnormalities.

Some clinicians present their fingers diagonally, one in the up-

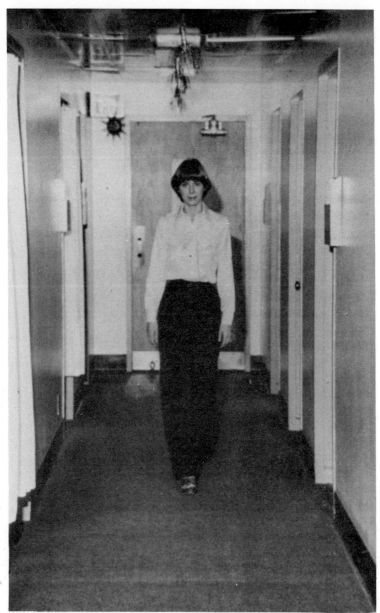

Figure 15-1. *Impressions about the patient and her diagnosis during the first few seconds.*

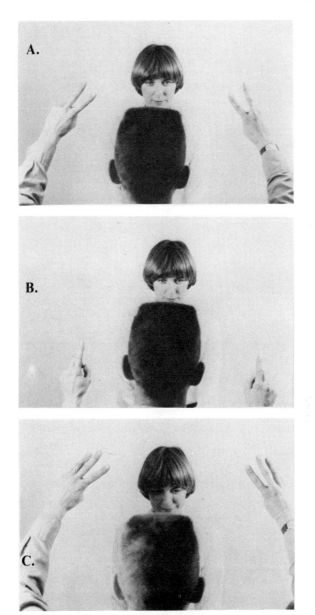

Figure 15-2. *Visual fields. (A) Middle fields. "Two." "Which side?" "Both". (B) Lower fields. "One." "Where?" "Both sides". (C) Upper fields. "Three.—Both sides!"*

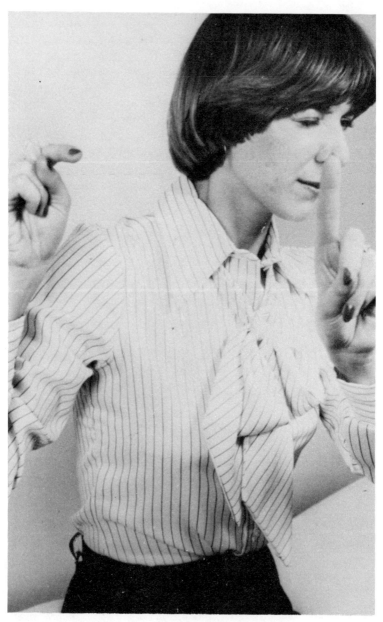

Figure 15-3. *The monocular visual field.*

per and the other in the opposite lower quadrant. This is at least theoretically disadvantageous, since it is not truly double simultaneous stimulation of the visual system. In some cases, stimuli that are presented bilaterally, synchronously, and symmetrically are missed by the patient, even though she may perceive all unilateral stimuli. If visual field examinations are performed diagonally, the stimuli are not truly symmetrical; and such patients could be passed as normal. Since there is absolutely no advantage to diagonal testing, do not take that small chance of missing a diagnosis. Test symmetrically and synchronously in the middle, lower, and then the upper fields.

The superior quadrants of vision are the least important to humans, and patients make their most frequent errors in this quadrant. I have a rule that if patients make more than this one error during the initial presentation of fingers, I go to more careful confrontation testing, using the shiny tips of ball point pens, brought slowly into the three quadrants of vision from behind. Most patients who make mistakes initially can demonstrate that their visual fields are intact during this procedure.

Examination of peripheral visual fields neglects central vision; but patients who have loss of visual acuity or central scotoma complain about it, so they automatically call for further testing that has been outlined in Chapter 4 (pp. 69-75).

Extraocular Muscles

During the initial examination of extraocular muscles, there are only two significant questions: 1) Does she have nystagmus? 2) Do her eyes move conjugately? Do not worry initially about what *kind* of nystagmus she might have, nor about which tract, nucleus, nerve, or muscle might be malfunctioning. Face those difficulties only if you must, and then go directly to detailed testing outlined in Chapter 5.

Nystagmus

If nystagmus is present on forward gaze, or within 30 degrees of forward gaze, it is pathological. "Terminal" or "end-point" nystagmus appears at further degrees of abduction, and this is normal. So take your patient only 30 degrees laterally and hold her there until you are certain that she does not have nystagmus (Figure 15-4). Then repeat the procedure to the opposite side.

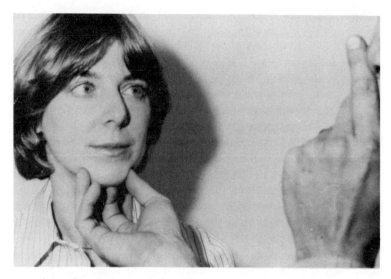

Figure 15-4. *Nystagmus. Abduct the patient's eyes **only** thirty degrees, and hold her there until you are certain.*

Conjugate Gaze

Once you have established that she does not have nystagmus, take her *rapidly* to left and right and up and down to the far extents of lateral and vertical gaze, and then have her converge, observing the pupillary reactions during accommodation as she converges her eyes (Figure 15-5).

Do not bother initially with six cardinal directions of gaze. If an eye muscle is weak, she will either have dysconjugate eye movements or restricted gaze in one or another direction, and then you can move to more specific testing techniques.

Remember as you bring her eyes far laterally, that the globe is normally abducted so far that no sclera, or only a small triangle of sclera is visible between the limbus of the cornea and the lateral canthus of the lids (Figure 15-6). If there is more than that visible, she has weakness of the lateral rectus muscle, partial or complete abducens palsy, or perhaps she is not trying as hard as she should! Some patients with high myopia leave a large triangle of sclera visible as they abduct the eyes. This may relate to the long anterior-posterior diameter of the myopic globe.

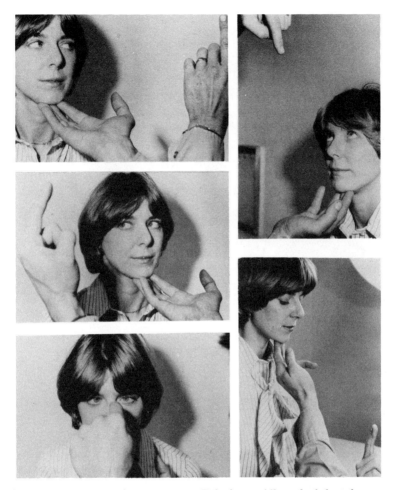

Figure 15-5. *Extraocular movements. Take her **rapidly** to far left, right, up, and down. Then have her converge and observe the pupils, too, as they constrict during accommodation.*

In Chapter 5, we discussed J. Lawton Smith's techniques for the discovery of minimal internuclear ophthalmoplegia (p. 90) This technique is useful whenever dysconjugate eye movements may be present. It is so simple that every clinician should know about it, even though it is not part of his screening examination. Hold your

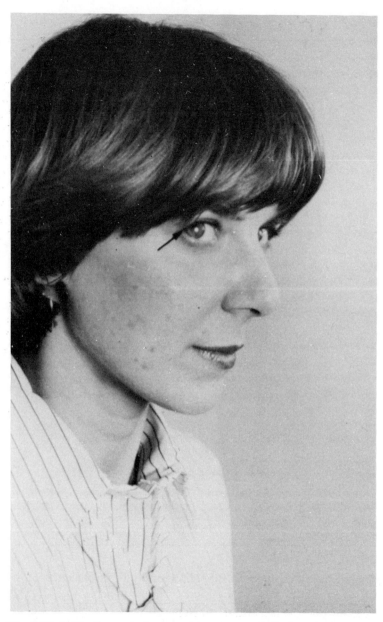

Figure 15-6. *She buries the limbus of the cornea behind the outer canthus of the lids.*

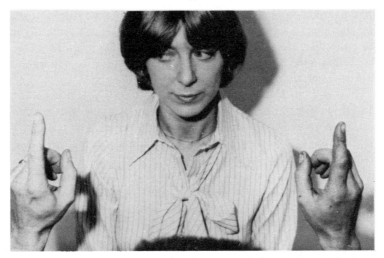

Figure 15-7. *Rapid gross saccades for minimal dysconjugate eye movements.*

testing fingers widely separated in front of the patient, and ask her to glance quickly back and forth between them (Figure 15-7). Then fix your *gaze* on the bridge of her nose and your *attention* on the two eyes. Note whether they truly move *together* with *equal velocity* in *both directions every time*. If they do not, they are abnormal and require accurate assessment.

Funduscopic Examination

Medical students usually learn funduscopy from ophthalmologists, who advise them to begin the examination from a distance and look for the red reflex. Then with the light still on, they are supposed to approach the eye and look in, turning the ophthalmoscope lenses accurately as they do, so as to examine the anterior chamber, the lens, the vitreous, and finally the retina. When they do this, students usually find themselves examining the eyebrow or the cheek; if they reach the fundus, they are frequently so disoriented that they cannot find the important structures there.

This procedure is unnecessarily complex. Ophthalmologists are interested in the red reflex because cataracts interrupt it; and since ophthalmologists remove cataracts, the absence of the red reflex is a valuable sign to them. But the rest of us are interested primarily in the optic disc, retinal blood vessels, and the retina itself, hence we should begin the examination there. If we cannot see in, then we can back off and discover what the trouble is.

It is easy to look directly at the optic disc if you first do two things: 1) estimate the patient's optical correction and add that correction to your own in the ophthalmoscope lenses. For instance if you are about two diopters near-sighted, and the patient wears moderately strong myopic lenses, set the machine on the red 5 or 6. 2) Remember that the optic disc is situated about fifteen degrees medial to the axis of vision on a horizontal plane in the globe.

Before you even *begin* to look in, aim the ophthalmoscope directly at the disc by asking the patient to look at something ahead, aiming the light beam horizontally and about fifteen degrees medially to the axis of vision. Stabilize your hand by placing your middle finger on her cheek, and then simply look in! Keep your other eye open to prevent your eyes from accommodating (Figure 15-8).

If you have done this correctly, you will always be within one disc diameter of the optic disc when you start.

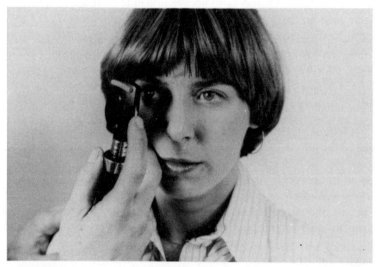

Figure 15-8. *Aim the ophthalmoscope directly at the optic disc—and then simply look in!*

Once you have found the disc, you can examine it, and then move about the retina in an orderly fashion to observe normal and pathological features that might be there.

Pupillary Reaction to Light

Now take your flashlight and look for the pupillary reaction to light (Figure 15-9). I use the otoscope head, which provides brighter illumination than the ophthalmoscope head. Because you have already observed the pupillary reaction during accommodation, this completes the examination of the pupils.

If you have reason to expect that there is damage to pupillary pathways, go directly to special techniques discussed in Chapter 4.

Palate and Tongue

I have designed the sequence of this examination for the efficient use of examination tools and the preservation of the examiner's energies. Now that you have the flashlight in hand, it makes sense to go directly to an examination of the palate and tongue, even though those nerves are not numbered in direct sequence with the pupils.

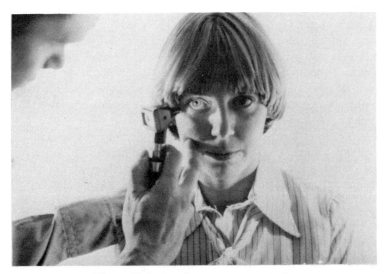

Figure 15-9. *Pupillary reaction to light.*

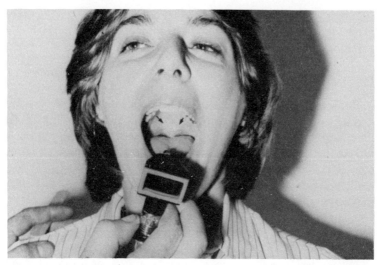

Figure 15-10. *Insertions of the levator veli palatini. No tongue blade is needed.*

The palatal examination is also misunderstood by many clinicians who have been taught to look at the uvula. The uvula is merely a piece of connective tissue surrounded by skin; it is completely irrelevant to this examination. The levator veli palatini muscle elevates the palate (Figure 15-10). It is innervated by the vagus nerve. It becomes paretic in hemiparesis and weak in various kinds of bulbar palsy. It inserts several centimeters anterior to the uvula, either as a broad arching band across the soft palate or as two sharp points near the median raphe.

Minor asymmetries of the palate are common if it is examined for this feature. Usually these are related to previous tonsillectomy or some other irrelevant cause. The important thing is that sometimes palatal paresis may be the first sign of hemiparesis. If the patient's complaints fit, and if face and tongue are also paretic, they form a definite beginning for the diagnosis.

Unless you suspect that your patient has amyotrophic lateral sclerosis or a brainstem lesion, do not spend much time looking for atrophy and fasciculations on the resting tongue. The protruded tongue is usually central to the examination, because the genioglossus muscle protrudes the tongue and receives its innervation from the opposite side of the brain. The tongue deviates toward the side of the weak or paretic genioglossus muscle.

Use your thumbnail, set perpendicular to the chin to give a precise middle line that can be identified despite the presence of a beard, facial asymmetry or absent teeth. Have her stick out her tongue (Figure 15-11)—"bleah!" Be enthusiastic in your instruction and be certain that her response is equally enthusiastic, or you will not observe the function of her genioglossus muscles!

Slight tongue deviations are also seen in some normal people but not as often as palatal asymmetries. The normal medical student in Figure 15-12 has several millimeters of tongue deflection, but she has no neurological complaints and no other abnormalities on her examination.

Examination of the Face

Central Facial Paresis

The normal medical student in Figure 15-13 has mild facial paresis on the left that is evident as he talks but largely disappears when he grimaces. Notice that the upper lip is slightly flatter on the left, and the lips are less widely separated than on the right. These are the first findings of facial paresis. If facial paresis becomes more severe, there is effacement of the nasolabial fold and even widening of the palpebral fissure on that side, but these are not the earliest signs of facial paresis.

If you observed asymmetrical facial function as the patient gave his history, you are free to ask him to grimace if you wish during the examination, but this should not teach you much if you have been observant during the entire interview.

Peripheral or Nuclear Facial Weakness

Because the top half of the face has bilateral cortical innervation to muscles of expression, there is little or no dysfunction above the mouth in patients with central facial paresis. But in Bell's palsy, Guillain-Barré syndrome, or in lesions that involve the facial nucleus, one entire side of the face becomes paralyzed, including lid closure and forehead elevation.

Ask the patient to close her eyes *tightly*! In Figure 15-14, she

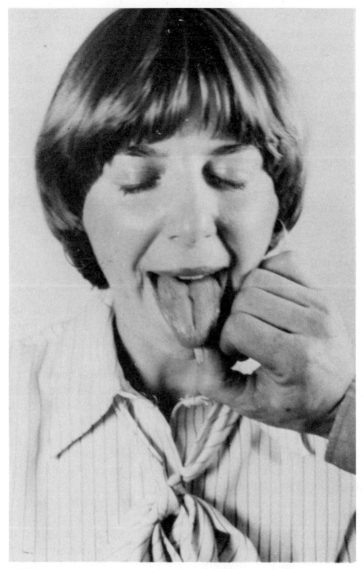

Figure 15-11. *Function of the genioglossus, and the thumbnail as a middle line.*

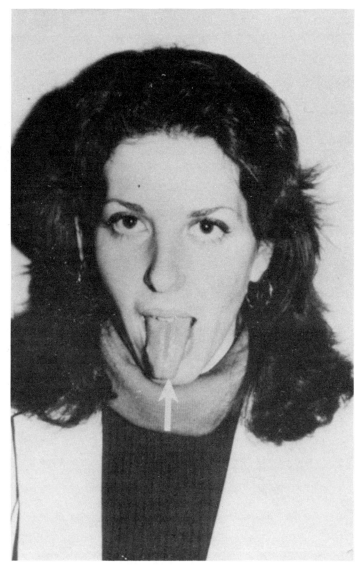

Figure 15-12. *Minimal tongue deviation to the right.*

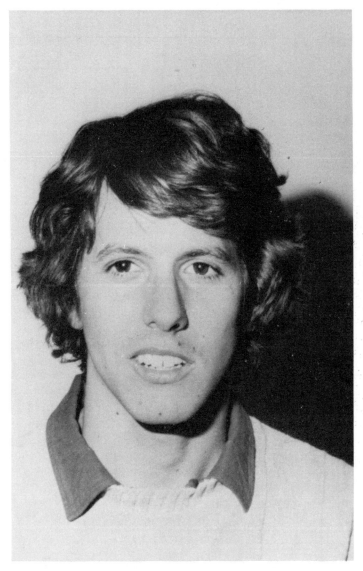

Figure 15-13. *Minimal left facial paresis. If you look for it, it is obvious and common among normal people.*

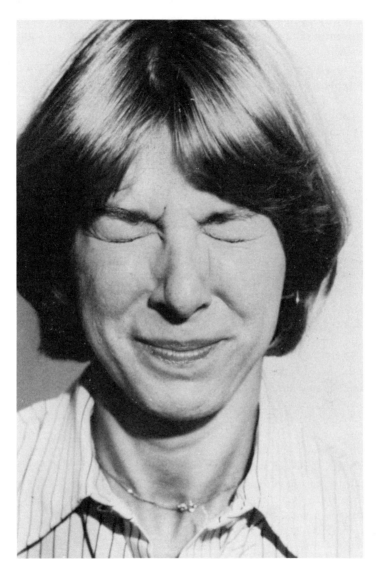

Figure 15-14. *She buries her eyelashes symmetrically, and we could not open her eyes, even with forcible pressure of our thumbs.*

has nearly completely buried her eyelashes. She would successfully resist any attempt we could make to open her eyes against resistance. But the nurse in Figure 15-15, who had Bell's palsy many years ago with incomplete recovery, buries her lashes only on the left. On the right, the eyelashes are clearly visible; the eye opens easily to upward pressure on the upper lid.

Guillain-Barré syndrome provides a major pitfall in the diagnosis of bilateral facial weakness because this condition is not disfiguring, since the face is always symmetrical. Inexperienced examiners fail to make the diagnosis because they forget to look specifically for facial weakness by having the patient close his eyes, noting the eyelashes, and trying to open the eyes against resistance.

Examination of these cranial nerves takes slightly more than a minute. During that time, you have observed intact visual functions. You have seen raw muscle power in the palate and tongue and watched coordinated movements of eyes and face. You know whether the pupils react to light and in accommodation, and you have actually examined the function of about a thousand grams of brain and brainstem, leaving only the cerebellum, spinal cord, and the peripheral neuromuscular systems to be examined; not bad for the first minute of your examination!

Examination of cranial nerve functions provides direct and highly specific information about brainstem nuclei, internuclear connections, and some motor and visual connections in the brain. The rest of the examination provides much less specific information.

When the patient does rapid gross or fine alternating movements, or finger to nose coordination, he displays the functions of the entire sensory and motor nervous system that relates to the upper extremities. Tests of gait and standing balance involve even broader neurological function, excluding only lower sacral segments of the spinal cord. Even the deep tendon reflexes provide unspecific information that must be evaluated by the examiner as he proceeds. Is the hyporeflexia at one joint caused by segmental sensory or motor neuron disease, muscular weakness, cerebellar disease, or rigidity? If they are asymmetrical, is the one side *hyper*-reflexic, or is the other *hypo*-reflexic? The clinician can answer these questions as he proceeds to each subsequent part of the examination. His answers will depend upon the aggregate results of the entire examination and

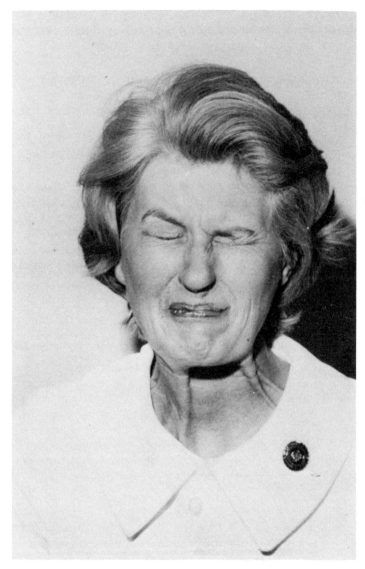

Figure 15-15. *The nurse pictured here had Bell's palsy on the right. The eyelashes are **not** well buried, and the eye opens easily to upward pressure from a thumb. Look at the eyebrow, too!*

his ability to analyze his results in terms of functional neuro-anatomy. Only Babinski's sign has specificity (for the pyramidal system), and there is no such thing as a "cerebellar test."

EXAMINATION OF THE UPPER EXTREMITIES

General Posture

Ask the patient to sit, arms outstretched, eyes closed (Figure 15-16). As she does this, *wait*. Fatigue and the passage of time are your friends here, because as she sits, one arm may begin to drift, or a tremor may appear. You may notice wasting of hand muscles, and certainly your examination of the hands reveals many things about her life activities. This initial maneuver merely points out which side may be abnormal. The *way* it is abnormal may suggest paresis, sensory loss, weakness, or imbalance. Make no firm conclusions about the pathological anatomy at this point, but go on to the rest of the examination.

Deltoids and Grip

While she still sits, arms outstretched, push down on her wrists

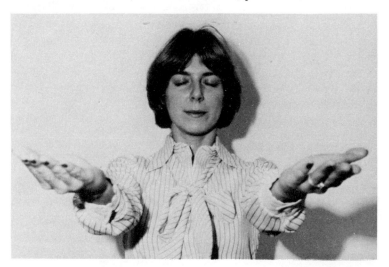

Figure 15-16. *The patient is seated, arms outstretched, eyes closed.*

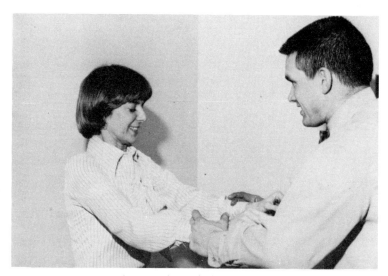

Figure 15-17. *Shoulder power.*

(Figure 15-17), asking her to "hold it!—tight!" Then test grip on each side and feel the power of her grip (Figure 15-18). Remember that the function of grip is to hold on, the test of grip is to escape, not merely to feel the pressure of fingers. If there is decreased power of grip, go directly to the finger pulling test described in Chapter 3 (pp. 45-47) to distinguish between upper motor neuron paresis and motor unit weakness.

During the fifteen seconds of testing deltoids and grip, you have examined a tremendous amount of the nervous system. Think of it! Each of these functions is directed from the cortex on the opposite side of the brain; connections descend through the internal capsule, through the base of the brainstem, and cross to the same side of the spinal cord, where they travel to specific segments to innervate anterior horn cells (Figure 15-19). Deltoid innervation comes from C5-6, and grip innervation comes from C8-T1. Each of these two functions uses a different part of the brachial plexus. The proximal position of the deltoid helps to distinguish weakness caused by primary muscle disease from that caused by other kinds of illness.

Actually, the only important cervical segmental innervation that is ignored during this fifteen seconds is C7. If you are not concerned

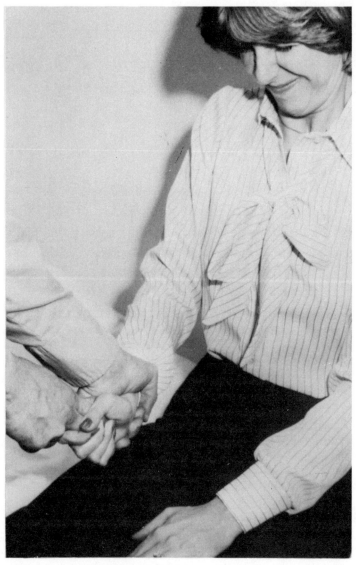

Figure 15-18. *Power of grip.*

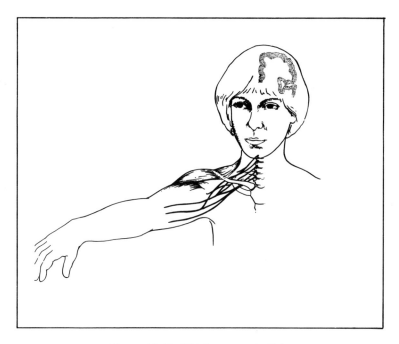

Figure 15-19. *Think anatomically!*

about cervical segmental disease, you can safely ignore that segment. Should you desire to test it, the triceps muscle, which straightens the elbow, is the best place to look. A formal examination of all muscles innervated by the cervical spinal cord is beyond the needs of the non-neurological clinician.

Finger to Nose

Patients are frequently confused, at least briefly, as they try to learn traditional finger to nose testing. Part of the trouble is that the clinician may try to explain the procedure in English, which is a relatively new form of communication. Nonverbal gestures provide much clearer directions in this situation.

A better test of finger to nose involves only one verbal command, "touch my finger!" As you say that, touch her right hand with your left and raise your left hand into the air, pointer finger extended. After the first touch, move your hand rapidly away, and say once more, "touch!" Then remain silent and move your target finger around the entire reachable space for her right upper extremity, alternating between a position close to her body and one far away. To examine her other upper extremity, simply drop your left hand, touch her left with your right, and raise the right hand. She will follow automatically (Figure 15-20).

There are pitfalls to this method. If you are lazy and move your target finger very little, you will not observe the *full range* of her arm movements through space, so you may miss mild dyssynergia or dysmetria. If you do not move *quickly* and *stress* your patient's abilities, you cannot stretch her function to its limits, so you will again miss mild dysfunction.

On the other hand, this technique offers tremendous advantages over traditional finger to nose testing, because it is always the clinician who determines when the patient will move. The moment her finger touches, the clinician moves, and she is kept constantly striving. During traditional finger to nose testing, when the patient has her finger on the nose, *she* decides when to move. Once her finger has reached the target, *she* returns her finger to a *predictable* position on her nose, so minimal degrees of dysfunction may be masked that become obvious during the stress of the more rapid and (for the patient) unpredictable technique.

This is also the place to consider the effect of nonverbal gestures. The reader has spent several minutes with a description in English that is complex and may sound difficult. However, if he performs the movements, they are really quite simple and easily learned. The same holds true for patients being examined. Spend as little time as you can speaking, and learn to demonstrate for your patient the moves she is to make. Once you have mastered techniques for nonverbal examination, your neurological "dance" will flow more smoothly and provide more and better information.

Rapid Gross Alternating Movements

Tell her "do this!" and then *show* her, by rapidly pronating and supinating your own hand on your own thigh. Once she is well-started, say "fast!" in a strained voice to encourage her to move as rapidly as she can. Always test each hand separately, never together,

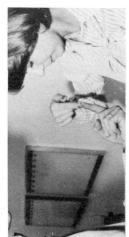
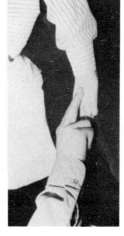
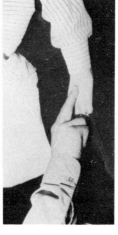
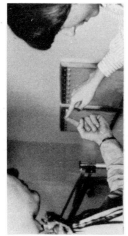
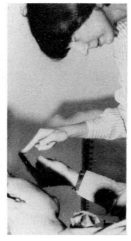
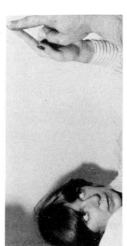

Figure 15-20. *A better way to do finger to nose testing. The examiner is in charge here.*

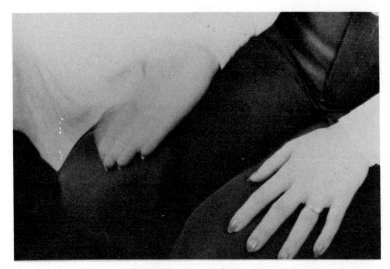

Figure 15-21. *Rapid gross alternating movements.*

because when the two hands are used together, the faster one slows down to match its partner; and small degrees of asymmetry disappear. When each hand is tested separately, small differences in coordination due to handedness are easily detected, and pathological degrees of asymmetry cannot be missed (Figure 15-21).

Rapid Fine Alternating Movements

Have the patient tap her third finger against the ball of her thumb. *Show* her and merely say "do this!" In addition to watching the *frequency* of tapping, note whether the *cadence* is smooth and *listen* to the regularity of audible taps. Observe whether wrist and elbow joints participate in the movements, because in most normal people, these joints are kept immobilized during finger tapping (Figure 15-22).

Avoid the more complex technique of having her tap her thumb sequentially against each finger. These movements are always done more slowly than finger tapping; they are more complex and more difficult to evaluate as you watch.

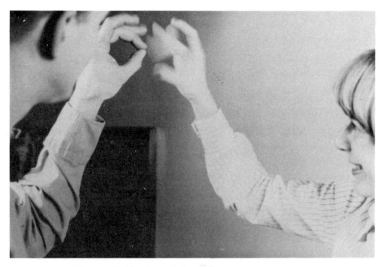

Figure 15-22. *Rapid fine alternating movements.*

EXAMINATION OF REFLEXES AND SENSATION

I ask patients to lie down for the reflex and sensory examinations, because even normal people may develop asymmetrical reflexes if they assume an asymmetrical sitting posture, and that is confusing (Figure 15-23). More importantly, the supine patient's body is all equidistant from the examiner, so we can examine her face and feet with equal facility and without unnecessary bending and straining. Once the reflex examination is finished, she can remain supine for the sensory examination, which may also cover all parts of her body. If you spend entire days examining patients, such economizing of your own effort becomes vitally important.

Deep Tendon Reflexes

Jaw Jerk

Begin the reflex examination with the jaw jerk. Have her open her mouth a bit. Place your finger on her lower jaw and strike your

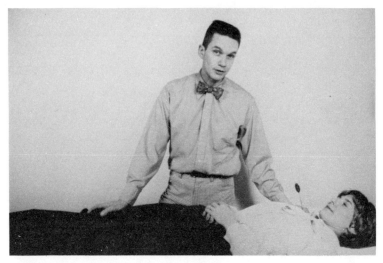

Figure 15-23. *Have the patient lie down for examination of reflexes and sensation.*

finger in a downward direction to open the jaw, not an inward direction that might hurt her dentures (Figure 15-24)! The jaw jerk is abnormal if it is extremely snappy or if there is jaw clonus. An abnormal jaw jerk signifies bilateral corticobulbar disease above the midbrain, so this is an important reflex, because its segmental origin is higher than that of any other reflex.

Pectoralis Reflex

Place your finger on the pectoralis tendon and strike it hard enough to get a response (Figure 15-25). Hospitalized patients frequently have intravenous therapy and occasionally restraints, so the pectoralis reflex may be the only deep tendon reflex in the upper extremities that can be performed symmetrically. Furthermore, the pectoralis reflex is the most proximal of all the limb reflexes, so it may be the only one left in patients with severe peripheral neuropathy. Because the pectoralis muscle receives innervation from several nerve roots, this reflex has little segmental localizing significance.

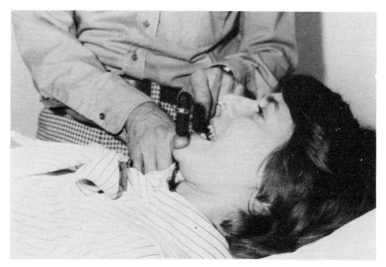

Figure 15-24. *Jaw jerk.*

Biceps Reflex (C5-6)

Place your thumb on the biceps tendon and hit it. The "off" biceps reflex is harder to learn than any of the others, because it feels awkward initially to bend over the patient, hit the reflex and miss her forearm and arm (Figure 15-26). Inexperienced clinicians may decide to walk around to the other side, or to have their patient sit up for the entire examination because of this difficulty. It is well worth your while to practice doing this technically difficult maneuver until it becomes easy for you, thus saving yourself trouble and fatigue for the remainder of your professional life.

Radioperiosteal Reflex (C5-6)

Radioperiosteal reflexes are frequently unresponsive. If that is so bilaterally, it is normal. Simply hit the radius with the broad side of your hammer and observe the result (Figure 15-27).

Trömner's Sign

Trömner's sign is an important adjunctive reflex that may be used to confirm impressions about other reflexes examined in the upper extremities. While it is truly a stretch reflex, the mode of acquisi-

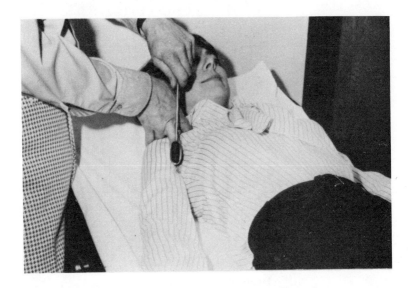

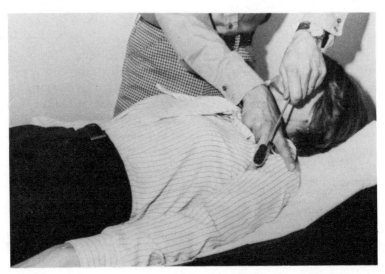

Figure 15-25. *Pectoralis reflexes.*

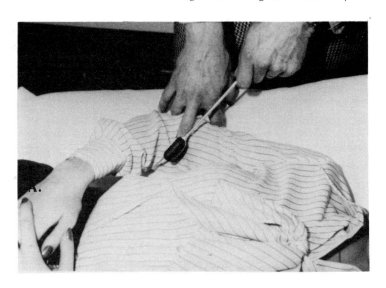

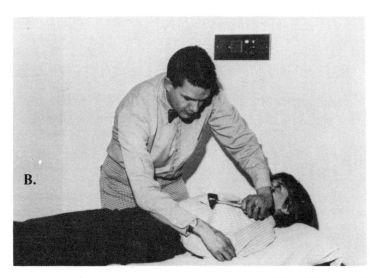

Figure 15-26. *(A) The right biceps reflex is easy. (B) The left biceps reflex feels awkward at first but becomes easy with practice.*

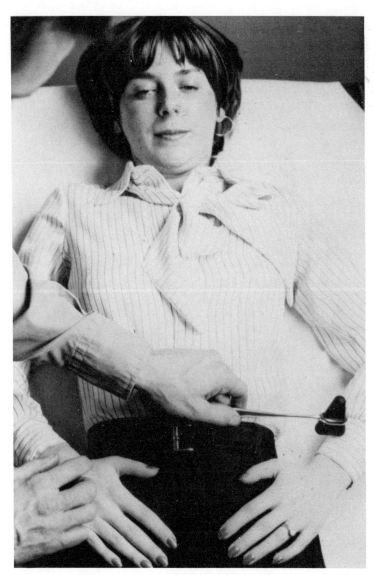

Figure 15-27. *Radioperiosteal reflexes.*

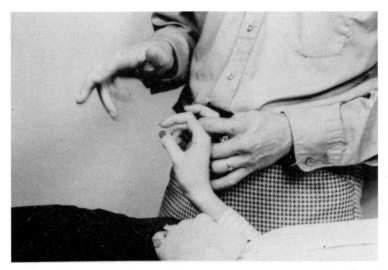

Figure 15-28. *Trömner's sign. The examiner is preparing to slap the patient's middle finger sharply upward from below.*

tion is different. Place your little finger in the small of her wrist, and your pointer finger under the first metacarpal of her middle finger. Then dorsiflex her wrist and immobilize her hand in this position. With your other hand, strike the palmar side of her middle finger abruptly upward with your own middle finger (Figure 15-28). Trömner's sign consists of flexion of the distal phalanx of her thumb. If spasticity is severe, other fingers join in the flexion movement.

Normal young people often have minimal Trömner sign responses, but they are symmetrical. If Trömner's sign is asymmetrical, or if there is more than a minimal gesture of thumb flexion, the response is abnormal and represents spasticity.

Practice doing Trömner's sign first with a patient who has significant spasticity. Demonstrate to your own satisfaction that dorsiflexion of the wrist is important, and that the sign disappears, even in the face of spasticity, when you allow the wrist to straighten or flex it in the opposite direction. Learn to deliver graded amounts of dorsiflexion flicks with your other middle finger that allow you to distinguish between various amounts of spasticity. Then practice on normal people and demonstrate that they may have minimal responses if you flick their fingers aggressively upward, especially if the patient is young, and even more so if he is nervous.

Because Trömner's sign is more aggressive and the stimulus can be of graded intensity, this is a much more valuable sign than the traditional Hoffmann's sign, which merely involves passive dorsiflexion of the middle finger after it is released.

Triceps Reflex (C6-7)

I do not routinely look for the triceps reflex unless I am concerned about segmental disease from the cervical region. In hemiparesis, the triceps reflex provides no more information than the others already examined, so the result is redundant.

Knee Jerk (L 2, 3, 4)

Knee jerks are best done with the knees held symmetrically. In this position, the examiner can easily alternate between the two sides to assess the symmetry of response (Figure 15-29).

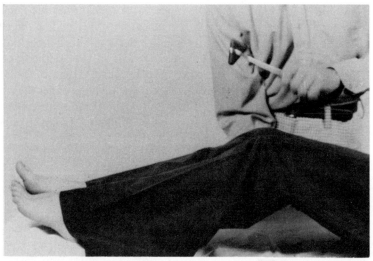

Figure 15-29. *Hold the patient's knees symmetrically, and then compare the responses on the two sides.*

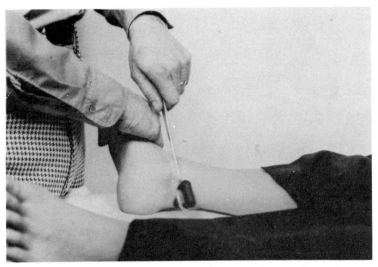

Figure 15-30. *Tilt the foot laterally, Wiggle it up and down a bit, and stop in the slightly dorsiflexed position—then hit it!*

Ankle Jerk (S1, 2)

Tilt the foot laterally, wiggle it up and down a bit, and stop in the slightly dorsiflexed position. Then simply hit the Achilles tendon and watch the response (Figure 15-30).

There is a pitfall here for the inexperienced examiner, because the reflex is best observed with the foot in a slightly dorsiflexed position. If the examiner simply pulls the foot into dorsiflexion, the patient will surely try to "help" by contracting the anterior tibial muscle. If she continues doing this as the reflex is struck, the response will be inaccurate. So watch the anterior tibial tendon (Figure 15-31). Be certain that it is relaxed before you do the reflex, and prevent your patient from "helping" by not telling her what you are about to do. Instead of pulling the foot into dorsiflexion, wiggle it up and down a bit and *stop* in dorsiflexion. Then the result will be valid.

Babinski's Sign

Bring a key or some other fairly sharp object slowly and firmly up the lateral aspect of the sole of the foot (Figure 15-32). Babinski's

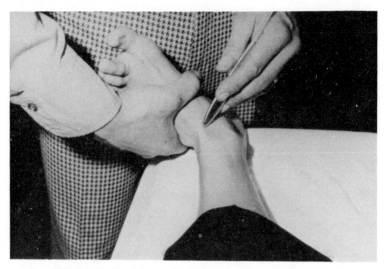

Figure 15-31. *The anterior tibial tendon. Be careful!*

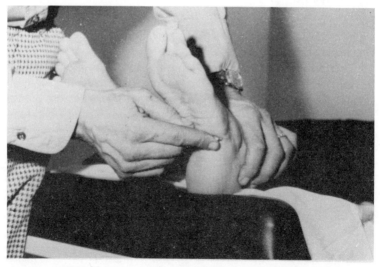

Figure 15-32. *Stay on the **lateral** side of the sole for Babinski's sign.*

sign is *present* (not positive) if the great toe dorsiflexes involuntarily.

Avoid the medial aspect of the sole, because the reflex is less active there; that area tickles more.

This is the first uncomfortable maneuver you have done, so warn her in advance; "I am going to be nasty to you now." Then she can get ready, not withdraw quite so much, and be pleased that you are concerned about her feelings as well as her reflexes.

Sensory Examination

The sensory examination is the most treacherous part of the entire neurological assessment. If the clinician is to acquire accurate information, his patient must be intelligent, alert, and truthful; many patients do not meet these criteria. Additionally, the clinician must pay special attention to his examination technique so the sensory examination may be an objective examination, even though sensation is purely an inner process. This is one part of the examination that may be omitted on occasion, and it is certainly an examination that should never be done without prior knowledge of the probable result! We have delayed this examination until late, because at this point, the clinician knows a great deal about his patient's nervous system and should find it easy to predict the probable sensory abnormalities. There are only six kinds of sensory loss to choose from, so that makes prediction considerably easier:

1) If disease is in the brain, the patient may have hemi-hypesthesia (Figure 15-33).

2) Crossed hypesthesia is characteristic of brainstem disease (Figure 15-34).

3) Spinal cord lesions produce sensory *levels*, depending on the segment that is involved (Figure 15-35). Also in spinal cord disease, "dissociated" sensory loss occurs because the spinothalamic tract is crossed while the posterior columns are not. Thus, the patient may have loss of pinprick on one side, but loss of position sense on the other, or segmental loss of pinprick and completely normal position sense.

4) Focal peripheral nerve lesions produce sensory (and motor) loss in their entire distribution distal to the lesion. Nerve roots or specifically named peripheral nerves may be affected (Figure 15-36).

5) Peripheral neuropathy produces symmetrical distal sensory

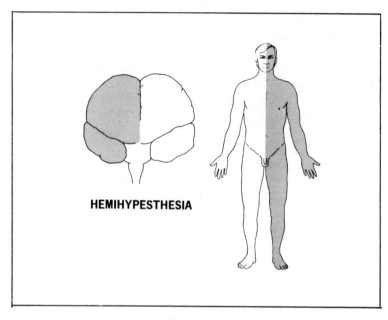

HEMIHYPESTHESIA

Figure 15-33.

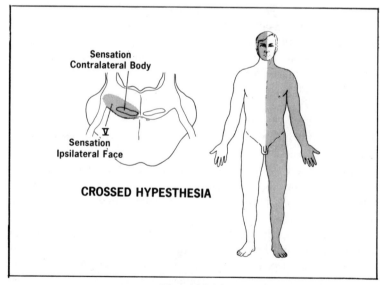

Sensation
Contralateral Body

Sensation
Ipsilateral Face

$\underline{V}$

CROSSED HYPESTHESIA

Figure 15-34.

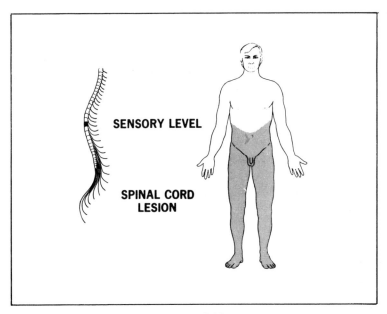

Figure 15-35.

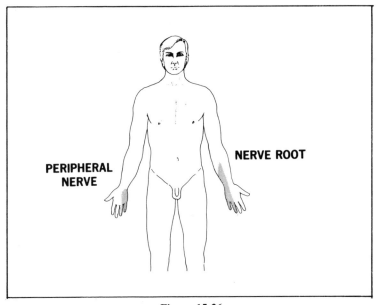

Figure 15-36.

loss (Figure 15-37). Remember that there is no sensory loss in the hands until numbness has ascended above the knees in patients with severe peripheral neuropathy. Thus, the patient with glove and nylon stocking hypesthesia has peripheral neuropathy (and absent knee and ankle jerks), while the patient with glove and bobby sox anesthesia is hysterical.

6) Hysterical anesthesia occurs anywhere in the body (Figure 15-38). The diagnosis rests on proof that the distribution does not follow known neuroanatomy, and the patient's method of presentation may also have suggested hysterical disability (pp. 9-11). It is dangerous for non-neurological clinicians to make a diagnosis of hysteria on the basis of neurological complaints unless they are fully familiar with the entire spectrum of organic neurological disease, so it might be appropriate to consult with a neurologist before making this decision.

Technique is terribly important during the sensory examination. The clinician must constantly guard against tainting his results by prior suggestion. When you are about to test pinprick sensation, hide

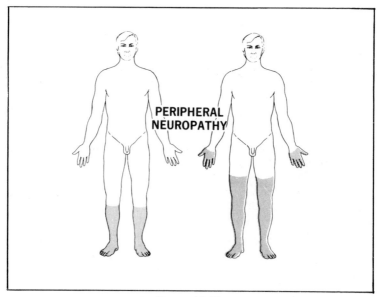

PERIPHERAL
NEUROPATHY

Figure 15-37.

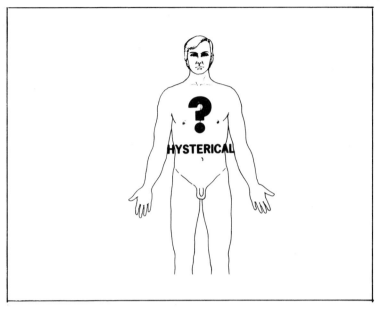

Figure 15-38.

the pin. Stick the patient *once* lightly on the ankle that is most likely to be hypesthetic and ask "What was that?" If you are testing vibration sense, strike the tuning fork *silently* and allow the vibration to die down some. Then place the fork on the medial malleolus and your finger on the lateral malleolus. Say "What does this feel like?" and if you can feel the vibration through the joint, expect your patient also to register it. Vibration sense is difficult for people to identify verbally. They sometimes make a to-and-fro gesture, may say "buzz," or may even say "bee"! In that case, ask "buzz or sting"? and let *them* tell *you* what they felt. Position sense is easily made objective, because the examiner knows precisely what has happened. Find the least excursions of the great toe that can accurately be identified. Young people detect a millimeter or two of movement in the great toe. Older people need a bit more movement. In the fingers, there is no threshold for position sense, because the fingers easily detect the smallest movement you can make.

Once your patient has identified a stimulus, you can compare the two sides with each other, or look for the sensory level or the distribution of peripheral nerve disease, according to your prior knowledge of the case.

EXAMINATION OF GAIT, STANDING BALANCE, AND MUSCLE POWER IN THE LOWER EXTREMITIES

Gait is the most complex function that we examine, so the formal examination of gait is last in the sequence. All levels of the nervous system contribute to normal gait except the lower sacral segments; disease at any level can alter gait in many ways.

We shall ask the patient to perform a series of increasingly difficult maneuvers that aid in grading her gait disturbance according to degrees of disability.

First she simply walks away, turns, and comes back. Then she walks on her heels, an activity that brings out arm swing and displays function of the anterior tibial muscles. Next she tandem walks one in front of the other, then stands tandem, heel immediately in front of toe. Then, in the same position, once she has her balance, she closes her eyes and stands in a more difficult modification of Romberg's maneuver. Last, she hops up and down in one place on one foot at a time eyes closed (Figure 15-39—15-42).

As she walks, note the breadth of gait and how she swings her arms. As she turns, does she do it with one step, or does she "walk around" to face you? Is her balance normal as she "walks the rail?" Some normal people cannot tandem stand, but normals can always hop up and down, eyes closed, in one place. Remember also, as she hops, that you are observing not only her balance, but the power and coordination of quadriceps and gastrocnemius muscles.

Patients with neurological disease have increasing difficulty as they progress along this series of moves, until they reach a level that is impossible for them. Patients with hysterical astasia-abasia may not be able to walk without displaying great difficulty but may later hop up and down unassisted, thus proving their diagnosis unequivocally.

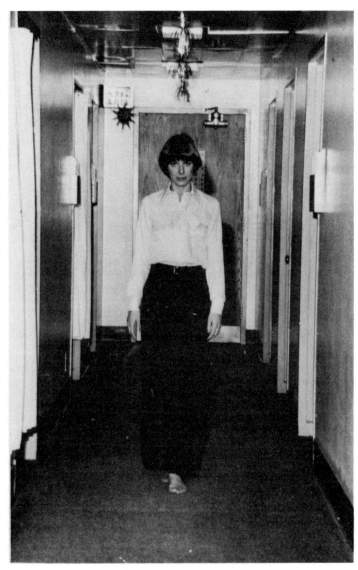

Figure 15-39. *First the patient walks.*

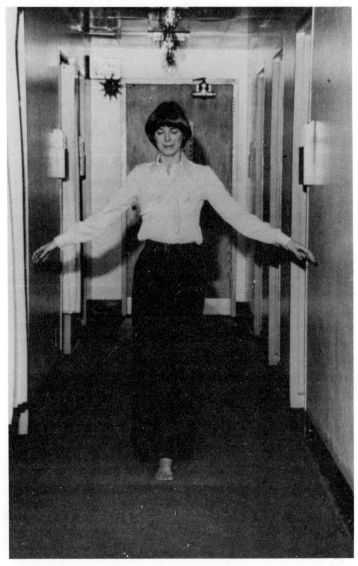

Figure 15-40. *Tandem walk.*

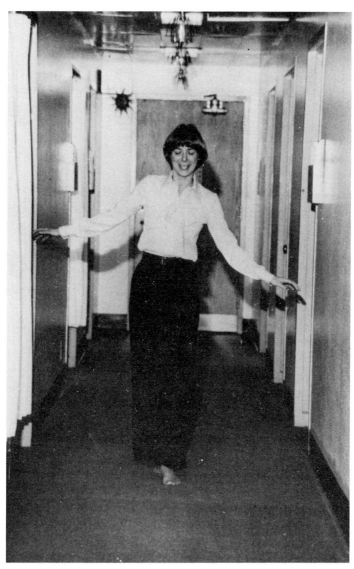

Figure 15-41. *Tandem stand, then do it with eyes closed.*

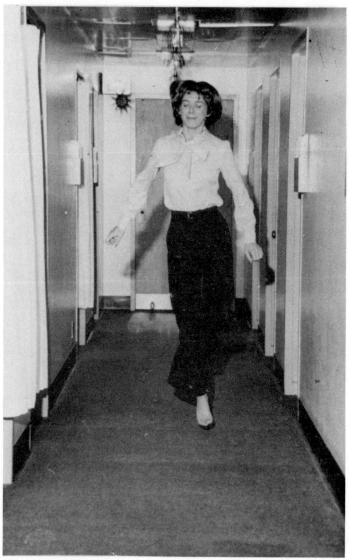

Figure 15-42. *Hop, one foot, one place, eyes closed.*

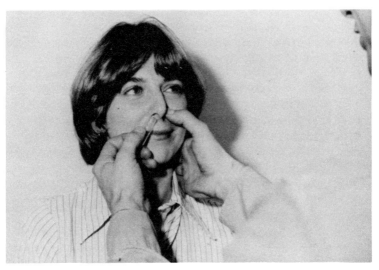

Figure 15-43. *Testing smell (obsolete).*

WHAT IS OMITTED?

We have omitted several relics from the nineteenth century neurologist, the testing of smell (Figure 15-43), and the Weber and Rinné tests of hearing. At one time, the olfactory tracts offered the best localizing information for lesions of the frontal and subfrontal regions, because that was the only testable cerebral function from that area. But now if the clinician becomes concerned about that region of the brain, he can order one or more of the exquisitely accurate radiographic examinations, such as the CT or nuclear brain scans, which can detect lesions in that area long before smell is ever affected. Rather than testing for smell, spend the time you saved thinking about the frontal region of the brain. Then decide whether it should be examined and order a diagnostic test.

In the same manner, the tuning fork was once the most accurate tool for testing hearing (Figure 15-44). Now we have competent audiology laboratories with equipment that can help to diagnose the site of hearing loss at all levels of the anatomy of hearing. If the presence or the kind of hearing loss is important to your neurological diagnosis, ask the audiology laboratory to help.

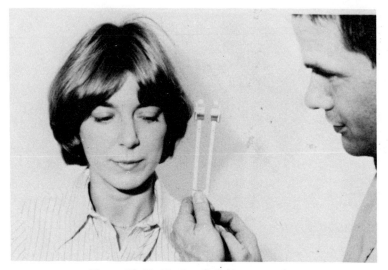

Figure 15-44. *Tuning fork (inaccurate).*

We have omitted three tests that do have anatomical validity and that can add important definition to the examination of certain patients, but these tests are uninformative in the usual screening examination because they are normal.

Corneal reflex and gag reflex add important information about the distribution of a brainstem lesion and should be performed if there is concern about such a lesion (Figure 15-45). But if the lesion

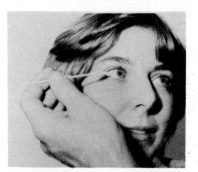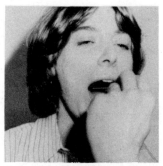

Figure 15-45. *Corneal and gag reflexes. (Redundant usually, because they are normal. Indispensable for brainstem or trigeminal, glossopharyngeal or vagal nerve lesions.)*

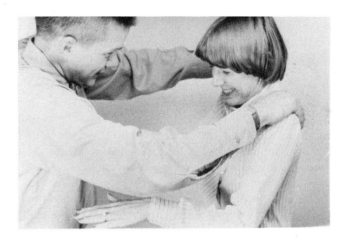

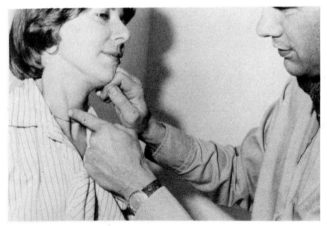

Figure 15-46. *Trapezius and sternomastoid power. (For stab wound in the neck, or other lesions that might interrupt the spinal accessory nerve in its peripheral course.)*

is elsewhere, or if the patient is normal, these tests are redundant.

We also did not examine trapezius and sternomastoid muscles in the screening examination. Testing of these muscles is important for the patient who has had a stab wound in the neck, or some other lesion that might interrupt the *peripheral* course of the spinal accessory nerve, but that patient is likely to tell you about such a lesion (Figure 15-46). In patients with lesions of the spinal cord or the medulla, examination of these two muscles is redundant, because you have already examined that area in the palate, the tongue, and the long sensory and motor tracts that course through the area.

This examination has advantages of simplicity and completeness. The three parts are easily remembered and easily learned: First, the patient sat up for examination of cranial nerves and the functions of her upper extremities. If we had wished, we could have examined her heart and lungs at the same time. Next, she lay down for an examination of reflexes and sensation, and we could have examined her abdomen. Last, she walked in a series of increasingly difficult tests of gait, standing balance and muscle power of the lower extremities, and the examination was complete. We have examined many aspects of function from the entire neuraxis. If we were astute, we performed the examination in such a way that our patient used her functions to the fullest during the examination, so we were able to detect the small asymmetrical functioning that occurs even in normal people, and we were highly unlikely to miss pathological degrees of malfunction.

Of course the crux of any examination is the clinician himself. Proper technique is indispensable; then the results must be analyzed in order to decide whether further physical examination is indicated, or whether the patient should have diagnostic radiographic or laboratory examinations. By that time, the patient is well on her way to an accurate diagnosis.

* * * * * * * * *

The author has prepared a 30-minute lecture demonstration, titled "A Neurological Screening Examination", as a supplement to the material in this chapter. The lecture-demonstration provides a vivid demonstration of examination techniques and allows the clinician to alternate freely between examinations of his own patients and the audiovisual demonstrations.

This program is available as a ¾ inch U-Matic videocassette. For further information, please write to:

Division of Educational Communications
SUNY—Upstate Medical Center
Syracuse, New York 13210

Index

Index